Nurses' Aids Series
SPECIAL INTEREST TEXT

CW01476983

ORTHOPAEDIC NURSING

NURSES' AIDS SERIES

SPECIAL INTEREST TEXTS

Nurses' Aids Series
SPECIAL INTEREST TEXT

Orthopaedic Nursing

Sixth edition revised by

Edward C. Pinney,

MBE, SRN, ONC, RNT

Senior Tutor, Nuffield Orthopaedic Centre, Oxford

BAILLIÈRE TINDALL · LONDON

Published by BAILLIÈRE TINDALL,
a division of Cassell Ltd,
1 St Anne's Rd, Eastbourne BN21 3UN

First published 1945
Fourth edition 1971
    Reprinted 1973, 1975
English Language Book Society edition 1973
Spanish translation (CECSA, Mexico)
Fifth edition 1978
Sixth edition 1983

British Library Cataloguing in Publication Data

Stone, Elizabeth
    Orthopaedics for nurses. — 6th ed. — (Nurses' aids series. Special interest texts)
    1. Orthopaedic nursing
    I. Title   II. Pinney, Edward C.   III. Series
    617'.3'024613   RD753

    ISBN 0 7020 0986 5

Typeset by Alan Sutton Publishing Limited, Gloucester.
Printed in Great Britain by Robert Hartnoll Ltd.

Contents

I DEDICATE THIS BOOK TO MY WIFE BARBARA IN
THANKS FOR HER DEVOTED COMPANIONSHIP

Preface

It has given me much pleasure to revise Orthopaedics for Nurses with a view to producing, within the scope of the Nurses' Aids Series Special Interest Text, a book which I hope will be helpful to students of general nursing, and also serve as an introduction to nurses starting their course for the Orthopaedic Nursing Certificate, or for physiotherapists engaged in orthopaedic work.

In revising this book I have taken into account not only the changes in orthopaedics but also those which have taken place in nursing practice. The good orthopaedic nurse must have a sound knowledge of the condition being treated and the needs of the patient — she will then be in a position to plan the appropriate care. Then with the other members of the team she will be able to give that care in a way that most benefits the patient.

Having carefully considered the contents of this new edition I have retained the chapter on Tuberculosis because, although it is not a major problem in this country, it still causes concern in some countries where this book will be read. In this country there are fewer people who have experience of this condition when it does occur. The chapter on Amputations has been extended together with the text on Rheumatoid Disease and Haemophilia. There is still no cure for these conditions but their management has been much improved. Replacement of the hip joint is now common place, and the problems of total knee replacement are better

understood. Trauma is still an important part of orthopaedics —
this section has been revised. David Bradley's Accident and
Emergency Nursing, a book in the same series, is recommended
for further reading. The chapter on Rehabilitation has been
extended to include the nurse's role in this very important area of
work. The nursing of children with orthopaedic conditions is still
one of the most important parts of the speciality, and one of the
most rewarding for the orthopaedic nurse.

July, 1982   EDWARD C. PINNEY

Acknowledgements

I would like to record my thanks to Miss E.M. Stone for her previous contribution to the text. Miss Stone was a previous Principal Tutor and later Matron of the Nuffield Orthopaedic Centre for many years. She had wide experience in teaching orthopaedic nursing. My thanks also to my colleagues at the Nuffield Orthopaedic Centre for their willing help and cooperation, especially the ward sisters for their help with the practical aspects of nursing care. I am also indebted to Messrs Matthew Thomas and Paul Cooper for their help with photography, and to Mr Nigel Webb for the illustrations. To Miss Gillian McCay for her advice on Rehabilitation; to Seaton Products for the illustration on stump bandaging; to my teaching colleagues who act as my sounding board for ideas; to Miss Elizabeth Henderson for permission to use some of her material on congenital talipes equino varus; and to Newton Aids Ltd for Fig. 161. My special thanks are extended to Professor Robert Duthie, Nuffield Professor of Orthopaedic Surgery, University of Oxford, and to the consultant medical staff for their advice and encouragement. Also for the invaluable help and advice given by Baillière Tindall in their careful production of this text book. I would also like to thank my wife for her patience and help, without which I do not think I could have finished the text.

EDWARD C. PINNEY

1 Introduction

The word orthopaedic, taken from the Greek word *orthos*, straight, and *pais*, child, is somewhat misleading as orthopaedic treatment covers a far wider field than is suggested by the expression 'straight child'. It deals with diseases and injuries of the locomotor system which affect the joints, bones, muscles, nerves and other soft tissues. These are the crippling diseases and when complete restoration of function is not possible and there remains a residual disability, every means, including education and vocational training, is used to enable the patient eventually to lead a happy and useful life. This is a complete contrast to the age-old attitude by which the cripple was regarded with fear and either treated with scorn and derision or smothered with sentimental pity. This change of attitude is due to the orthopaedic progress of the last 50 years.

At the beginning of this century anaesthesia and antisepsis had greatly increased the scope of surgery, nevertheless operations were performed under conditions which seem appalling compared with those in a modern operating theatre.

In 1894 Sir William Arbuthnot Lane (1856 to 1943) for the first time in Britain performed an open reduction and internal fixation with metal for a fractured tibia. It became clear to him that in bone and joint work the introduction of outside infection was more disastrous than was the case in other tissues. He increased the aseptic precautions and perfected the non-touch technique. After more than 50 years, and despite the advance of chemotherapy, this rigorous technique is still an essential part of orthopaedic surgery. It is now aided by a much better operating environment provided by a system of lamina air flow pioneered by Sir John Charnley. The continuing advances in physiology, dietetics, biochemistry, antibiotics, radiography and new synthetic materials have all widened the scope of orthopaedic work. In the nineteenth century two pioneers were W. J. Little (1810 to 1894) of the London Hospital known as the 'apostle of tenotomy' and Hugh Owen Thomas (1834 to 1891) of Liverpool, who was the pioneer of conservative orthopaedic treatment with emphasis on 'rest — enforced, uninterrupted'. Little and Thomas founded the two schools of orthopaedic thought, the London and the Liverpool. When the eccentric H. O. Thomas died he was greatly mourned by the general public of Liverpool, but his work was unrecognized by the medical profession of his own time. It was left to his pupil and nephew, Sir Robert Jones, to make Thomas's principles accept-able to the profession and known throughout the world. Sir Robert did this by the charm and force of his personality and established orthopaedics as a special branch of surgery. As a lifelong friend of Thurston Holland, the pioneer in radiology, he helped to produce the first radiograph in Britain. Sir Robert realized that the crippled child was a social as well as a surgical problem, and required treatment in a special type of hospital. With the help of some Liverpool philanthropists the Royal Coun-try Hospital for Children was opened at Heswall in 1900. Here treatment was based on rest, fresh air and surgery. Nine months later, and quite independently, the Baschurch Home in Shropshire for open-air treatment of cripple children was opened by that dauntless woman Agnes Hunt. The story of Dame Agnes Hunt and her work for cripples is well known. She was herself crippled from childhood by a suppurative arthritis of the hip. Combating a great many difficulties, she trained as a nurse and part of her training was taken at the Royal Alexander Hospital, Rhyl. This small hospital, founded by Miss Vizard and Miss Graham of the Great Ormond Street Hospital for Sick Children, had H. O. Thomas as honorary consulting surgeon, and was probably one of the first institutions to advocate fresh air as part of the treatment. Fresh air and happiness in the management of patients with

chronic illness were the two principles that impressed Dame
Agnes. In 1904, because of increased pain in her hips, she
consulted Sir Robert, and a close and enduring friendship started.
He joined the Baschurch staff and in that year performed the first
operation by candlelight in the dining-room. In 1921 the Baschurch Home moved to its present site and was renamed the
Shropshire Orthopaedic Hospital. After Sir Robert's death it was
again renamed The Robert Jones and Agnes Hunt Orthopaedic
Hospital. Today it stands as a modern orthopaedic hospital of 500
beds, although it originated in the ramshackle buildings of Baschurch.

In 1903, under conditions that would have daunted the average
person, Mrs Kimmins and Miss Renrie started the Heritage Craft
School in Sussex, and in 1907 the Sisters of St Vincent de Paul
opened a house at Clapham with the object of educating and
teaching trades to crippled boys. It was soon realized that surgical
treatment was also needed. From this modest beginning, under the
guidance of Sister Teresa Fraser together with Mr McCrae Aitken
and Sir Robert Jones the present Orthopaedic Hospital Training
School, now at Pinner, Middlesex, was started. In 1908 the
Children Act was passed by which penalties could be imposed on
parents who neglected to obtain treatment for their children when
it was needed. In the same year the Lord Mayor Treloar Hospital
and College were founded at Alton, Hampshire, in the charge of
Sir Henry Gauvain. At all these hospitals long-stay patients
received not only surgical and medical care but also education.
The example of these hospitals and an increased awareness of
crippling as a social problem resulted in the formation of more
voluntary organizations, and several new hospitals such as the
Royal National Orthopaedic Hospital, Great Portland Street,
were opened before the First World War. The problem was
increased owing to the numbers of disabled ex-service men of the
1914 to 1918 War and in the 1920s orthopaedic hospitals were
instituted throughout the country. Today an orthopaedic service is
available in all regions.

After the 1914 to 1918 War, on the recommendation and
encouragement of Sir Robert Jones, Gathorne R. Girdlestone
organized the Oxford Orthopaedic Region and later its peripheral
clinics. The founding of The Central Council for the Care of
Cripples, played an outstanding part in the creation of the open-air

country hospitals attached to the main London hospitals such as those at Stanmore and Pyrford, and later with other orthopaedic surgeons, formed the British Orthopaedic Association. In 1937 the Oxford Chair of Orthopaedic Surgery was created, and G. R. Girdlestone was appointed its first occupant, having his headquarters at the hospital he created — The Wingfield-Morris. In 1958 because of the financial help given by Lord Nuffield during his lifetime the hospital was renamed the Nuffield Orthopaedic Centre.

In the early days patients were often readmitted with broken splints and other signs of neglect that made after-care supervision essential. In 1909 Dame Agnes sent out the first after-care sister, who rode a secondhand motor bicycle. This started the pattern of after-care that was followed all over the country. A notable example occurred at Exeter, where the scheme was due to the untiring work of Dame Georgina Buller. From a central hospital were created centres which are now regularly visited by a team of trained orthopaedic nurses and physiotherapists with a fleet of cars and, less frequently, by surgeons from staff of the parent hospital. In this way early cases are detected, and long periods of supervision are carried out.

During the First World War Sir Robert Jones discovered the value of organized fracture treatment which segregated fracture cases and gave continuous treatment from the time of injury to complete recovery. This lesson was neglected and the surgeons who started fracture clinics during the interwar years met with considerable opposition. The need for a more comprehensive accident service to treat fractures and soft tissue injuries was emphasized during the Second World War. Subsequently residential rehabilitation centres were founded to bridge the gap between hospital treatment and return to work. Many hospitals now have a combined orthopaedic and accident department.

Under the present-day code of social welfare and the National Health Act of 1946 it is hard for anyone to realize how meagre was the provision for the disabled at the turn of the century. Since that time various Acts of Parliament dealing with health, hygiene and education have much reduced the suffering caused by disease and injury. Schemes for the rehabilitation and resettlement of the disabled as part of the community are now provided by the State and local government. This would not be so if pioneer work had not been undertaken voluntarily by people of vision. In 1926 Dame Agnes Hunt established the Derwen Cripples Training College at Oswestry. Ninety per cent of Derwen trainees earn their own living, some in the workshops of the College but most in the open market.

Dame Georgina Buller founded the Queen Elizabeth Training College at Leatherhead in 1935, and, two years later, St Loyes at Exeter. These two colleges were not restricted to young persons but also included trained disabled persons. They provided instruction in skilled operations which could be followed in industry itself. At first there was much criticism but the colleges proved so successful that government training centres have since been modelled on their pattern.

There have been advances and many changes during the century; hardly any other speciality has developed so rapidly.

During this time a wider sense of public responsibility has replaced the old ideas that originated in the Poor Law. Scientific knowledge and improved techniques have also increased. But for the work of great men and women, surgeons of the immediate past and present, orthopaedic sisters, physiotherapists, secretaries and experienced voluntary workers, there would have been no progress in orthopaedics.

In recent years the clinical problems in an orthopaedic hospital have altered. The gross deformities of rickets, untreated anterior poliomyelitis and neglected congenital deformities are rarely seen. Tuberculosis is being attacked from many angles and brought under under control. There are fewer children in an orthopaedic hospital. Far more help is now given to adults with osteo-arthritis, rheumatoid arthritis and sciatic pains. The patients in an orthopaedic hospital or clinic may vary from a baby a few days old with talipes, to a woman of over 80 years with a fractured femur. Among the elderly, many will now be admitted for joint replacement.

The speciality of orthopaedics includes the study and treatment of diseases, deformities and injuries of the locomotor system. Prior to the First World War this branch of surgery was included in the expertise of the general surgeon but the advent of war which produced casualties on a scale hitherto unknown was responsible for the creation of an orthopaedic service by Sir Robert Jones. Many of the well-known names in the field of orthopaedics worked with him at that time. Later, on the cessation of hostilities, there followed the formation of the British Orthopaedics Association with Sir Robert as their first President. Orthopaedic hospitals soon became established in various parts of the United Kingdom.

The common orthopaedic conditions treated some 40 years ago included tuberculosis of bone and joint, deformities associated with poliomyelitis and osteomyelitis. Today these conditions have ceased to be surgical problems due mainly to the advent of chemotherapy, improved standards of living and a National Health Service which integrates all aspects of medical care from childhood to the aged. In the present time we are dealing with degenerative conditions of bones and joints in elderly patients together with a tremendous increase in the number of injuries associated with road traffic accidents. There are now further developments in the treatment of rheumatoid arthritis in liaison with the physician in the orthopaedic centres together with the establishment of research facilities for the rehabilitation of the handicapped under the direction of a consultant in physical medicine.

Together with these changes orthopaedic surgical procedures have developed correspondingly as indeed have anaesthetic techniques, together with a practical appreciation of fluid and blood replacement.

The orthopaedic team consists of experts in their own fields, governed by the orthopaedic surgeon who is primarily responsible for the treatment ordered throughout. The nurse must appreciate the necessity to be conversant with the work of the other members of the team, physiotherapists, occupational therapists, medico-social workers and after-care sisters. The latter not only cares for the patient after discharge but looks after patients before possible admission and in some cases can prevent admission to hospital, e.g. early cases of club feet or the congenital dislocated hip in liaison with local maternity departments.

Orthopaedic nursing demands a good basic understanding of the anatomy of the skeleton and how it is activated, for much of the work involves appreciation and recognition of the abnormal and the ability to observe and report. Once the essential principles of treatment have been grasped the nurse will discover that among the fascinations of orthopaedic nursing are the various ways in which these principles are applied to each individual. This is learned not from a textbook but from practical experience under the guidance of a well-versed orthopaedic sister. An orthopaedic nurse needs to be strong and healthy, with a balanced and stable outlook. The day-to-day work of the orthopaedic nurse may seem less dramatic than some other forms of nursing, but to help a human being back to a normal physical and mental life is a most rewarding experience.

During the early years when the speciality of orthopaedics was developing, the orthopaedic nurse had plenty of time to know her patients, to find out their likes and dislikes and to assess their needs. Although the stay in hospital is much shorter now, it is just as important as it ever was to make a plan of care which will meet them, in fact it is even more urgent now because of the reduced time.

Orthopaedic nurses must appreciate that they are members of a team of people who are contributing to the patient's care. It would be easy to think, because others such as surgeons, physiotherapists, occupational therapists, social workers, etc. have a role to play in the treatment of the patient, that together these people constitute a team. This is only so when all are working towards a common aim and the work is coordinated for the benefit of the patient. Some overlap between different members of the team is inevitable and even desirable, but gaps in the treatment or care due to lack of proper communication are not acceptable.

Not only are our patients in hospital for a shorter time but nurses work fewer hours. The pattern of treatment is also changing. Often patients spend a period of time in hospital and are then discharged and their care is continued in the community, sometimes by after-care sisters but most likely by the family supported by the community nursing service. For these reasons it is essential to know the social background of the patient so that the treatment and care are continuous, whether the patient is at home or in hospital.

For these reasons it is important that discussion time is devoted to making a proper assessment of the needs of the individual patient, and that a plan of care is produced based on these needs. If the details are recorded accurately, they will be available to all members of the team who are concerned with the patient's welfare whether they are in the hospital or home. It will contribute greatly to the continuity of care, and not least to the rewards of the nurse who is responsible for that care. She will be able to follow up her patients and be in a better position to see that the plans drawn up for their care are working, and if not, to see what changes are necessary.

This approach to patient care will link up the best of established orthopaedic nursing with the changing methods being put forward as a result of nursing research in recent years.

THE ORTHOPAEDIC WARD

'Good management is the precondition of good care'. This quotation is from the Report of the Committee on Nursing *(Briggs Report 1972)*. Dr Pembrey in her book *The Ward Sister — Key to Nursing* (1980) examines the role of the ward sister and its relationship to care. She stresses the need for good organization, together with proper accountability of the nurse to the person in charge of the ward.

The ward sister must not only be a good manager, she must also be the expert in orthopaedic nursing, and an educator. *(DHSS 1980)* The manager appreciates the need to delegate the work to those competent to do it. The clinical aspect of her work gives the ward sister an appreciation of the condition which the patient suffers, together with the treatment and nursing care that is needed. The educational aspects of the role emphasize the need to be aware of the training opportunities which exist at the time. The ward will then provide the environment where the patient can be treated and cared for, and at the same time nurses will be trained to give that individualized care which is the common aim of the team.

Patients with diseases of the locomotor system will be admitted into a suitable bed. Observations will be recorded on the patient's condition – these will include temperature, pulse and respiration, blood pressure, the condition of the skin, and the general condition of the patient. Special observations may be needed in certain conditions such as head injuries. All of these should be properly recorded. During the initial period the nurse will have an opportunity to get to know her patients by asking some questions, by observation, and by talking to them when carrying out such procedures as blanket bathing. This is essential in order to be able to assess their needs. With this knowledge a plan can be prepared to include the treatment ordered by the surgeon, and the care which is required of the nurse. It will need to take into account the contribution that other members of the tream will make so that all aspects of care may be co-ordinated.

2 Joint structures and movements

A good general knowledge of anatomy and physiology is essential and this is assumed for the purposes of this book. Only those points especially relevant to the subject are mentioned here. The

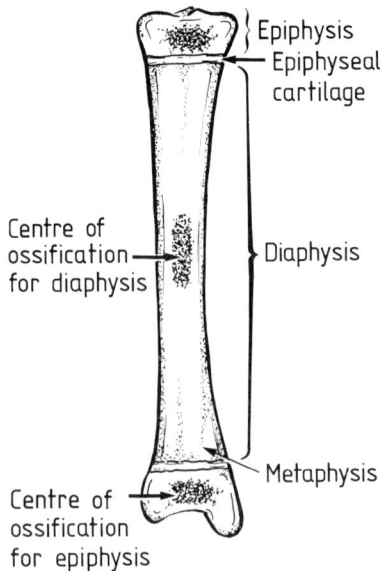

Fig. 1. *Long bone.*

knowledge must be such that it can be applied. It is not enough for the nurse to know where the great trochanter of the femur can be found on a classroom skeleton. She must be able to locate it on the human body and must practise finding bony points on her fellow students so that she may be able to locate them on the patients. This knowledge will enable her to apply splints correctly.

JOINTS

When two bone ends are adapted in such a way as to form a freely movable or synovial joint, certain structures are essential for perfect mechanism. There is often fibrocartilage, such as the glenoid cartilage of the shoulder joint or the meniscus of the knee joint which, by deepening the socket, helps the fitting of one bone to another. In order to prevent friction, the ends of the bone are

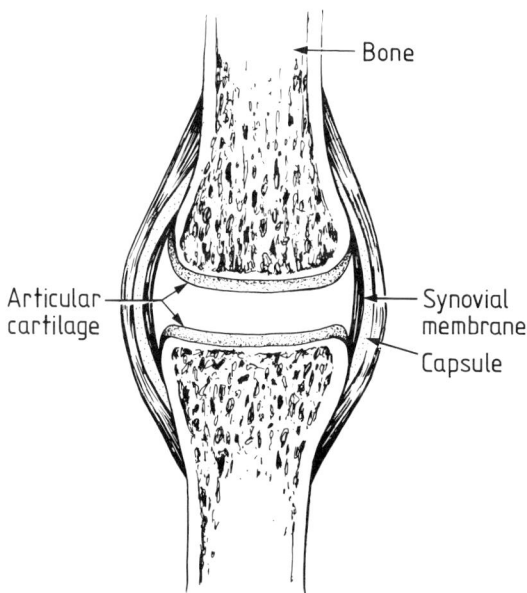

Fig. 2. *A freely movable joint.*

covered with smooth hyaline cartilage (Fig. 2). Continuous with the periosteum there is a strong sleeve of fibrous tissue which encloses the joint and is called the capsule. In the hip joint this is firm; in the shoulder joint it is comparatively slack in order to allow for greater movement. The capsule is strengthened by bands and cords of fibrous tissue — the extra-articular ligaments, e.g. the Y-shaped ligaments of the hip joint, which limit extension. Some joints also have intracapsular ligaments which increase stability and also limit movement in one direction. The anterior cruciate ligament of the knee joint prevents a forward displacement of the tibia, and the posterior cruciate ligament prevents a backward displacement of the tibia. The capsule is lined with synovial membrane, which secretes just enough synovial fluid to lubricate the joint; it also helps to nourish the articular cartilage. The most extensive synovial membrane is found in the knee joint. Around some joints are closed sacs of synovial fluid called bursae. These are most numerous around the knee joint, but there is a sub-deltoid bursa of the shoulder and an olecranon bursa of the elbow and bursae at other joints. Each joint has a nerve and blood supply. The movements of the joints are limited by the following:

1. Ligaments
2. Contact with other structures
3. The shape of bones
4. Resistance of muscles.

MOVEMENT OF JOINTS

Joints are capable of the following movements:

1. Flexion — bending
2. Extension — straightening
3. Abduction — moving away from the median line
4. Adduction — moving towards the median line
5. External and internal rotation — rolling in or out
6. Circumduction — moving through a circle, a combination of all movements.

The shoulder joint is a ball and socket joint of great mobility. Movements are flexion, extension, abduction, adduction, internal and external rotation and circumduction. Elevation of the arm above the shoulder level, when the shoulder girdle as a whole moves, is carried out by muscles moving the scapula. Muscles moving the scapula greatly assist movements of the arm and because of this a wide range of movement can be developed after an arthrodesis (fixation of a joint by operation). The stability of the joint depends on the muscles that cross the joint, especially the deltoid which is regarded as the 'key' muscle. This joint is easily dislocated because of the shallow glenoid cavity and very lax capsule.

The elbow joint is a hinge joint permitting flexion and extension. Supination (turning the forearm and palm upwards) and pronation (turning the forearm and palm downwards) take place at the radio-ulnar joint, which is a pivot joint.

The wrist is a double-hinge joint allowing for flexion and extension, abduction and adduction. The flexor and extensor muscles on the ulnar side adduct, and the flexors and extensors on the radial side abduct.

The carpo-metacarpal joint of the thumb. This joint, owing to the shape of its bones and the muscles of the thenar eminence, has a very wide range of movement. It has flexion, extension, abduction, adduction and it also has the movement of opposition, that is, of bringing the thumb across the palm towards the little finger. This is unique to the human hand.

The hip joint is a ball and socket joint with a very firm extracapsular ligament. Because of this, and the shape of the bones, it is a very stable joint, and a dislocation is rare. The movements are flexion, extension, abduction, adduction, external and internal rotation and circumduction.

The knee is an atypical hinge joint with the movements of flexion and extension. There is some degree of rotation when the joint is flexed, and its stability depends not only on the extracapsular ligaments and the intracapsular cruciate ligaments, but on the muscles, especially the quadriceps, which waste rapidly when the joint is injured or diseased.

The ankle is a hinge joint with movements of dorsiflexion, or bringing the foot up towards the body, and plantar flexion, moving the foot down away from the body. The movements of inversion — turning the sole of the foot in — and eversion — turning the sole of the foot out — take place at the joints formed by the tarsal bones.

MUSCLES

Muscles are the general stabilizing factor of the joint. A joint, unless controlled by muscles, is useless. The skeletal or striped muscles, which usually pass over a joint, are made up of bundles of muscle fibres. These fibres shorten or contract to the fullest possible extent when stimulated by a nerve impulse, thus bringing about movement of the joint. When resistance is increased, for example when the weight being lifted is made heavier, more fibres are contracted. Because of the continuous discharge of impulses from the central nervous system some fibres are always contracted. This is known as muscle tone, and is an important factor in maintaining the posture of the body. The tone of the abdominal muscles keeps the viscera in place. The tone of the deep muscles of the calf maintains the arches of the foot. Muscles are attached to the bone by bands of fibrous tissue known as tendons.

The cord-like tendons around the wrist and ankle are enclosed in synovial sheaths. These sheaths serve a double purpose. The tendons can move smoothly in them and their pulley-like action ensures that the effort is concentrated in the right direction.

Muscles always work in groups. Those muscles which initiate the movement are known as the prime movers, and always have another opposing group known as the antagonists. For example, when the elbow is flexed by the brachialis, biceps and brachioradialis, the triceps relaxes by an automatic action of the central nervous system. If the elbow is extended, the triceps contracts, and the brachioradialis and biceps relax.

There are always two opposing groups, such as:
1. Flexors — extensors
2. Abductors — adductors
3. Pronators — supinators
4. External and internal rotators.

The attachments of muscles to bone are known as the origin and the insertion. When a muscle contracts, the origin and insertion are brought nearer together. The origin usually refers to the more fixed point. Muscles, as is well known, can work 'with their origin and insertion reversed'. For example, the latissimus dorsi adducts the shoulder by bringing the arm to the body, but if the arms are fixed, as when hanging on the ribstalls, the latissimus dorsi helps to draw the trunk upwards. Again, the ilio-psoas is a prime flexor of the hip, but when a person lying flat on his back sits up with his arm folded, this muscle flexes the spine and the insertion into the lesser trochanter becomes the fixed point.

Muscles are said to contract statically when they contract without moving a joint. They do this to hold a starting position thus allowing the prime movers to work, and are known then as fixators. Patients when immobilized, are taught to contract statically certain muscle groups at regular intervals, so that muscle tone is maintained: for example, static contractions of the quadriceps are ordered following meniscectomy or a fracture of the femur.

Synergists

Prime movers may cross over more than one joint and, to prevent unwanted movement, muscles acting as synergists, fix the adjacent joint. In flexing the fingers, the extensors of the wrist contract so that the flexors can work more powerfully. A firm grasp is not possible with the wrist in flexion. An important point to remember when dealing with flaccid paralysis of muscles is their range of movement. The whole range is from the greatest possible lengthening to the greatest possible shortening. Weak or paralysed muscles are usually kept in middle or inner range, and should not be stretched. When splinting a paralysed limb, preference is given to the antigravity group. The best way of learning about muscles is to pick out their points of attachment on a skeleton and demonstrate the muscle working on a living body. To do this, get a colleague to contract a muscle against resistance. Ask her to abduct her arm and try to prevent this with one hand, placing the other hand on the deltoid which can be felt contracting.

THE VERTEBRAL COLUMN

The spine is made up of strong bones almost impossible to break, except by direct injury, a fall or an accident which severely bends, twists or crushes. The vertebral column is composed of seven cervical, twelve thoracic, five lumbar, five fused sacral vertebrae and the coccyx. Each vertebra consists of a body, two pedicles, four articular processes, two laminae, two transverse processes and a spinous process. The mobility of the column is maintained by the presence of the intervertebral discs and the adjacent articular facets which are true synovial joints, together with the

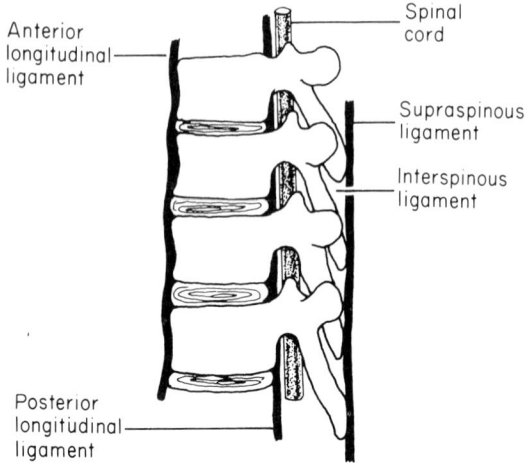

Fig. 3. *Lateral view of vertebrae showing ligaments.*

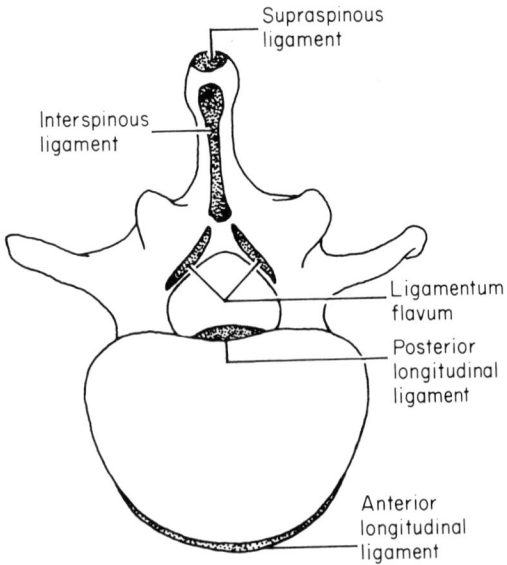

Fig. 4. *Superior view of a vertebra showing ligaments.*

ligaments which bind the bones together and the musculature. All these provide stability of the column.

The anterior and posterior longitudinal ligaments, the musculature and the intervertebral discs hold the bodies together (Fig. 3). The spinous and transverse processes give attachment to ligaments and muscles (Fig. 4). The larger transverse processes of the

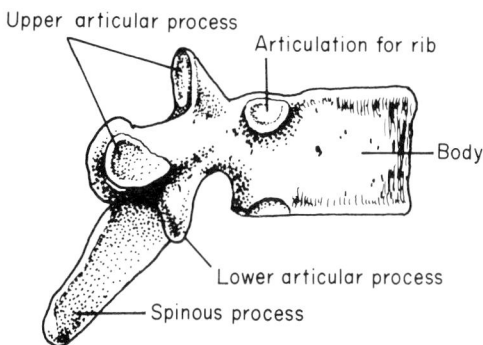

Fig. 5. *A vertebra.*

thoracic region articulate with the ribs (Fig. 5). Between each pair of individual vertebrae movement is slight, but the spine as a whole moves freely because the joints are numerous and close together. The movements are flexion, extension, lateral flexion and rotation. Movement is not so free in the thoracic region because of the ribs.

Curves of the spine

There are two primary curves present at birth which are in the thoracic and sacral region and are both concave forward.

There are two secondary curves both convex forwards. The cervical curve begins after the child starts to hold up his head at about six months. The lumbar curve develops when the child sits right up, and becomes more marked when walking starts at about 12 months. The shape of the curves depends largely on the intervertebral discs, as they are wedge-shaped on section. In the thoracic region they are thicker behind but in the lumbar region they are thicker in front.

GLOSSARY OF ORTHOPAEDIC TERMS

Adhesion	An abnormal attachment of structures limiting movement
Ankylosis	Spontaneous fusion of a joint either by fibrous tissue or bone
Arthrodesis	Surgical fusion of a joint
Arthroplasty	The formation of a new joint
Atrophy	Wasting, usually of muscle
Avulsion	Forcible separation
Biopsy	The surgical removal of tissue for investigation
Bursitis	Inflammation of a bursa
Chondromalacia	Erosion of articular cartilage
Coxa	Relating to the hip
Cubitas	Relating to the elbow
Diaphysis	Shaft of a long bone
Dislocation	The displacement of joint surfaces
Distraction	Excessive pulling on a broken bone
Eburnation	Dense bone formed when the cartilage is worn away
Epiphysis	Growth nucleus at bone ends
Equinus	Plantar flexion of the foot
Exostosis	A bony out-growth
Ganglion	A small cystic swelling near a joint
Haemarthrosis	A collection of blood in a joint
Hallux	The big toe
Idiopathic	Cause unknown
Involucrum	New bone laid down outside of existing bone
Ischaemia	Inadequate or deficient blood supply to a part of the body caused by constriction or blockage of the arteries to the part
Kyphosis	Excessive forward curvature of the spine
Loose bodies	Fragments of joint structures free inside the capsule
Lordosis	Excessive backward curvature of the spine

Movements of joints
  Active   Performed by the patient's own efforts
  Passive   Performed by the physiotherapist
                    without help of the patient's own
                    muscles
Metatarsalgia   Pain associated with the metatarsus of
                    the foot
Motor neurones
  Upper   Motor cells whose axons extend from
                    the cerebral cortex to end in the
                    anterior horn of the spinal cord
  Lower   Motor cells in the anterior horn of the
                    spinal cord whose axons transmit to
                    the periphery
Myelitis   Inflammation of the spinal cord
Myositis   Inflammation of muscle
Neuroma   A tumour involving a nerve
Osteochondritis   *(osteo — bone; chondro — cartilage;
                    itis — inflammation)* An inflamma-
                    tory affection of bone and cartilage
Osteophytes   New bone formation at the margin of a
                    joint due to a degenerative condi-
                    tion of the articular surfaces
Osteoporosis   Rarefaction of bone
Osteotomy   Surgical division of a bone
Prosthesis   An artificial part used to replace a
                    diseased or damaged portion of the
                    body
Pseudarthrosis   The formation of a false fibrous joint
Scoliosis   Lateral curvature of the spine
Spondylitis   Inflammation of the spine
Spondylosis   Disease of the spine, e.g. ankylosis
Subluxation   An incomplete dislocation
Talipes   Deformity at the tarsal joints
Tenosynovitis   Inflammation of the lining of the ten-
                    don sheath
Torticollis   Drawing of the head to one side and
                    twisting of the neck
Valgus   The bone beyond the joint which
                    qualifies the term is directed away

from the mid-line of the body, e.g.
coxa valgus — an increase in the
neck angle of the femur; *cubitas
valgus* — increase in the carrying
angle at the elbow; *genu valgus* —
knock-knees; *hallux valgus* — big
toe pointing outwards

Varus   The bone beyond the joint which
qualifies the term is directed to-
wards the mid-line of the body, e.g.
coxa varus — decrease in the neck
angle of the femur; *genu varus* bow
legs

SOME SPECIAL TESTS USED IN DIAGNOSIS

Real and apparent shortening. A disparity in leg lengths may be
due to:
1. The position in which the leg is held; for example when the
   hip is held in adduction — this is an apparent shortening.
2. When there is destruction of the joint or pathological
   dislocation there is true or real shortening.

Measurements for apparent shortening are taken from the
umbilicus to the sole of the heel with legs lying side by side in line
with the trunk.

Real shortening is measured from the anterior superior iliac
spines to the tip of the medial malleolus on the same side with the
pelvic spines horizontal.

Arthrogram
An arthrogram is a radiograph of a joint. An opaque substance is
injected into the joint to show up the outline and the articular
surfaces.

Queckenstedt's test
When a lumbar puncture is being performed pressure is applied to
the jugular vein which normally causes a rise of pressure of the
cerebrospinal fluid. Failure indicates a blockage due to some
spinal lesion.

Thomas test

The Thomas test is used for demonstrating a hip flexion deformity, which if present is indicative of joint irritability.

With the patient lying flat the sound knee and hip are flexed towards the abdomen which obliterates all lumbar lordosis. The patient is then asked to lay the other leg flat on the table. If he attempts to do so, and cannot, some fixed flexion is present and the test is positive.

The Lasegne test

The Lasegne test is used in cases of low back pain for determining the degree of severity of irritation of the sciatic nerve.

With the patient lying flat the leg is raised off the table with knees straight; in acute sciatica the amount of straight leg raising is limited and painful.

Myelogram

A myelogram is a radiograph of the spinal cord and subarachnoid space made after injection of an opaque substance by lumbar puncture. Myelography may be used to reveal the presence of a prolapsed intervertebral disc.

3 Principles of orthopaedic nursing

TYPES OF BEDS

In an orthopaedic hospital beds may vary, but it is always essential to have a type of bed that is easily moved (Fig. 6) so that the patient can be taken to plaster room, X-ray and other departments without interfering with appliances. Beds should also be made to stand up to all weather conditions, and usually have a full-length slatted fracture board. It is also necessary to be able to move them easily in and out of the ward. Beds often have to be moved for school. The education of the child is essential from every point of view and there should be cooperation between the teaching and nursing staff. Patients in orthopaedic hospitals are allowed more latitude than those with acute conditions, and the art of running an orthopaedic ward is to keep a happy balance between discipline and freedom. If the patient is to progress he must be happy and take an interest in things outside as well as taking an intelligent interest in his own condition.

SPLINTS AND APPLIANCES

The nurse should have a clear understanding of the principles and use of splints, the purpose for which they are designed, and why it is sometimes necessary to modify or alter the splint to suit the needs of a particular patient.

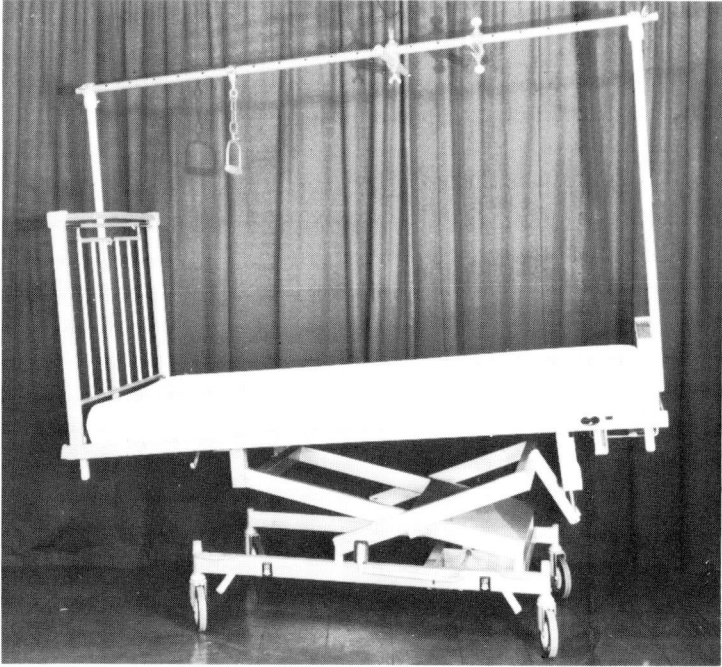

Fig. 6. *King's Fund bed. This type can be raised and tipped and is easily moveable.*

REASONS FOR SPLINTING

Splinting is employed for the following purposes:

1. To immobilize a part after injury in order to repair damaged tissues or to enforce the 'rest' principle in inflammation. Hugh Owen Thomas, who designed many splints to ensure this principle in tuberculosis and other pyogenic infections of joints, laid down the law 'rest enforced, uninterrupted and prolonged'.

2. To prevent deformities, when there is muscle imbalance, as in anterior poliomyelitis, or peripheral nerve injuries, when one group of muscles works without an opposing muscle group.

3. To correct deformities which is usually done by holding the part in an over-corrected position, e.g. Denis Browne splints for club feet.

4. To protect a joint or limb in the healing stage, e.g. wearing a

caliper in the ambulatory stage when tuberculosis of the knee is quiescent, or after a fractured femur has united but not yet consolidated.

5. To compensate for the loss of paralysed muscles, e.g. the wearing of a caliper to keep the knee straight when the quadriceps muscles are unable to control the joint.

6. To overcome muscle spasm, that is the continual uncontrolled contraction of muscles due to pain or other irritation. This type of spasm is often present in a lesion of the upper motor neurone.

7. To splint the paralysed group of muscles, at the same time allow the opposing group to function, e.g. a radial nerve splint.

8. Splints play a very important part in the application of traction.

9. Spinal splints or braces, as they are more usually called, prevent and sometimes corrrect spinal deformities.

Splints are made of leather, wood, metal, plaster of Paris and plastics. Most splints have to be made for the individual and the patient lying on a firm bed or plinth is measured from bony point to bony point. Measurements should be checked, where possible, by a second person. A plaster cast may be required or the splint maker, using malleable wire, may take a tracing. Measurements vary slightly with different surgeons and splint makers, but the essentials are the same, namely:

1. The splint must fulfil the purpose for which it is applied.

2. The fit must be perfect — an ill-fitting, badly applied splint is not only useless but dangerous. If the part is not sufficiently rested, healing is delayed, pain and muscle spasm are uncontrolled and the patient is made thoroughly uncomfortable. When a splint is bandaged in place, the bandage is applied to maintain the position and must be firm. Often the classic rules for bandaging must be ignored in order to fix the position first. This is so, for instance, when applying a back splint after a meniscectomy when, in order to keep the knee from flexing, the knee must be fixed with a figure of eight bandage.

Splints need constant observation, especially at first. Before being discharged the patient must be taught to manage the splint.

A limb in a splint should be kept warm and the extremities should be watched. Any failure in circulation or loss of power must be reported. This especially applies to splints that hold the arm or legs in a wide abduction. Splints, after removal, must be reapplied exactly as they were, unless otherwise ordered, using the same slots and tensions. While changing a splint the position must be maintained and the traction kept up manually.

Splint sores, like bed sores, are caused by local areas of pressure which result in gangrene and destruction. They occur when the splint does not fit or has been incorrectly applied. Too small or too tight a splint causes pressure. Too large or too loose a splint causes friction. The leather may be hard and cracked, or part of the splint may need repairing. Loose screws and damaged buckles and straps should be immediately repaired.

THE PREVENTION OF COMPLICATIONS

The patient should be told to complain and the nurse must not ignore complaints of pressure or burning pain. Very young children do not complain but will be fretful and restless especially at night. The skin and splint must be kept quite clean and the leather part of the splint should be kept pliable and clean with saddle soap. Areas liable to pressure should be carefully washed with soap and water and thoroughly dried. Pads can be used to relieve, but not directly, over the points of pressure.

When immobilizing a joint, it is essential that the other joints should be freely exercised:
1. To maintain circulation in the limbs and prevent venous stasis and oedema and the forming of adhesions.
2. To prevent muscle atrophy.

These principles apply especially to fingers and toes when the limbs are in splints or plaster. When the wrist is immobilized following Colles fracture, the elbow, shoulder and fingers should be moved frequently to their full range. If the tendons passing over the wrist joint are moved, subsequent stiffness of the wrist is very much reduced.

OPTIMUM POSITION

When it is necessary to immobilize a joint, whether it is normal, or injured or infected and unlikely to recover, the immobilization is carried out in the optimum position which is the position of physiological rest, ordinarily the position of maximum useful function. The surgeon always keeps this in mind when the

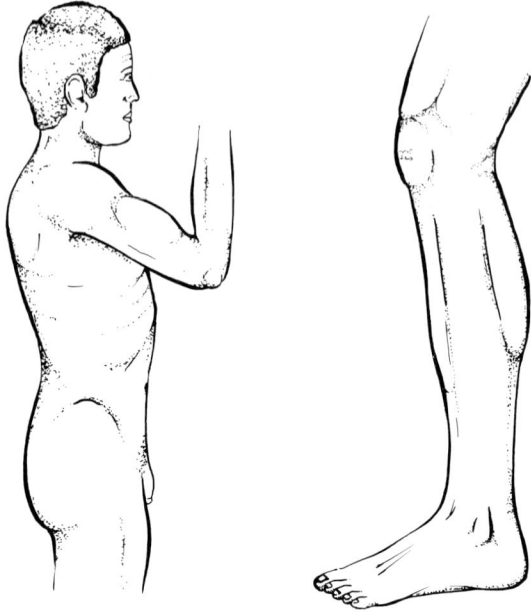

Fig. 7. *Optimum positions for elbow, knee and ankle.*

operation of arthrodesis (making a stiff joint) is performed.

The optimum positions of the main joints (Fig. 7) are as follows:

The hip is put 5° to 10° of abduction, or enough to compensate true shortening, and 30° of flexion, which allows the patient to sit if there is compensatory movement of the lumbar spine.

The knee is very slightly flexed, i.e. in a position just short of full extension.

The ankle is placed in plantar grade, that is the position that the foot normally takes when standing, although some plantar flexion is allowed for the heels of shoes. A neutral position between inversion and eversion is also maintained.

The toes. The metatarso-phalangeal joints are slightly flexed and the interphalangeal joints extended.

The shoulder is fixed in 60° abduction, 30° flexion, and external rotation, which is sufficient to allow the patient to bring his hand to his mouth when the elbow is flexed.

The elbow is placed at just over a right angle with the forearm, but the position is varied with the occupation of the patient because a more acute angle is easier for clerical work. If both elbows are stiffened one is fixed at a lesser angle.

The wrist is placed in 30° dorsal flexion which is a neutral position as regards deviation and allows the patient to grasp. *The fingers and the thumb* are placed in a semigrasp position such as a hand holding a tumbler.

TRACTION

PRINCIPLES OF TRACTION

The skeleton is the basic framework of the body and joint movement is controlled by the balanced action of opposing groups of muscles. If any part of the framework is broken that part becomes unstable and the pull of the muscle over the distal fragment may cause overlapping and consequent shortening or deformity.

If a joint is damaged or infected, muscles controlling the joint immediately go into spasm, which holds the joint in the position of greatest comfort, preventing friction of joint surfaces which would otherwise occur in movement. This is useful in that it rests the joint, but if prolonged it will lead to fixed deformities, e.g. contraction or even ankylosis in a bad or abnormal position.

Traction therefore is used to overcome muscle spasm and to reduce or prevent deformity.

Traction is applied when it is needed:

1. To secure immobility in the desired position when the bone structure is affected as in Perthes's disease of the hip joint or tuberculosis of the hip. This is done to prevent the surrounding muscles from pulling the joint into an unwanted position by protective muscle spasm. An untreated acute tuberculosis of the knee due to spasm of the hamstrings acquires a deformity of flexion accompanied by a pathological subluxation.

2. To secure immobilization and prevent overriding of fragments and faulty alignment in fractures, especially in long bones such as the shaft of the femur when the fracture line is oblique and the muscles are powerful. Efficient traction and immobilization stops muscle spasm and pain. A patient who has been thus fixed should have immediate relief and should require little or no

sedation. If he still complains, the immobilization and traction must be checked.

FIXED TRACTION

Traction is 'fixed' when it is attached to a stationary point, e.g. if an extension is tied to the end of Thomas's splint with the ring against the ischial tuberosity as a point of counter-traction, the limb is described as being in fixed traction (Fig. 8).

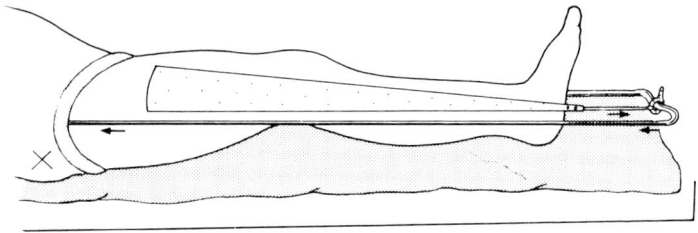

Fig. 8. *Fixed traction. Extension tapes are tied to the end of Thomas's splint and the ring of the splint presses against the ischial tuberosity.*

The Jones-Thomas abduction frame is another form of fixed traction, when traction is held by extension tapes tied to the end of the splint while the groin strap is the fixed point. The same principle is applied with a simple incline. Extension tapes are tied to the foot of the bed. This is raised and the weight of the patient, plus gravity, exercises the pull.

Advantages. The advantage of this type of traction is that it facilitates transportation, the limb remaining undisturbed.

Disadvantages. The disadvantages of fixed traction are the greatly restricted movements in bed and the difficulty in preventing pressure sores occurring under the ring especially in very fat or very thin patients; therefore it is important that the splint ring fits perfectly. If too tight it will cause constriction, if too loose it will produce friction and may slip right over the ischial tuberosity instead of resting against it.

The area of skin related to the ring must always be kept clean and powdered and the skin under the ring moved two or three times daily to prevent subjection to pressure.

PRINCIPLES OF BALANCED OR CONTINUOUS TRACTION

If a force is applied to pull an object in one direction, there must be equal force to pull in the opposite direction, i.e. traction must be combined with counter-traction; this can be effected by using a weight and pulley system.

When traction is applied to the leg, counter-traction can be produced by elevating the bottom end of the bed, the body weight then slides by force of gravity in the opposite direction. It is essential that the traction and counter-traction are balanced. The greater the weight applied, the higher the bed will require to be elevated (Fig. 9). Thomas's splint is most commonly used for supporting the limb. The splint plays no part in the actual traction but facilitates suspension of the limb (Fig. 10).

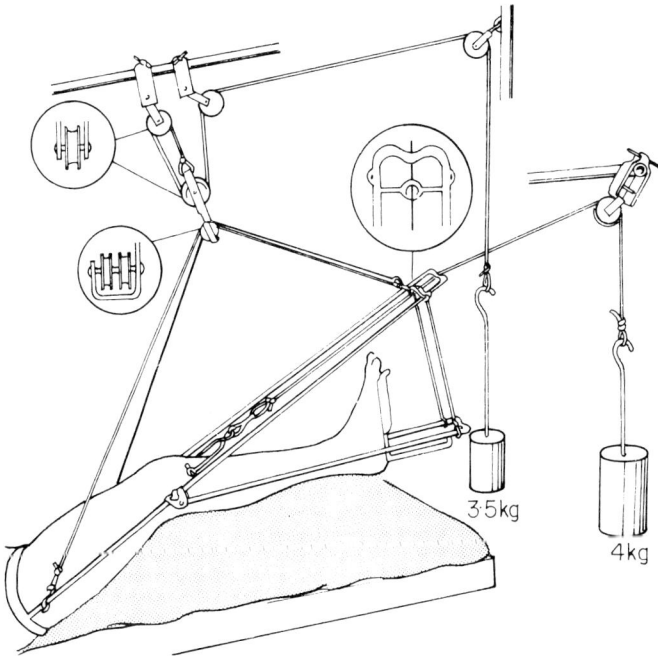

Fig. 9. *Balanced traction using Steinmann's pin (skeletal traction) through the tibial tubercle. The leg is supported in a Thomas's splint with a Pearson knee flexion piece attached.*

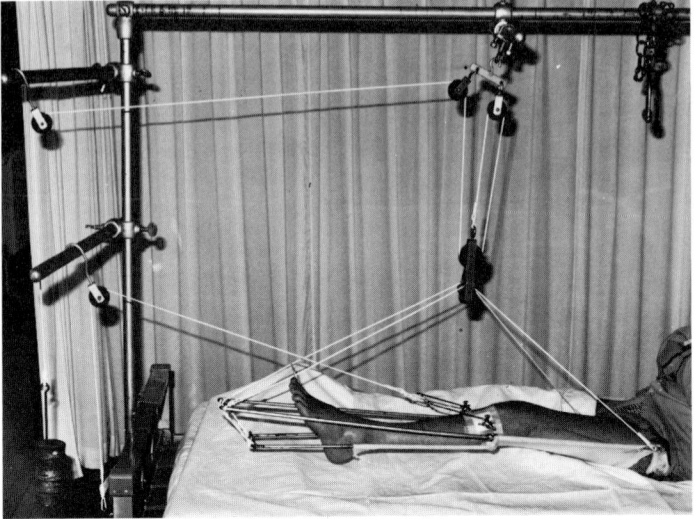

Fig. 10. *Pulley arrangement for elevating Thomas's splint.*

Advantages. The advantages of continuous traction are numerous. Provided the apparatus is properly applied, the patient can move relatively freely without interfering with the efficiency of the traction. The mobility diminishes joint stiffness, muscle wasting, decalcification, pressure sores and all other complications associated with immobilization.

The following points should be noted:

The pulleys should be smooth-running.

The cords should run in straight lines and without knots. Friction on bed bars should be prevented.

The limb should be able to move freely, i.e. no obstruction from sandbags, bedclothes, cradles and the like.

Never allow weights to rest on the bed, chairs or the floor. Simple adjustment of the cord will prevent this.

Elevation of the bottom of the bed must be maintained at all times so that traction and counter-traction are continuous.

HAMILTON-RUSSELL TRACTION

Hamilton-Russell traction represents a type of balanced traction which can be used after arthroplasty operation of the hip or a fracture of the neck of the femur. There is a beam over the bed. The limb is supported on a pillow to prevent backward sagging, and skin extensions are applied to the lower leg, with a sling placed under the knee. From the knee sling a cord is taken to a pulley fixed to the beam (A). From this pulley the cord is taken to another pulley on a frame at the foot of the bed (B), and then to a third pulley which is attached to a spreader separating the skin extensions (C). Finally the cord passes over another pulley at the foot of the bed (B) and its end is attached to a weight. The resultant pull is in direct line with the femur. Only moderate weight is required, about 3.5 to 4.5 kg for an adult and about 0.25 to 2.25 kg for a child (Fig. 11).

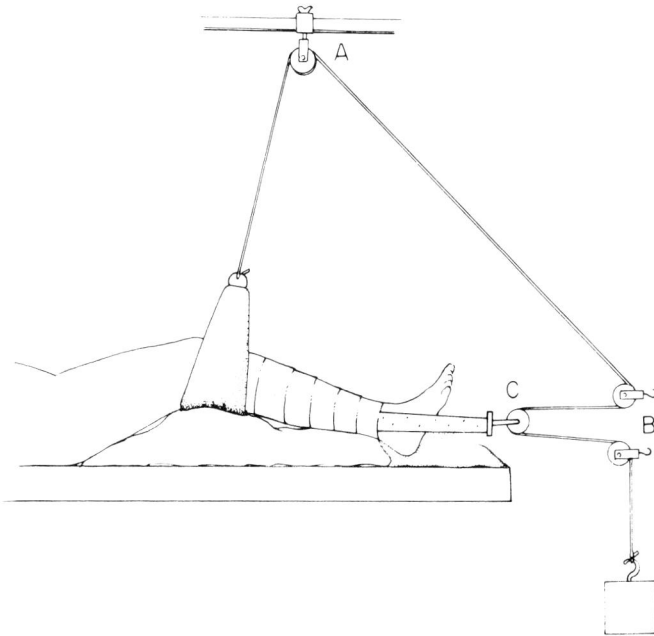

Fig. 11. *Hamilton-Russell traction.*

Points to note when nursing a patient on Hamilton-Russell traction:
  1. See that the heel clears the bed.

2. Too much weight will cause a flexion deformity of the hip and knee.
3. See that the bandage below the knee is not creased and causing sores, and is not so tight that it causes a venous thrombosis.

In addition to the above slings, a crêpe bandage may be applied below the knee and tied to a cord leading to another pulley to check external rotation. See that this is loosely applied and not pressing upon the lateral popliteal nerve.

METHODS OF APPLYING TRACTION

Traction may be applied in three ways:
1. Skin traction
2. Skeletal traction
3. Pulp traction.

Skin traction
Extensions are made from Taylor's perforated zinc oxide strapping or zinc oxide plaster. A method now also being tried is tubular gauze.

Method of application. Two straps are cut to fit the limb for the purpose required. At the end of the strapping a length of webbing or lampwick is stitched with the addition of a square of lint to prevent friction on the malleoli, or the webbing or lampwick may be applied as a small loop through which another length is tied using a bow-tied knot, keeping the smooth surface on the inner side. On either side the strapping is notched so that it can be moulded around the limb. Adhesive plaster and Taylor's strapping should not be unwound before use. Prior to application, the skin is shaved and painted with compound tincture of benzoin because this lessens the irritating effect that strapping has on some sensitive skins. The limb is firmly and gently steadied by one nurse. A limb that requires an extension should never be subjected to rough handling. The strapping should be applied smoothly since wrinkles are another cause of extension sores. The two straps may overlap at the back but bony points, such as the malleoli, the anterior border of the tibia and the patella should be left uncovered. The strapping is held in place by a circular openwove bandage in a spiral turn and fixed by stitching. For fractures, adhesive plaster is often used. The extensions should end above and behind the malleoli, not only in order to prevent pressure but so as to allow free movement of the ankle joint. The foot is supported by gallows in the plantar grade position, but the ankle joint and toes should be exercised in full range frequently and regularly. Although they must be protected from the weight of the bedclothes, they must be kept warm especially if the legs are in wide abduction. Traction must be maintained 24 hours of the day, and released only by order of the surgeon. When a skin extension is being renewed, traction must be maintained by a nurse grasping the heel with one hand, and the forefoot with the other, and exerting a steady hold the whole time. The sudden cessation of traction irritates diseased joints, causes displacement in a fracture and is very painful for the patient. The extension should be observed at least twice a day to see that the pull is in the right direction, that there are no moist spots, which would indicate a sore, and that the strapping is not slipping. Weights should hang away from the bed and everybody in the ward, including auxiliaries and domestic staff, should be warned not to knock against them or pull them up.

Skeletal traction

Skeletal traction is obtained by inserting a pin through the bone. It is used generally for the treatment of fractures. Common sites for introducing the pins are the condyles of the femur, tubercle of the tibia and the calcaneum. Three common methods are:

1. Steinmann's pin
2. Denman's pin
3. Kirschner's wire.

Steinmann's pin is a rigid steel pin driven through the bone and attached to a special stirrup. Denman's pin is similar to Steinmann's pin but with a screw thread in the centre. It is used in the same way. Because of the stirrup, the surgeon can alter the line of the pull without turning the pin. This is important because movement might cause infection.

Kirschner's wire is a narrow steel wire which is not rigid until pulled out by the stirrup. A rotary movement of the stirrup can move the wire and cause infection. For this reason it is not as commonly used as Steinmann's pin. When the pins for skeletal traction are introduced through a prepared skin with all aseptic precautions, the risk of infection is negligible, but they are foreign bodies and need careful watching. The area of skin around the point where the pin or wire has been introduced is covered with sterile gauze. The points of the wire are fitted with corks to protect bedclothes and the nurses' fingers. Much more weight can be used with this type of traction and there is no danger of it slipping. Whichever type of pin is used the assistant must hold the leg in a position of mid rotation with the toes pointing upwards. Failure to do so will alter the line of pull.

Pulp traction
Pulp traction is used for displaced phalangeal, metacarpal and metatarsal fractures. A suture or Broch's pin is put through the pulp of the finger and fastened to an extension wire which is incorporated in plaster.

SOME PRACTICAL POINTS IN THE USE OF TRACTION

1. Traction may be fixed, sliding or a combination of the two as when the traction cords are tied to the end of the splint (fixed traction), which is then pulled on by a cord passing over a pulley to a suspended weight at the end of the bed — sliding traction enough to relieve the pressure from the ring that fixed traction necessarily imposes upon the ischial tuberosity.

2. The ring should be a *little too large* when Thomas's splint is applied to a fresh fracture as the thigh may continue to swell for 24 hours.

3. Skeletal traction has the advantage of not harming the skin and of leaving the leg free from bandages but it can give trouble from sores and infection, especially with fat legs and thin, soft, old bones.

Requirements for skeletal traction
Swabs and cleansing material
Sterile towels, waterproof sheet and dressings
Towel clips
Collodion (used with wool to seal the puncture wounds round the wire or pin)
2 gallipots. Small scalpel or tenotome
10 ml syringe, needles and local anaesthetic
Kirschner's wires and apparatus for their insertion or Stein-

mann's pin and handle

Stirrup

Cord, Thomas's splint, slings and clips

If general anaesthesia is used, as when the fracture has to be manipulated, the syringe, needles and local anaesthetic are not required.

4. Skin traction can be used for long periods but it is liable to slip if much weight is used and can cause serious blistering if the strapping has wrinkles in it or if the circulation and nutrition of the skin have been impaired by diseased veins or arteriosclerosis. The strapping must be secured by soft bandages, never by strapping.

Requirements for skin traction. Two people are required, one to hold the limb and one to apply the splint and traction apparatus. Everything that is to be used should be prepared before the limb is handled as it is then possible to lift the limb clear of the couch or bed and hold it quite still while the traction appliances are applied. The less the limb is moved the less discomfort the patient is required to tolerate.

1. If necessary, the limb is shaved, washed and dried thoroughly, after clothing has been removed tincture of benzoin is often painted on the skin to protect it.

2. Adhesive felt pads are applied *around* and *not over* the malleoli so as to protect them from pressure (Fig. 12, top). Alternatively a spreader (Fig. 12, bottom) can be used or the cords can be passed round the side bars of the splint. The strapping is thus made to diverge and clear the malleoli.

3. The strapping is applied up to the level of the fracture, or to the knee with fractures of the tibia, on each side of the limb. The strapping should be applied a little behind the middle of the limb on the outer side and a little in front of it on the inner side to help counteract the tendency of the limb to roll onto its outer side. If a spreader is used the strapping should be applied as a long U, otherwise a separate strip is applied on each side.

4. The strapping is bandaged securely in place and it must be ensured that it is free from wrinkles. Bandages of crêpe or flannelette, never strapping, should be used for this purpose. Care must be taken not to start the bandage too near the ankle or a pressure sore may form (Fig. 13).

5. The Thomas's splint, with slings and clips already in place, is slid over the limb.

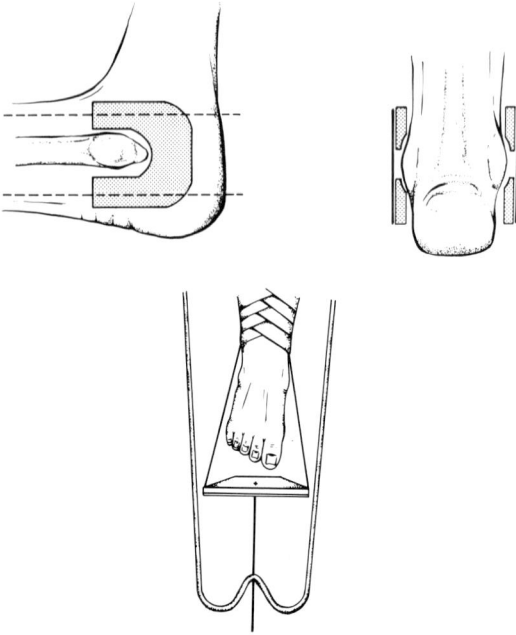

Fig. 12. *Surface and sectional views to show correct use of malleolar pads (top) and a spreader (bottom).*

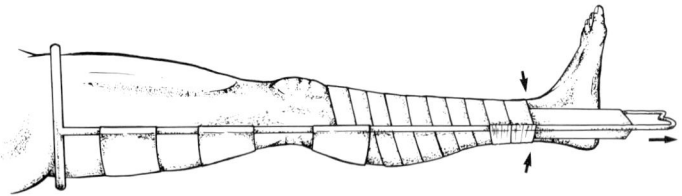

Fig. 13. *Pressure zones at the ankle.*

6. The spreader is then inserted or the traction cords are applied. If a spreader is used a single cord is passed through its central hole and knotted to keep it from slipping through.

7. The cord(s) must be attached to the end of the splint with sufficient tension to steady the limb.

8. The tension of the slings is adjusted and it must be ascertained that they are free from wrinkles and that sharp edges do not press on the skin, especially above the heel (Fig. 12). The slings behind the calf and knee should be tight enough to keep half or two-thirds of this part of the limb above the side bars. The slings for the thigh should be taut enough to support it firmly as it passes upwards from the ring to the knee.

The limb and traction apparatus must be examined frequently for swelling of the foot, wrinkling of slings, looseness of the cords and slipping of bandages and strapping.

Crutchfield caliper

Crutchfield calipers are a method of applying traction to the skull in cases of fracture, dislocation of cervical spine, or for dislocation of the cervical spine in rheumatoid arthritis. The area of skin on either side of the head is shaved, having explained the procedure to the patient. A small hole is drilled through the outer table of the skull, usually under local anaesthetic. The cord from the caliper is extended over a pulley at the end of the bed. Elevation of the head of the bed ensures that the weight of the body provides the counter pull. Nursing care includes reassuring the patient, correct positioning of the head with pillows or sandbags, and care of the pin holes, which should be dressed with strict aseptic precautions to prevent infection being transmitted to the bone. Antiseptic cream may be applied and the dressing changed daily, some surgeons prefer less frequent changes.

GENERAL CARE OF THE PATIENT ON TRACTION

This form of splintage and immobilization is often extended over a period of time. As well as the observation of the splints and pulleys the nurse must be aware of the whole patient — their diet, state of skin, fluid balance, their bowels, together with their general well-being. Young people on traction can get very bored, and a cheerful nurse and occupational therapy can do much to counteract this state.

4 Nursing care of amputations

Amputation of a limb is performed for the following reasons:

1. For peripheral vascular disease as in senile arteriosclerosis or diabetes. This is the largest group of patients needing amputation most of whom will be aged, thus increasing the risk of complications and adding to the problems of management.
2. For acute infection where amputation may be a life-saving measure, e.g. gas gangrene.
3. For chronic infection which is endangering the general health of the patient causing long periods of incapacity and subjecting the patient to many operations and much pain.
4. For malignant neoplasm, e.g. osteosarcoma.
5. For trauma where there is extensive tissue damage especially to the blood supply.
6. For deformity that is not correctable, when the patient would be able to lead a more active life with a prosthesis and have a better cosmetic result.
7. For a flail, useless limb following a brachial plexus injury, amputation may be accompanied by arthrodesis of the shoulder.

GROUPS OF PATIENTS REQUIRING SPECIAL CONSIDERATION

Children. Amputation in the case of children is usually performed on the lower limb for gross deformity such as congenitally absent tibia. It will allow a prosthesis to be fitted early, in some cases when the child is still crawling. He will then begin to stand and start walking as normally as possible. The results are good, both functionally and cosmetically.

Preparation of the parents as well as the child is needed. To be able to show them children with a similar condition is helpful. Time is needed in order to establish a proper relationship with members of the team, and the child and parents.

Adolescent. This group often need an amputation for osteosarcoma. This is one of the most malignant of new growths. Since the operation is likely to be performed as soon as possible after the diagnosis is made, there is little time to establish the sort of relationships needed. As neither the adolescent nor the parents have time to adjust to the situation, it must be pointed out to them that the operation is a life-saving measure, and that it is possible to lead a full and active life with an artificial limb.

Young adults. This group usually require amputations for severe trauma. It may be part of the initial treatment which gives them no time to prepare or adjust to the idea of amputation. They do, however, usually make a good recovery if the team maintains a good positive approach.

The elderly. It has been estimated that 60 per cent of all amputees are over 60 years of age, and that the amputation is performed for ischaemia. This increases the risk of complications. However, with help and encouragement many of them will lead a good life, even if it is a little more restricted than it was before.

Double amputees. To have to amputate both lower limbs is a serious disability. If one is below-knee the situation is a little better than both mid-thigh, but even these patients, if they are young and well motivated, can lead very useful and full lives.

AMPUTATION SITES

Sites chosen for amputation may be as follows:

Lower Limb

1. Symes amputation through the ankle joint using the heel pad as a weight-bearing area.
2. Below-knee amputation. A prosthesis fitted in this case should cause a minimum of restriction to the patient's activity.
3. Through-knee amputation. This is not favoured by the limb-fitter because the joint mechanism is attached to the outside of the prosthesis.
4. Mid-thigh amputation. This is the most likely site when the amputation is for peripheral vascular disease in the elderly.
5. The hip. Disarticulation of the hip is performed for malignant disease when the whole of the affected bone needs to be removed.
6. Hind-quarter amputation is a much more radical procedure involving hind-quarter removal of one side of the pelvis invariably for malignant disease.

Upper limb

Usually as much as possible of the limb is preserved especially if the amputation is for trauma leaving a reasonable length of stump to fit the prosthesis. In the case of amputation for a brachial plexus lesion, control is achieved by shoulder girdle movement.

POSSIBLE COMPLICATIONS AFTER AMPUTATION

Complications which may occur following amputation are:

General complications

Pneumonia
Thrombosis
Pulmonary embolism
Pressure sores.

The elderly with vascular disease are particularly prone to these complications:

Local complications
    Flexion deformity at the neighbouring joint
    Infection which may follow a haematoma
    Misshapen stump which may be caused by a wrongly applied
    bandage
    Skin sores which could be caused by an ill-fitting prosthesis.

TREATMENT

The aims of treatment are:
    To encourage early mobilization and restoration of function
    To prevent complications.
In order to achieve these aims it is essential to have a cheerful
positive approach to patients needing, or having had, an amputation. 'Amputation is a treatment, not a tragedy.' The treatment is
to replace the limb which is of no further use and may be
endangering life.

Pre-operative management
The decision to amputate will be taken by the surgeon in consulta-
tion with the patient, and in the case of a child with the parents. It
is essential that the team realize why the decision was taken in
order that support may be given to the patient to enable them to
make the necessary adjustments to their lives — most will need
comfort and reassurance. The nurse has a special role to play at
this stage.

Preparation for theatre
Preparation will be determined by the reasons for amputation. If it
is an emergency such as trauma there may be no opportunity for
special preparation of the limb. In the case of gangrene a clean
dressing is applied, and the limb usually wrapped in a sterile towel.
If for diabetic gangrene, etc. necessary adjustment of the insulin
routine will be necessary.

Post-operative care
Special consideration should be given to:

    Prevention of pressure sore
    Prevention of flexion deformities in hospital and home

Appropriate heights — bed, chair, toilet
Opportunity to react to loss
Care of other leg — chiropody if necessary

The patient should be received into a warm bed with fracture boards. This allows proper positioning of the patient, and makes it easier for movement to take place. Observations will include temperature, pulse, respiration, blood pressure, care of the transfusion and stump drains. Sandbags may be used for a short period to keep the stump steady. If so it is essential that they are placed on the bed and not resting against any part of the patient which could further damage the blood supply. Sand bags left in place too long limit the patient's mobility and increase the risk of pressure sores, especially in the elderly patients with ischaemia.

The patient can be moved from side to side, but care must be given to support the stump in a position of extension. Other measures to prevent flexion deformity will include lying the patient prone. Later the patient will be shown how to do exercises by the physiotherapist which will increase the power of the extensor and abductor muscles. Sheepskins for the patient to sit on and under the heels are helpful in preventing pressure sores; this must be combined with a regular two-hourly movement routine.

In the early post-operative period the physiotherapist will encourage the patient to breathe deeply thus decreasing the risk of chest complication. The nurse must be able to continue to encourage the patient to carry out these exercises when the physiotherapist is not able to be present.

Other measures which will increase the patient's well-being and prevent complication are a well-balanced nourishing diet, and activities which will stimulate movement of the whole body, especially the upper-limbs which will be important later on when the patient is using crutches.

Control of pain

Professor Hayward in his research on pain shows there is a relationship between anxiety and pain; uncertainty increases anxiety. The nurse who spends time explaining procedures to her patients and listening to their worries will make a positive contribution to reducing the level of anxiety and so help to relieve pain. Pain can also be reduced by careful handling of the stump. A firm grasp is essential — this will limit movement and movement causes pain. The stump should be placed in a comfortable position for the patient but avoiding flexion.

Phantom pains often continue for some time after the operation — it is best to warn the patient of this but to reassure him that they usually subside with time.

Care of the stump
Observation in the early stage to determine excessive blood loss, and removal of the drain as requested by the surgeon 24 or 48 hours after surgery. A dressing of non adherent substance such as *tulle gras* is applied in theatre. The patient may return to theatre for the first change of dressing to be carried out under anaesthetic. Sutures are removed 10 to 14 days post-operatively.

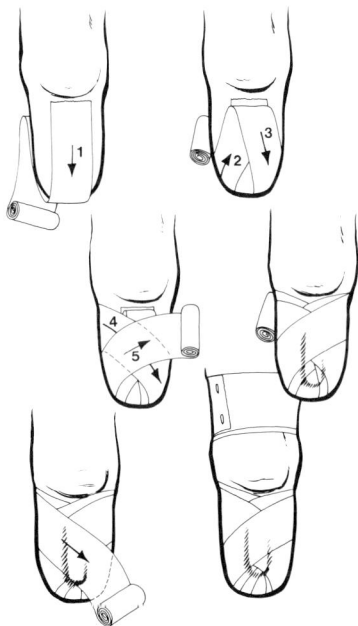

Fig. 14. *Below knee stump bandaging (by courtesy of Seton Products).*

Bandaging the stump in the post-operative period will help to reduce swelling and may help to shape the stump, but this shaping

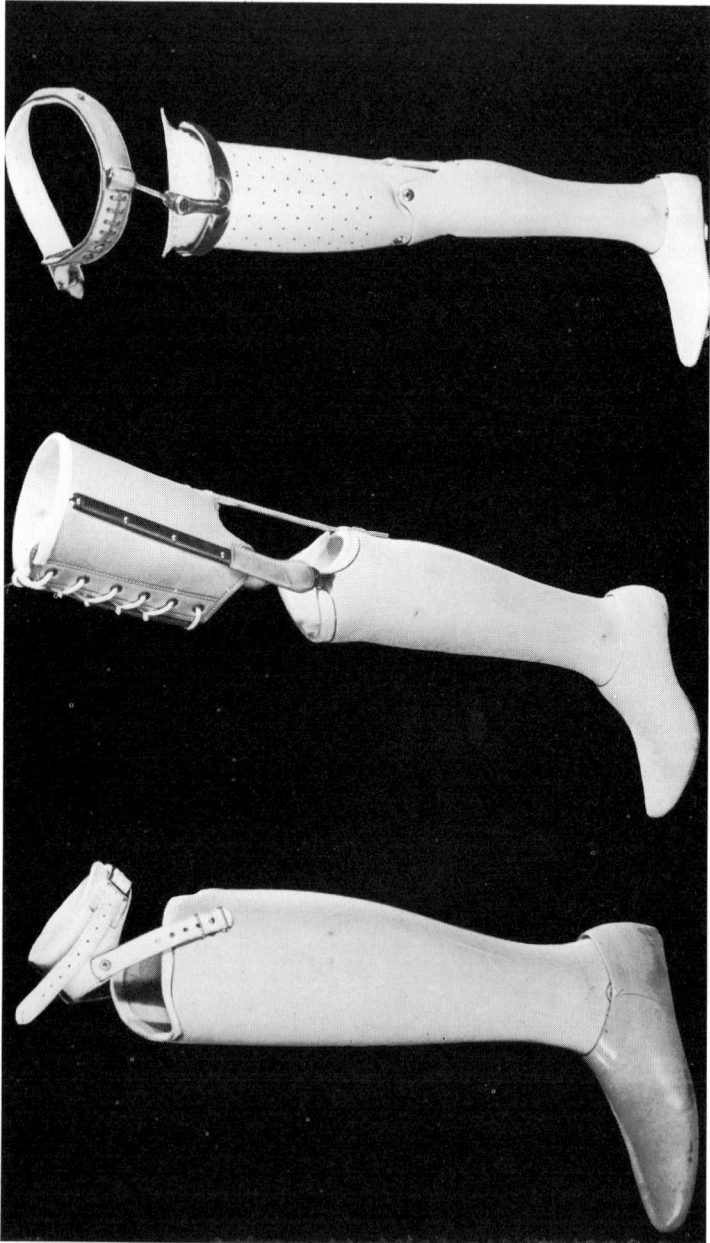

Fig. 15. *Lower limb prosthesis: below-knee patella bearing (left); below-knee corset topped (middle); above-knee showing pelvic band (right). The patient can flex and abduct the hip.*

is better done by the newer methods of amputation so called myoplasty. Some surgeons do not advocate bandaging because of the risk of further damaging the blood supply, and a bandage badly applied could produce a misshapen stump which will cause problems when fitting the prosthesis. A 10 to 15 cm crepe or elastic bandage is used. The bandage is applied at the extremity of the stump. It is applied firmly taking several turns round and then under the end of the stump. Bandaging is continued in an upward direction, using slightly less pressure so that the tightest turns are at the end of the stump (Fig. 14).

In the case of an above-knee amputation the bandage is extended to the top of the thigh. For a below-knee amputation it is taken as far as, but not above, the knee joint.

Although care of the stump is important it is vital not to neglect the so-called good leg. This will inevitably have more work to do, and a careful watch must be kept on the circulation, the state of the skin and the nails. Chiropody may be necessary as well as physiotherapy to strengthen the musculature.

Opportunity to react to loss
There is bound to be reaction to the loss of a limb. An amputation is a mutilating operation, and in the case of a hind-quarter amputation very much so. Whether it is worse for the different age groups is difficult to say. The patient can be helped by members of the team; the medical social worker has a specially important role to play, so too do the relatives. The long-term aim is to get the patient back home living as normal a life as possible, all — including the patient — contributing.

Fitting the prosthesis (Fig. 15)
The patient may be measured for a pylon before, or very soon after, the amputation. The fitting of this simple prosthesis will enable the patient to mobilize early after operation thus helping to prevent complications. The limb-fitter, physiotherapist, occupational therapist and the nurse all have an important role to play in getting the patient to accept the artificial limb, to see that it is properly fitted, to teach him how to care for the stump, and to see that he resumes normal activity as soon as possible. In order to achieve this aim it is better for the patient to be admitted to a ward near to the Artificial Limb and Appliance Centre. This enables the

limb-fitter, physiotherapist and occupational therapist to work together to provide for the patient's needs.

Liaison with the community services
Before discharge it will have been necessary to liaise with the community services in order to consider whether there is a necessity for home helps, home adaption, occupational therapy or aids such as a wheel chair or walking aids to be supplied. The relatives will need to know what is expected of them, and the general practitioner will need to be informed of the progress of the patient, as well as the plan of future visits to the Artificial Limb and Appliance Centre.

5 Splints (orthoses), their use and management

THOMAS'S BED KNEE SPLINT

Thomas's splint (Fig. 16) is one of many designed by Hugh Owen Thomas of Liverpool, who is known as the father of orthopaedic surgery. It is made of two rigid bars joined above to a ring of the same material. The ring is padded with felt and covered with soft leather. It is ovoid in shape and the outer side is at a slightly higher level than the inner. The back half, made to fit the back of the thigh, is larger, as can be seen by holding a tape across between points where the bars meet the ring. This determines whether the splint is for the left or right leg.

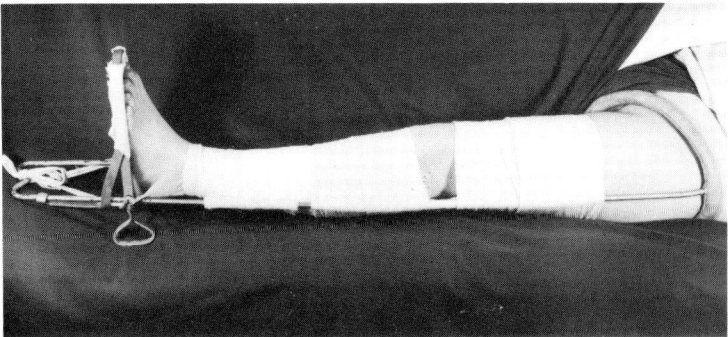

Fig. 16. *Thomas's bed knee splint.*

The great advantage of this splint is that the patient can be lifted with the limb supported, and the limb can be raised from the bed without disturbance by means of counter-weights and pulleys going to an overhead beam. The cords are tied to the splint and are quite separate from the traction weights. Because it is possible to lift a limb in a Thomas's splint, it is frequently put on over the clothes, with a clove hitch as an extension, as a first-aid treatment for a fractured femur. A common use of this splint is to immobilize the knee joint with fixed traction. It is the standard method of treating an acute tuberculosis of the knee, though it is used for any infective condition of the knee joint. When used like this the ring should fit snugly around the groin and press on the tuberosity of the ischium which is the fixed point. It can also be used for any condition when it is necessary to keep the knee in extension, as in a spastic paralysis.

Below-knee extensions are applied and the extension tapes are taken over the outside bar and under the inside bar and pulled and tied to the W-shaped junction. Tension can be increased by using some type of windlass, a rigid bar the size of a large nail. The ring must fit. Too large a ring causes pressure on the perineum. Too tight a ring causes pressure on the inner side of the groin. The leg is supported by slings of soft leather, flannel or domette, which are attached to the side bars and held by clips, stitching or pins. They should overlap so that even pressure is exerted on the traumatized tissue. In treating fractures the tension of these slings is often adjusted to correct alignment. For further immobilization, a metal gutter splint or gutter-like plaster slab may be placed between the slings and the limb, extending from the upper part of the thigh to 7.5 cm above the malleoli, so that two-thirds of the leg is above the level of the side bars.

Lateral guarding splints of plaster or metal may be used if the condition is very acute. The knee must be kept slightly flexed and the upper end of the tibia supported by a pad of wool to prevent subluxation. Care must be taken that the distal sling leaves the heel free and does not press on the Achilles tendon which would cause a sore. A cradle is added to keep the weight of the bedclothes off and support the foot in the plantar grade position. It also keeps the heel off the bed. The whole limb is covered with wool and then bandaged, the knee being fixed first. It is desirable to end the bandage at the upper border of the patella in order to avoid pressure on the quadriceps. If this is not practicable, generous use should be made of the wool and it must be ensured that there is no pressure on the lateral popliteal nerve where it winds around the head of the fibula. When there is much swelling in the knee joint, a ring with a buckle is used which makes it possible to have a well-fitting ring when a ring without a buckle would not go over the joint.

Care of the patient
At first, the skin under the ring will require four-hourly treatment. The area is washed and rubbed well with the lather of a good soap, easing the skin under the ring and leaving the part dry and powdered lightly. Incontinent and old patients can have the part rubbed with a mixture of zinc ointment and castor oil. Do not use anything like petroleum jelly that causes the ring to adhere to the skin.

This splint is used not only for 'fixed' traction but to 'cradle' the limb for sliding traction. Like this it is used for a fractured femur and for the postoperative treatment of an arthroplasty of hip. An arthrodesis of knee in plaster can be 'cradled' in a Thomas's splint and it is used sometimes for paralysis of the quadriceps.

Pearson flexion piece
The flexion piece may be hinged to the bars of a Thomas's knee splint and can be adjusted to any angle. It is used for a supra-condylar fracture of the femur. It is useful for post-operative knee exercises and for the correction of flexion deformity of the knee.

To measure for a Thomas's bed knee splint
The patient lies on a firm bed with the foot in dorsi-flexion and the leg is measured as follows:

Obliquely around the thigh at the level of the adductor tendon. From the adductor tendon to the heel. Allow 20 to 30 cm for extension irons.

WALKING CALIPER

A walking caliper is similar to a Thomas's bed knee splint, but the side bars terminate by being turned at right angles to form a spur.

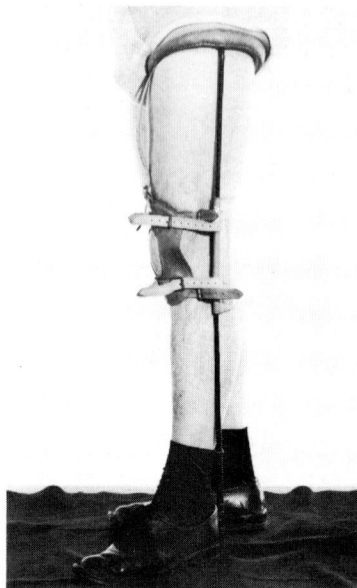

Fig. 17. *Ring caliper applied to patient.*

The spurs fit into sockets made in the heels of the shoes.

A caliper is worn either to take weight off the lower limb or to keep the knee in extension when the joint is unstable (Fig. 17). A weight-relieving caliper may be ordered for tuberculosis of the knee or any other inflammatory condition in the quiescent stage. The ring must fit well against the tuberosity of the ischium and the caliper must be long enough to allow the heel to rest lightly in the shoe without pressure, although the toes are in contact with the ground. The greater part of the body weight is transmitted from the tuberosity of the ischium down the bars to the heel of the shoe. These calipers are sometimes referred to as 'long' calipers. The 'short' caliper is of the same design, but the heel fits normally into the shoe. The ring fits comfortably around the groin or is replaced by a leather cuff.

For old people or those who will wear a caliper indefinitely, instead of a ring, a moulded leather 'bucket top' is used (Fig. 18). This is taken from a plaster cast and can be weight-relieving or non-weight-relieving. There is a leather sling at the back of the

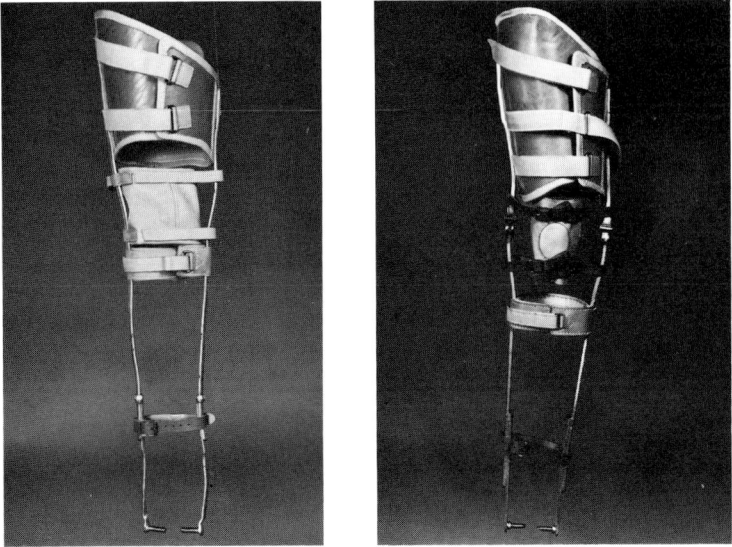

Fig. 18. *Bucket topped caliper.*

thigh and another behind the head of the tibia to prevent subluxation of the knee joint. Flexion of the knee is allowed by the addition of a knee joint in all adult calipers. A leather heel strap is provided to prevent the spurs slipping out of the sockets. The heel sockets can be square or round with the spurs to fit. A round socket allows movement at the ankle joint.

A square socket prevents normal plantar- and dorsi-flexion of the ankle and has been used for a flail foot. This, however, is very rigid and it has been found better to have, in conjunction with square sockets, hinges at the level of the ankle joint. This device allows the patient to make full use of any muscles that are unaffected and to develop weak ones. If there is muscle imbalance, movement can be checked by anterior or posterior stops or a toe-raising spring can be used (see Double Irons, p. 56). For children, the ends of the calipers are adjustable so that they can be lengthened with growth. The caliper bars can be bowed, if necessary, to accommodate a distended knee. The shoes worn with a caliper should be of the laced type with a firm leather upper and flat heel. Boots are often preferred, especially if there is any spasm, and the heels have a tendency to rise out of a shoe.

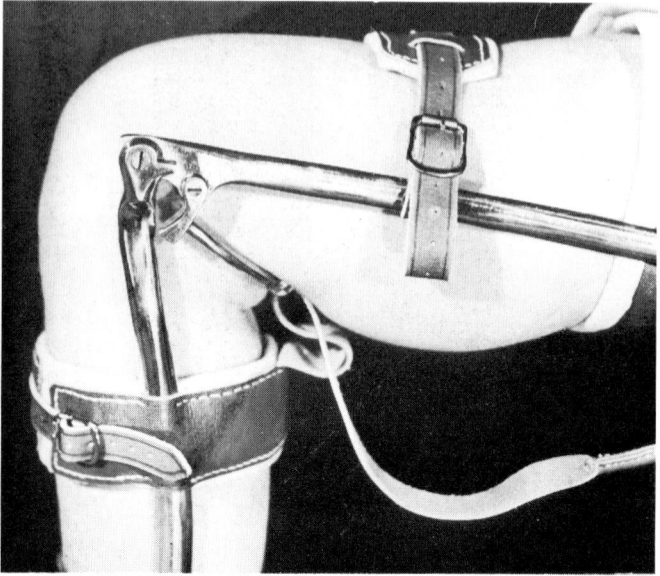

Fig. 19. *Caliper hinge allowing flexion of the knee joint.*

A permanent caliper may be fitted with a locking device that can be manipulated by the patient (Fig. 19). This allows the patient to sit and is used for residual paralysis of the quadriceps following anterior poliomyelitis and for osteo-arthritis of the knee.

Care of the caliper
If the calipers are worn continuously the shoes can be covered with canvas bags to protect the bedclothes. Pressure areas under the ring may be treated by washing and drying thoroughly, dusting with powder and then moving the skin backwards and forwards and massaging gently. A thin layer of sponge rubber in the shoe is sometimes helpful. The patient should be first taught to stand with the weight evenly distributed on both feet, which are apart as far as the width of the shoulders. A slight raising on the heel of the shoe on the sound leg may be necessary. When the patient can stand correctly he should start walking lifting the leg forward and not clutching furniture or swinging the caliper outward.

When the patient is discharged, definite instructions should be

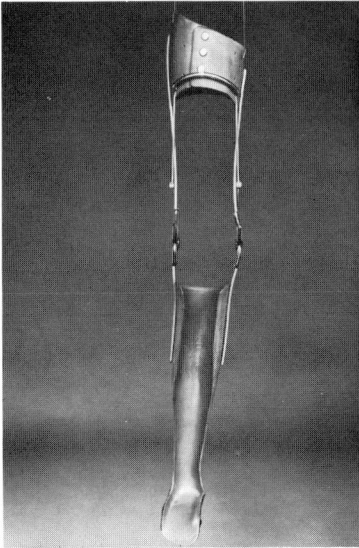

Fig. 20. *A cosmetic caliper.*

given regarding the care of the skin and application of night splints. The leather should be kept soft with saddle soap, a thin oil in small quantities should be applied to the hinges, and repairs should be seen to when required.

To measure for a caliper
Measure straight around the thigh at the level of the adductor tendons.

For length measure from the ischial tuberosity to the plantar surface or the heel with the foot in dorsi-flexion.

State whether the splint is right or left leg and send the correct shoe, clearly labelled, for tubing.

THOMAS'S PATTEN-ENDED CALIPER

The side bars of the Thomas's patten-ended caliper do not fit into the heels of the shoe, but continue below the heel and are fitted into a circular metal base, which has a rubber under-surface. Usually this caliper is about 7.5 cm longer than a caliper taking an

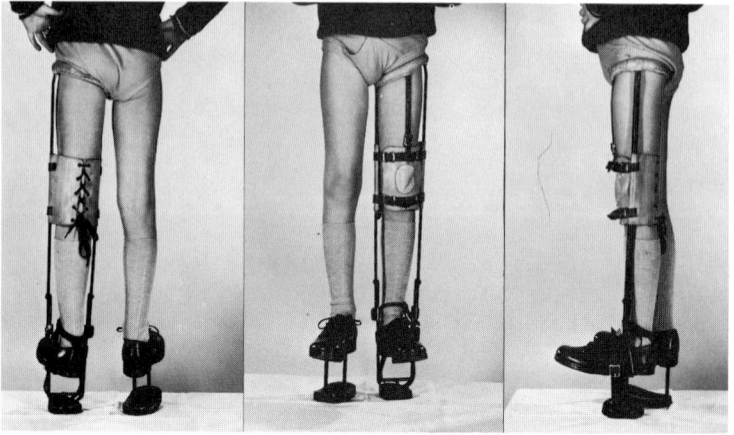

Fig. 21. *Patten-ended weight-relieving caliper with compensatory patten to right foot.*

ischial tuberosity bearing (Fig. 21). A compensatory patten is fixed to the heel of the opposite boot. As the foot is off the ground the weight is taken completely off the leg. In addition to the back sling and knee shield, a soft leather anklet is fitted over the boot and buckled around the splint to hold the foot in position. A webbing strap is fixed around the ring and carried over to the opposite shoulder. See that a child does not wedge books, toys, and the like between the boot and the patten, and so make it weight-bearing. This splint is used for tuberculosis and other inflammatory conditions of the ankle, such as osteomyelitis, and in Perthes's disease of the hip joint.

Measurements that should be taken for this splint are the same as for walking caliper with the length of the patten, as ordered by the surgeon.

KNEE CAGE

A knee cage is used for an unstable knee that is non-paralytic. The condition may be due to torn crucial ligaments. The cage has two side bars hinged at the knee joint level which are attached to metal and leather bands around the thigh and ankle. One bar terminates in a spur fitting into tubing of the heel of the shoe. The leather bands are laced so that the patient can easily put on or take off the cage. This splint allows full weight-bearing, but gives a certain degree of protection to a painful knee with osteo-arthritis or an unstable knee.

A similar splint to give protection and limit mobility is sometimes ordered for the elbow joint. For an accurate fit these splints are usually made from a tracing or plaster cast as measurements are not satisfactory.

BELOW-KNEE IRONS AND T-STRAPS

Below-knee irons and T-straps are bars of metal (steel or Duralumin) which are attached above to a metal band which is padded, covered with leather and buckled just below the knee on the outside of the leg and slightly to the front. There is a slight curve over the malleolus and the end is a round or square spur fitting into the heel of the boot as a caliper does.

They are used to prevent deformity due to muscle imbalance when a calcaneous, equinus, inversion or eversion is liable to occur. They are commonly used for anterior poliomyelitis.

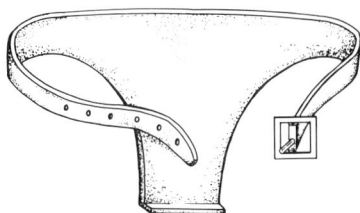

Fig. 22. *T-strap.*

An essential part is the T-strap (Fig. 22) which is made of leather and is attached to the side of the shoe between the sole and the upper, and straps around the boot to be buckled round the iron on the opposite side. The strap provides stability and compensates for weak invertor or evertor muscles. Increased stability is obtained if the tongue of the strap is elongated and passed through a buckle on both sides. T-straps are used with calipers, double and single irons (Fig. 23).

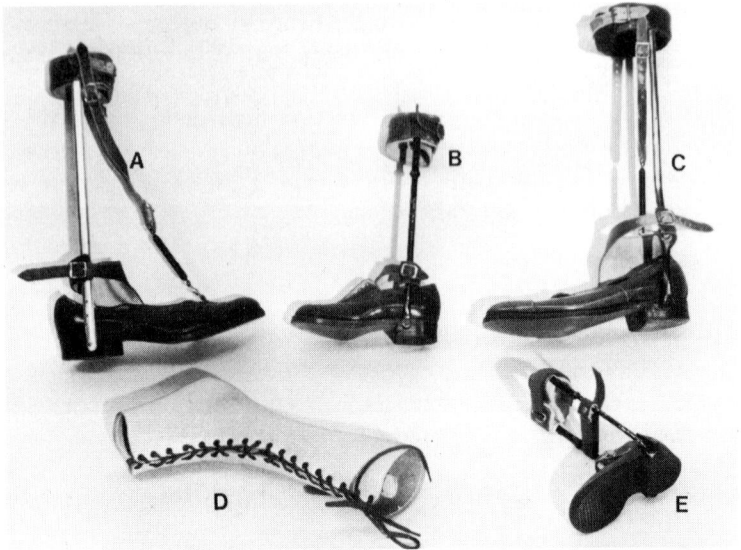

Fig. 23. *(a). Inside, T-strap, outside iron with centre toe-raising spring;* (b) *inside T-strap, outside iron;* (c) *inside T-strap outside iron with flat socket ankle joint and side spring to help the dropped everted foot;* (d) *moulded leather anklet to give stability to the ankle joint;* (e) *double below-knee iron to give stability to the ankle.*

SINGLE IRONS

The iron is always on the side to which the foot is turned and the T-strap on the opposite side. An *outside iron* and inside T-strap is used to correct a valgus (away from the mid-line) deformity due to weak invertors and overaction of the evertors due to anterior poliomyelitis or spasmodic flat foot. An *inside iron* and outside T-strap is used for a varus (towards the mid-line) deformity due to weak evertors and strong invertors and for talipes equinovarus in the ambulatory stage (Fig. 24).

DOUBLE IRONS

Double irons are used to prevent movement at the ankle joint. If no movement at all is wanted, square sockets may be used or a stop placed in front of one heel tubing and behind the other. These are known as contrary stops.

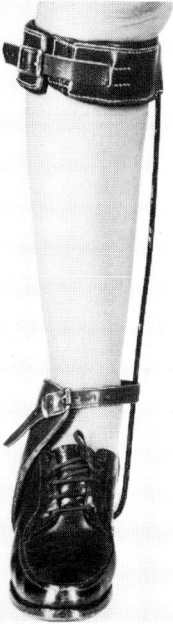

Fig. 24. *Inside iron and outside T-strap to aid eversion; the reverse consequently helps inversion.*

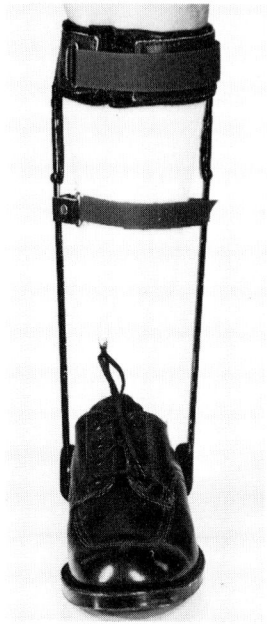

Fig. 25. *Double below-knee iron with back-check stops to prevent plantar flexion.*

When the calf muscles (posterior tibial group) are affected, a stop is placed in front of each socket (anterior stops) to prevent the stronger anterior group lifting the foot off the ground. When the anterior tibial group is weak, the overaction of the calf muscles, together with gravity, causes a plantar-flexion deformity and posterior stops (drop-foot stops) are used. They are employed in order to overcome drop-foot in anterior poliomyelitis, spastic paralysis or following injury to the lateral popliteal nerve (Fig. 25).

Alternatively, a toe-raising spring may be used, attached to the calf band by two leather straps. Two other leather straps are fixed to the spring and to the side of the shoe between the sole and the upper. This is preferable to a spring attached to the toe of the shoe which pulls on the toes and makes them feel cramped. In mild cases the spring can be attached laterally. Another method is the coiled spring, using the Exeter coils.

To measure for a short iron

Measure the circumference of the limb, around the tibial tuberosity. Measure the length from the head of the fibula to heel, with the foot in dorsi-flexion. Allow for the heel of the shoe. State whether the iron is for the right or left leg. Send the shoe for fitting the T-strap.

ALTERATIONS TO BOOTS AND SHOES

The shoes must be of the firm walking type that are laced and have a wide heel. They should have a straight inner border and be wide enough to accommodate the toes without cramping them, but it is necessary that they should fit closely especially around the heel so that alterations of tilt can be transmitted to the foot and ankle and not just slide the foot over to one side.

Inside raising to the heel

An inside raising to the heel is used to alter the line of weight-bearing in a weak abducted foot. It is also used to correct knock knees in children and to take the strain off the internal ligament of the knee joint and make walking far easier after a period of prolonged recumbency (Fig. 26).

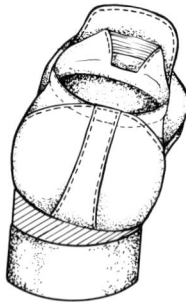

Fig. 26. *Inside raising to heel.*

The wedge may be placed between the upper and the sole. The thickness varies from 3 to 12 mm according to the size of the patient and the orders of the surgeon. With wedges in this position, the shoes can be repaired by any shoemaker. This is known as a 'crooked' heel. The heel is sometimes floated out to the opposite side of the wedge to prevent a tendency to bulge on the outer side and increase the weight-bearing area.

A cork wedge and a leather sock can be placed inside the shoe and used for more than one pair. When the inner margin is brought forward 12 mm or so more than the outer edge, there is more control of the tarsal region and greater inversion. This is the classic Thomas heel — the 'crooked elongated heel' (Fig. 27).

Outside raising to the heel
Outside raisings to the heel are applied in the same way and used to correct and preveent a varus deformity such as a talipes equinovarus when the foot has been corrected and the child is walking. They are also used to take the strain off the external lateral ligament of the knee joint.

As well as altering the heel, wedges or flappers may be added to the outer half of the sole to correct inversion (varus) or to the inner half to correct eversion (valgus) (Fig. 28).

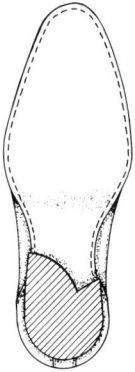

Fig. 27. *Thomas heel.*   Fig. 28. *Wedge.*

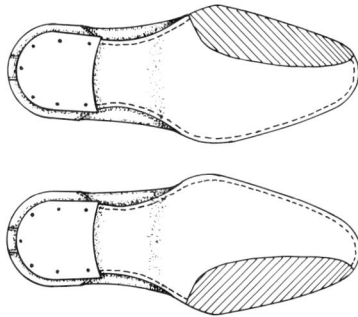

Shoe alterations to compensate for shortening
Apparent shortening is due to pelvic tilt and indicates adduction of the hip. *Apparent lengthening* is due to abduction of the hip. *Real* shortening is due to destruction of bone or failure of growth, such as the short leg of anterior poliomyelitis or the arrested growth at the epiphyses above and below the knee joint following prolonged recumbency.

The shortening is measured by laying the patient flat and measuring from the anterior superior iliac spine to the internal malleolus. This is academic and the practical way to estimate the amount of raising required is to have a collection of wooden blocks varying in thickness from 0.6 to 7.6 cm. The foot of the affected side is placed on blocks of increasing thickness until the anterior superior iliac spines are level.

Most surgeons do not consider it necessary to compensate for shortening of 1.2 cm or less.

When there is slight shortening, 1.8 cm or so, the heel is raaised and bars are placed on the sole one behind the tread and one about 5 cm from the toe of the shoe.

For greater shortening, the heel and sole are removed and the shoe built up with layers of cork. This is not quite so high at the toes and is shaped to give a rocker action (Fig. 29). The cork is covered with the same leather as the shoe and the sole and heel replaced. This type of shoe is very satisfactory from a cosmetic point of view. A patten can be used, but the gait is not so normal and it looks clumsy. It is used as a temporary measure.

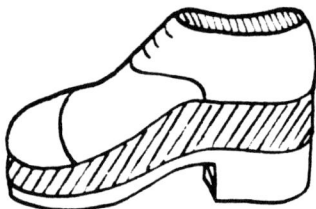

Fig. 29. *Universal raising.*

Metatarsal bar

A metatarsal bar is used to take the weight off painful metatarsal heads (Fig. 30). It is used for claw foot and hallux valgus and is a bar of leather about 0.6 cm thick and 2.5 cm wide, placed obliquely across the sole behind the metatarsal heads. It gives no relief if it is too far forward, but if well placed should take the weight as the foot is plantar-flexed in walking.

Metartarsal insoles

The pain of dropped metatarsal heads can be relieved by a sponge rubber pad on a leather insole. Care must be taken to ensure that

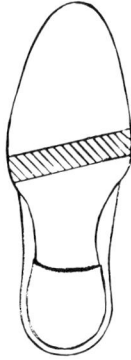

Fig. 30. *Metatarsal bar.*

the pad is not too far forward and so putting pressure on the head of the first metatarsal. To get the fit, a little petroleum jelly is placed behind the metatarsal heads and the patient stands on a piece of blank paper. A tracing of the foot is taken with the pencil held upright. The mark left by the petroleum jelly must be outlined in pencil before it spreads. Sponge rubber pads covered with chamois leather and mounted on broad elastic bands are often useful, because the elastic gives support to the foot. These can be kept in stock. The same effect can be obtained with felt and zinc oxide plaster, but this method is not so convenient.

Supports for the internal longitudinal arch must be firm and resilient, and made for the individual foot. For these reasons many of the commercial types are not satisfactory. The most comfortable types are made from built-up layers of felt or sponge rubber. A plaster cast is taken of the foot when a metal or moulded leather insole is ordered. This is when a permanent support is needed, as in chronic flat foot, when there are arthritic changes in the tarsal joints, or to support the calcaneo-cuboid joint after the operation, known as stabilization, performed in order to prevent the boat-shaped sole.

SPLINTS FOR WRIST AND FINGERS

The handicap of stiff fingers and the importance of keeping the hand in a functional position has been so stressed of recent years

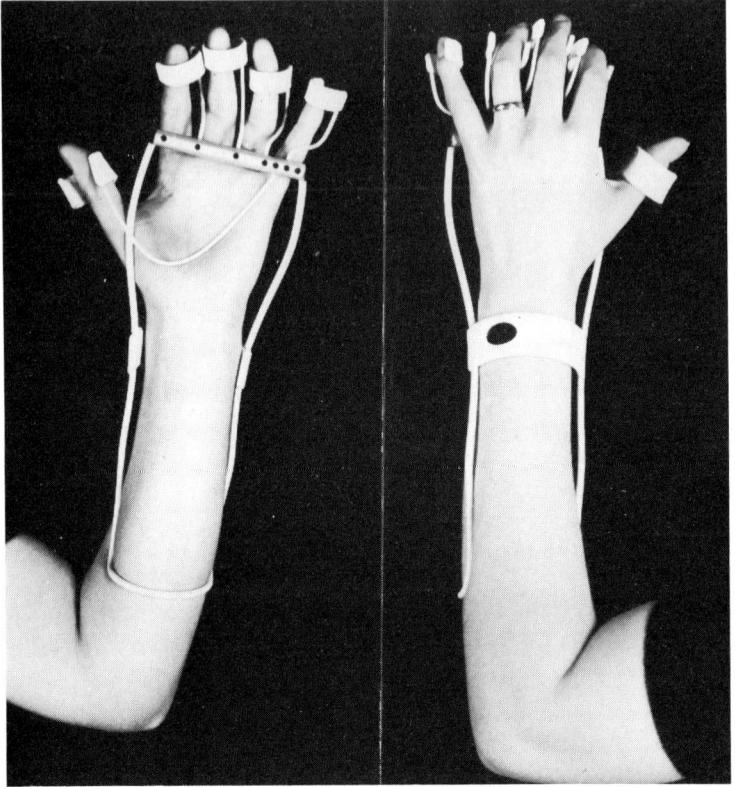

Fig. 31. *A lively splint for radial nerve injury.*

that the long cock-up wrist splint that kept the fingers extended and obliterated the arches of the palm has almost disappeared.

A radial nerve injury splint permitting movement of the inter-phalangeal and metacarpal joints is effective (Fig. 31) and a short cock-up splint of metal or plaster (Fig. 32) to keep the wrist at rest in 30° dorsi-flexion, leaving the fingers free, is now used. Metal splints of this type can be kept in stock. When applied, the splint should extend from the proximal palmar crease to the middle of the forearm.

Innumerable hand splints have been designed with springs, levers, elastic bands and the like for conditions such as poliomyelitis,

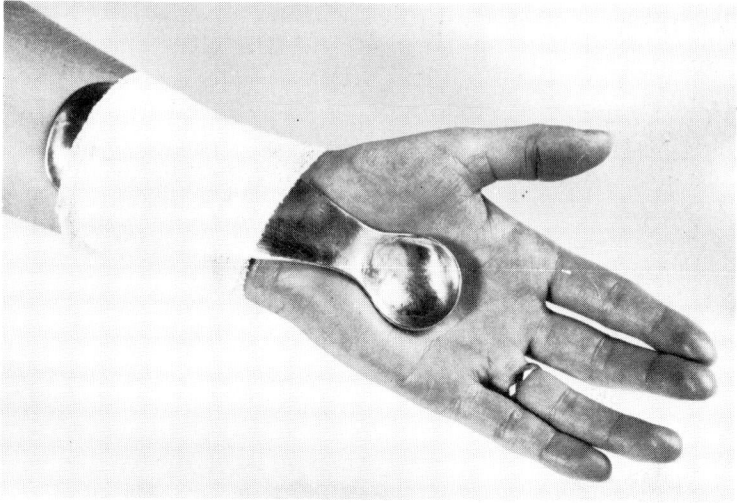

Fig. 32. *Short cock-up splint for the wrist.*

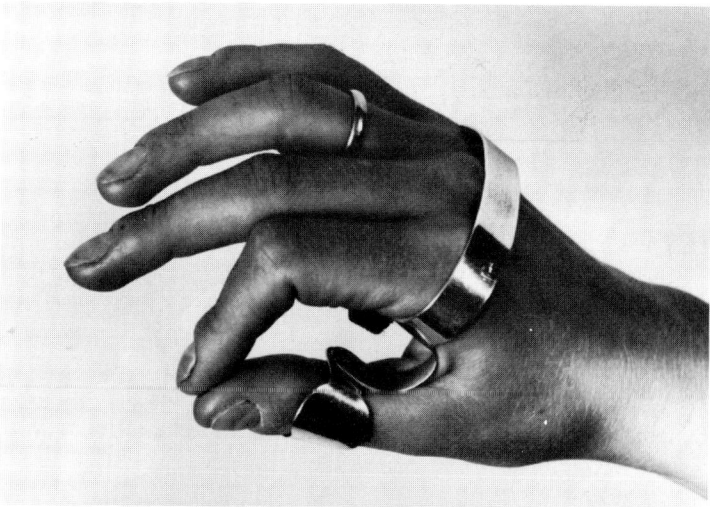

Fig. 33. *Opponens splint with ulnar adaptation.*

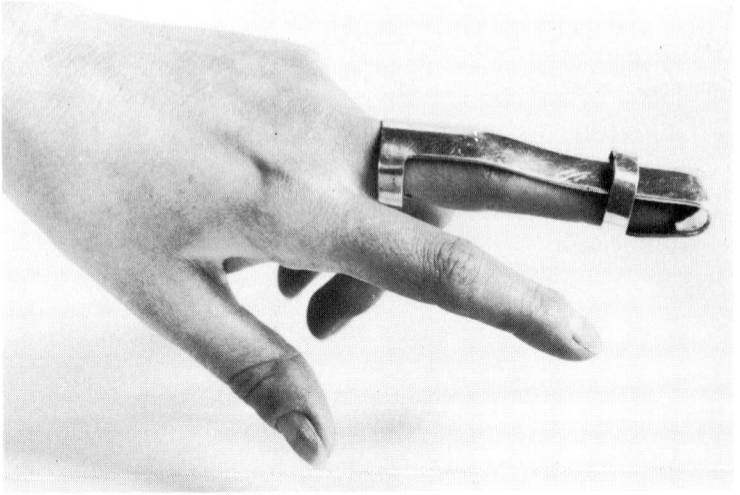

Fig. 34. *Mallet finger splint for ruptured extensor tendon showing the extension of the distal phalangeal joint.*

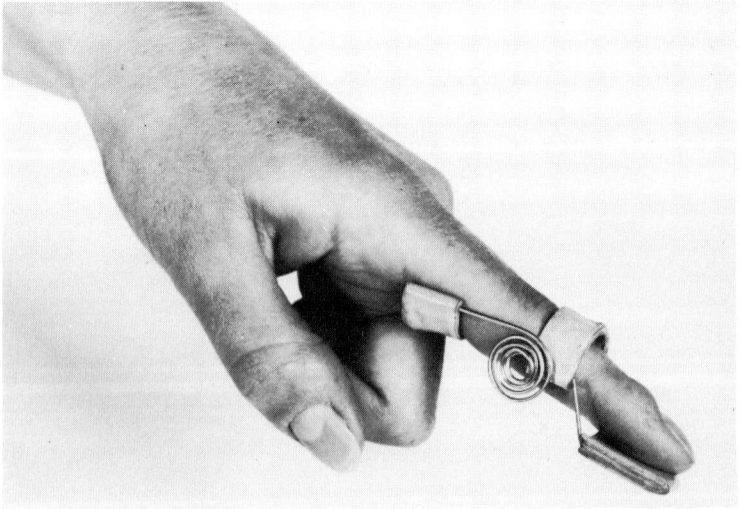

Fig. 35. *Exeter splint for extension of the metacarpal joint.*

peripheral nerve and tendon injuries, not only to immobilize but also to restore function, e.g. the ulnar nerve splint (Fig. 33); the mallet finger splint (Fig. 34). The Exeter splint (Fig. 35) is the Exeter adaptation of the mallet splint.

SHOULDER ABDUCTION SPLINT

The shoulder abduction splint (Fig. 36) is designed to keep the arm in abduction following injuries to the shoulder girdle or brachial plexus and also following anterior poliomyelitis, especially when the deltoid is affected. It is also used for tuberculosis and other inflammatory conditions of the shoulder and circumflex nerve injuries.

The shoulder is usually placed in slight forward flexion. The degree of rotation can easily be varied if the splint is designed with a hinge at the elbow. External rotation is obtained by flexing the elbow with the hand in supination. The splint is constructed of tubular steel connected at the bottom by a padded metal band moulded to fit the pelvis below the line of the crest. This finishes at the midline both in front and at the back and is completed with a webbing band.

The weight of the splint should rest mainly on the pelvis but is also taken by a webbing strap at the centre of the splint on the same side, another higher up to the opposite side, and one on the shoulder which should be padded at the neck. The arm rests on leather slings. Care must be taken that there is no pressure on the ulnar nerve. This splint is often worn over the clothes and care must be taken that it fits on the pelvis and that when walking the patient does not lean continually over onto the splint. The hand must be kept warm.

To measure for a shoulder abduction splint
Holding the arm of the patient in abduction, measure:
The circumference of the trunk at the iliac crest.
The circumference of the trunk at the nipple line.
From the symphysis pubis to the suprasternal notch.
From the suprasternal notch to the shoulder joint anteriorly.
From shoulder to the point of the elbow and from the elbow to the hand.
Finally outline the hand with the palm flat on paper.

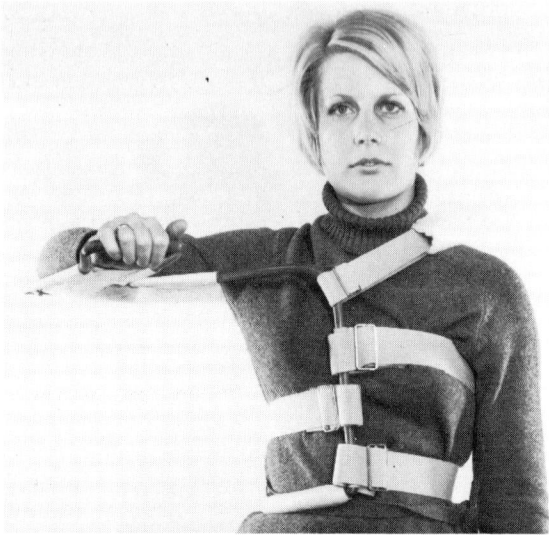

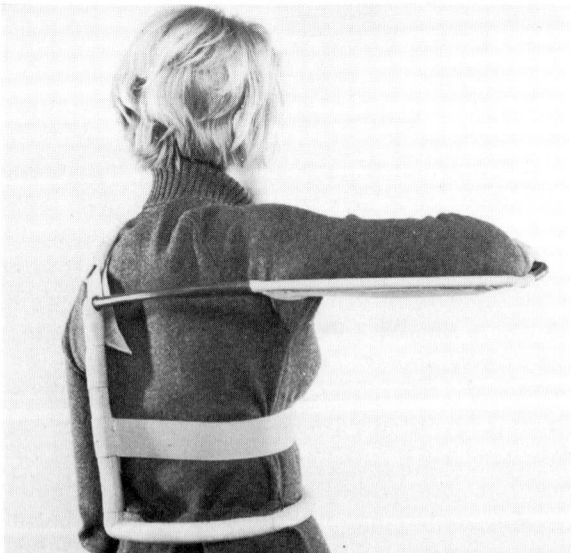

Fig. 36. *Aeroplane splint or shoulder abduction splint.*

GUTTER SPLINTS

Gutter splints are slightly curved metal splints in many sizes. They are frequently used in conjunction with other splints (see Thomas's Bed Knee Splint, p. 47) or as temporary splints.

When used to keep the knee joint in extension, the splint should extend well up the thigh to control the hamstring muscles and end just above the Achilles tendon.

CRUTCHES

When using crutches, the weight should be taken on the hands and not on the axillae. For this reason crutches with adjustable hand pieces are better. It is convenient to have a stock of crutches that can be adjusted in length. The axillary supports should be well padded with felt or sponge rubber. The pneumatic type now used are very comfortable. Pressure of the axillae means pressure on the musculospiral (radial) nerve which supplies the extensors of the wrist, and a dropped wrist results. This should be watched for and the crutches temporarily discarded if the patient complains of inability to grip. The hand pieces are padded for comfort and rubber tips are placed on the bottom of the crutches to prevent slipping.

Walking on crutches

The patient is first taught to stand and acquire a sense of balance. If he can put only one foot on the ground, both crutches are brought forward simultaneously, then the leg is brought forward. If he can put both feet on the ground a 'four point' walk is used. To begin with, the patient, without moving forward, lifts first one foot and then the other off the ground to gain confidence. Then in short steps of even length he advances forward like a quadruped: *Right crutch forward, Left foot forward, Left crutch forward, Right foot forward.* Then he begins again with right crutch forward.

The same method is used with arm crutches or walking sticks which should not be used singly, or tripod crutches which are a steady form of walking stick, but rather clumsy to use.

Tripod walking is used for paralysis of the lower limbs. The legs are controlled by some type of caliper. The two crutches are brought forward and slightly out and the legs simultaneously drawn forward.

To measure for crutches

Measure from the axilla to a point 20 cm outward from the lateral side of the patient's boot.

COLLAR AND CUFF SLING

The collar and cuff sling is more used in orthopaedic work than is the classic sling (Fig. 37). It is made of two leather guards, with

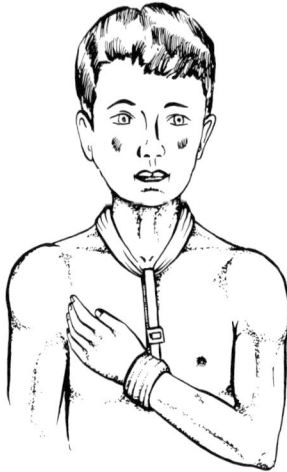

Fig. 37. *Collar and cuff sling.*

short lengths of bandage passed through them, or a more comfortable method is to make guards of flannel with a lining of splint wool. One is tied around the neck, the other around the wrist and the two are held together by a third bandage. It is used to keep the elbow flexed at the degree of flexion ordered by the surgeon when treating a supracondylar fracture of the humerus, or a fractured shaft of the humerus and to support the arm when the elbow is immobilized in plaster of Paris. It is vital that a constant watch should be kept on the circulation and sensation of the fingers. For the first 24 hours the pulse should be taken every half an hour because of the dangerous complication Volkmann's ischaemic contracture. Finger movements should be maintained the whole time of fixation and attention given to make certain that there is no chafing from the bandage at the back of the neck. The antecubital fossa tends to become sore from perspiration, especially in warm weather. This part should be kept dry and powdered.

BÖHLER-BRAUN FRAME

The Böhler-Braun frame is used for fracture of the tibia, and sometimes of the femur when skeletal traction is required (Fig. 38). It is also useful to elevate the very swollen foot that results from a fracture of the os calcis. The limb is supported by flannel wound completely around the metal frame and securely held by strong safety pins. The flannel should be taut except for the part supporting the calf which should be slacker to avoid pressure on these muscles. A padded board for the patient to press his sound foot against aids movement in bed.

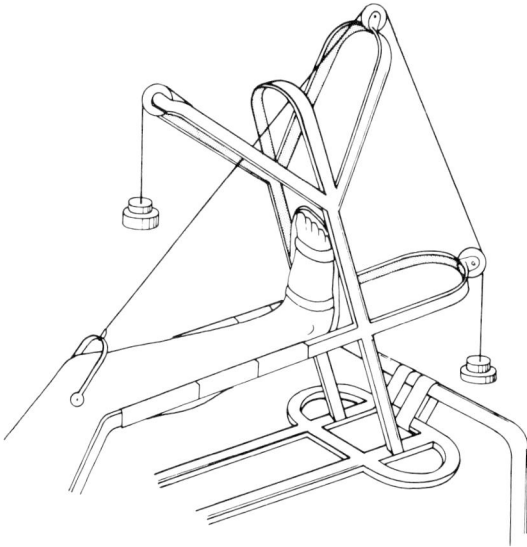

Fig. 38. *Skeletal traction with a Böhler-Braun frame.*

COCKIN SPLINT

The Cockin splint is an adaptation of the Thomas's knee bed splint. It is easily assembled and encourages movement (Fig. 39).

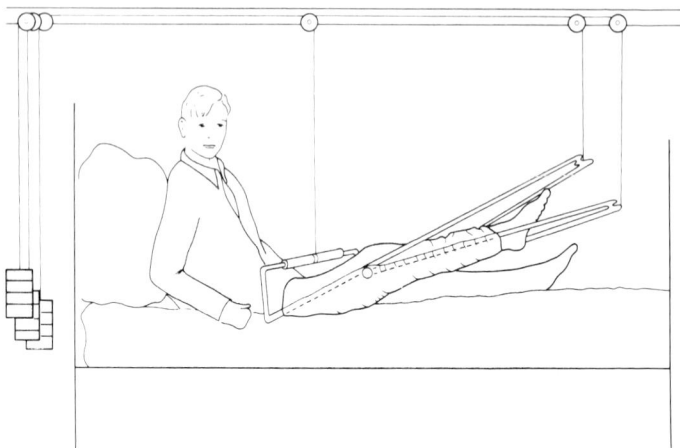

Fig. 39. *Cockin splint which allows movement of the hip and knee. It can be used following surgery of the hip.*

ORTHOPAEDIC FRAMES

Orthopaedic frames (Figs 40 and 41) have been developed from the original spinal frame designed by Hugh Owen Thomas to apply the principles of 'rest, uninterrupted and prolonged', and for tuberculosis of the spine. Sir Robert Jones later added a hinge so that any degree of leg abduction that was desired could be obtained when treating an inflammatory condition of the hip. There have since been many modifications but nurses should understand the working of each type so that they can use it to the best advantage. The advantages of a frame are that it can hold the affected part accurately without undue pressure on soft tissues. The bony points will groove themselves into the padded leather saddle. It allows a large area of the body to be exposed to light and air. It avoids secondary deformities and can compensate for those already present. The whole frame can be lifted and tilted without disturbing the patient. It is easy to give bedpans and keep the patient clean, dry and comfortable, even if he is paralysed, incontinent or has spasm.

Conditions for which the straight frame is used
Conditions for which the straight frame is used include the resting

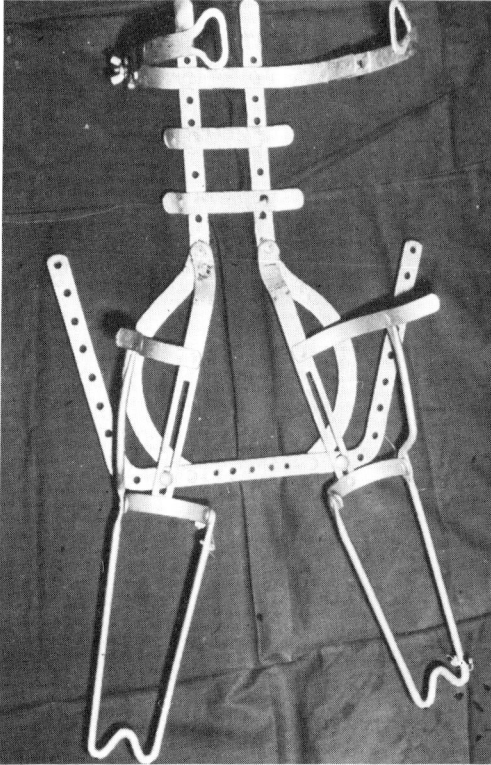

Fig. 40. *Metal framework of a double abduction frame.*

of inflammatory conditions of the spine, such as tuberculosis and osteomyelitis; the correction and prevention of spinal deformities such as ankylosing spondylitis and adolescent kyphosis; and in the treatment of anterior poliomyelitis when there is involvement of the abdominal and spinal muscles.

Basic construction of frames

A frame is constructed of two parallel bars of metal which run down the back from the level of the seventh cervical vertebra to just above the ankle. The bars are parallel until they reach the posterior superior iliac spine where they diverge at an angle of 15° to support the leg. At the level of the gluteal fold there is a slight

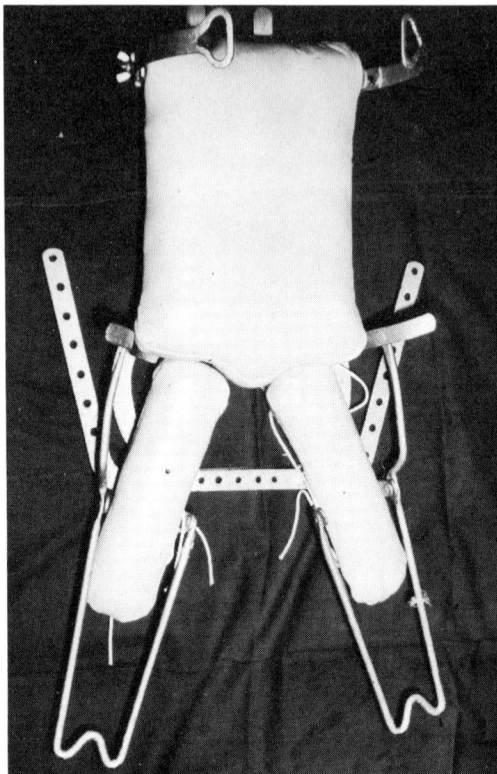

Fig. 41. *Double abduction frame with saddle.*

bend in the metal to give a more accurate fitting of the saddle
around the buttocks and ischial tuberosities. The knock-knee bar
is joined by a small bar to the bar that supports the leg and to the
ankle piece. The knock-knee bar must extend from the upper part
of the thigh and be in line with the horizontal axis of the femur. Its
purpose is to prevent knock knee which could be brought about by
spasm of the adductors, if the leg was held only at the ankle piece.
It also holds the thigh and saddle in place. The lower end of the
femur must be bandaged with the patella facing forwards. For an
adult the bandage should not extend more than a knock-knee
bandage if deformity and muscle wasting are to be avoided. These
bandages should be checked twice a day at least. Children need

more extensive bandaging. The position of the leg must always be noted and bandaging done over adequate quantities of wool. The ankle piece is a semi-circular rigid bar 0.3 to 2.2 cm wide and is padded and covered with chamois leather. It should touch the skin on either side to control rotation but it should not grip too tightly and, being above the malleoli, there is free foot movement. Pelvic and nipple bars are either held in position by 0.6 cm wing nuts or are welded. They are adjusted by means of a wrench. When the patient is first placed on the frame it is necessary then to make these bars fit because it is a very difficult task to correct them when they have been twisted out of shape. The pelvic bars are to prevent lateral pelvic movement and pelvic tilting. They should be moulded around the saddle and the patient. They are fitted with studs to which a groin strap can be fixed. The two pelvic bars are often held together by a firm cross-strap to prevent possible distortion by the groin strap. The nipple bars are also moulded around the patient and the saddle. They prevent lateral movement without hampering respiration. Each has a perforated end through which the shoulder strap from the opposite side is passed, this being first knotted before being tied across to the opposite side.

The shoulder strap is a length of calico bandage tied on the underside of the nipple bar. A length passes over each shoulder and across the chest. The bandage is covered with soft leather guards to prevent chafing over the shoulder. Unless they are knotted before being tied across, the patient will slip down the saddle.

There is also a strengthening transverse bar joining the leg pieces and, in the Wingfield Morris type, a transverse loin bar to prevent sagging of the saddle.

Foot pieces are added to keep the weight of the bedclothes off the feet. Unless the feet are splinted, foot exercises are carried out regularly, and the importance of foot movements should be explained to the patient.

The frame is raised off the bed by means of grooved blocks or metal stands, unless a special frame bed is used. Whichever method is employed, a bedpan can be given without disturbing the patient and left in situ if he is incontinent.

The saddle

The body of the saddle should extend from the seventh cervical vertebra to the tip of the coccyx, and the leg pieces end just below the knee joint. The front surface of the saddle should be covered with soft good quality leather. The back surface is covered with canvas or a cheaper leather. It is packed with lambswool or blanket combings. If there is not enough packing it is uncomfortable, if there is too much, the patient's body will not groove itself in, but will move about. The saddle is tied to the frame by tapes.

To measure for orthopaedic frames

The patient is measured in the neutral prone position with 20° abduction at the hips:

Measure the length from the top of the head to the base of the heel.

Measure the distance from the top of the head to the coccyx.

Measure the distance from the top of the head to the point of the lesion if the frame is to be angulated.

Measure the width of the frame between the outer side of the shoulders.

Measure for the pelvic belt to be worn with the frame.

Measure the circumference of the abdomen at the umbilicus.

JONES'S ABDUCTION FRAME

To immobilize the hip joint when treating an acute inflammatory condition, there must be traction because the powerful muscles around the hip joint go into spasm. One method of obtaining immobility for an acute condition of the hip is the single abduction frame. The abduction frame is used for any inflammatory condition of the hip, such as tuberculosis, acute infective arthritis, as well as for Perthes's disease and adolescent coxa vara (slipped femoral epiphysis). In construction it is similar to the straight frame. Beyond the ankle pieces extend extension bars which are the same as the foot end of a Thomas's bed knee splint. These are sometimes fixed to the end of a straight frame for the convenience of having something to which to fix the gallows. Just above the gluteal fold, on the longitudinal bar, a joint is made to form a hinge. The lower transverse bar is fitted with a series of holes and screws. Hinges and screws can be adjusted to obtain the degree of abduction ordered by the surgeon. When adjusting the degree of abduction before use, the frame must be placed on a straight line along the whole length so that the line cuts the transverse bars exactly in the centre at a right angle. It is then easy to see if the leg pieces are equally abducted to the correct degree. Abduction is usually ordered for both legs at 20°, but occasionally one leg may have wider abduction.

Groin straps are made of felt and covered with soft leather. At each end is a strip of firmer leather pierced with holes. These strips are fixed by one of these holes to the pelvic bar stud behind and passed under the frame along the groin and fitted over another stud on the front of the pelvic bar. They are a vital part of the abduction frame as they supply the fixed point for traction. Skin extensions are applied to both legs. If possible, this is done the day before. When the patient is on the frame, the groin strap, as the fixed point, must be fixed first. Then the extensions are tied. Both groin straps should fit firmly and comfortably, and extensions taut to be effective. The skin of the groin should be washed, dried thoroughly, powdered and may be gently massaged.

Later this treatment can be done once or twice daily. Two important points to remember:

1. The skin must be scrupulously clean
2. The skin must be kept dry.

Before undoing the groin strap, the foot of the bed must be elevated to give counter-traction. The groin strap should never be released until this has been done. Not only must the skin be left dry, but the groin strap must be dry and free from cracks. If it gets wet it should be dried slowly and cleaned with saddle soap. A spare groin strap should be at hand so that a wet one can be changed. When giving a bedpan, the groin strap should not be released or the foot of the bed elevated since this could cause the patient a considerable amount of discomfort. It is usual to have the groin strap on the unaffected side. This should be remembered when the skin of the groin is slightly red, and relief from pressure is given by temporarily removing the groin strap and elevating the foot of the bed. A localized area of pressure can be relieved by placing a small roll of lint either side of it before replacing the groin strap on the unaffected side, but for restless patients, two groin straps may be used. Groin straps can be used even without traction for a restless child with a lumbar spine lesion. The extensions must be kept tight and checked at least twice a day. The patient must be kept straight on the frame. This is checked by seeing that the anterior superior iliac spines are kept level. If the patient slips down and the ischial tuberosities are over the bend of the frame, the bandages must be undone. Traction is then held manually while the patient is put back in position.

The double abduction frame for treatment of congenital dislocation of the hip is used to obtain gradual wide abduction in congenital dislocation of the hip (see Chapter 12).

CARE OF THE PATIENT ON A FRAME

Placing the patient on a frame

The patient should be prepared by lying recumbent on a firm bed, for a few days before fixation. The reasons for fixation and immobilization should be explained to the patient. The appearance of the apparatus is alarming to the unaccustomed eye and the patient may be very frightened. If possible let the new patient be next to a patient who is already well settled. Suppositories to ensure a good bowel action should be given. Sedation is usually necessary for a few days prior to fixation, and until the patient has settled. The hair should be short, the patient blanket bathed and an enema given. The patient is taken into a warm room, as he will be wearing only a groin slip, and placed on the frame in the morning. It is undesirable to start frame fixation in the evening. The patient should be lifted steadily, first onto the saddle and then the saddle and patient are lifted onto the frame, to which the saddle tapes are then tied. The following points must be checked:

1. That the pelvis is level
2. That the tip of the coccyx is at the fork of the saddle, and that saddle and patient are in the correct position on the frame
3. That the ankle pieces, nipple and pelvic bars and head pieces fit and are comfortable.

General care of the patient on a frame

The following points should be observed daily. Patients who have a lesion below the sixth dorsal vertebra can wash themselves and should be encouraged to do so as far as possible. When a nurse washes the patient, nipple bars, pelvic bars and leg bandages are undone separately, and the exposed parts washed one at a time. Special attention should be given to the genitalia and anal region. The latter should be washed every time the patient has a bedpan.

Before giving a bedpan, pack the fork of the saddle with tow. The patient wears an open-backed gown tied around the frame, and a cardigan is worn back to front. A thin blanket or flannelette sheet is wrapped around the frame and a pair of woollen socks is worn.

Plaster turning cases
To avoid moving the spine and yet to inspect the back, a plaster turning case is made. The leg bandages are loosened, the bars bent back and the case made while the patient is on the frame, moulding over the clavicles and extending it to the ankle. It is made like a plaster bed, but, because it is shallower, the patient should not be in it too long. If it is necessary to keep the head still for a cervical lesion, metal bars are incorporated and a head sling fitted over the brow. A thin piece of plaster, moulded over the chin, will hold the head sufficiently if the lesion is a high dorsal one.

Turning the patient
The bars are bent back, the restraining bandages removed and the turning case fitted over the patient with enough splint wool to make it comfortable and take off the chill. Straps are buckled around the trunk and each leg with the buckles at the side. A child can be turned by four nurses, but a Cullen turning crane makes it easier for an adult.

When the patient is over, the back is inspected and washed. The frame is overhauled and the saddle cleaned and exposed to the air. The patient can be left quite safely for two or three months without turning, but should be turned without hesitation if there is any complaint of pain or pressure, if the saddle is soiled or the pelvic or nipple bars broken. More frequent turnings are done to improve the skin before operation, and when back raising and knee flexion exercises are ordered.

If a child is on a Bradford frame, or there is no turning case available, a turning can be done by the same technique using webbing straps and horse hair pillows, or another straight Bradford frame.

A turning case can be used for the abduction frame incorporating extension irons in the plaster. The foot of the bed is elevated and the extensions tied to the extension irons, before the straps are applied.

COMPLICATIONS OF RECUMBENCY

Recumbency is essential for the treatment of some conditions, but it is regarded as a necessary evil, because many complications, apart from the disease itself, may occur. The nurse must be aware of the latter and observe and report early signs and symptoms. Complications from the treatment, mentioned below, can be prevented by taking the necessary precautions and by good nursing.

Constipation

Two to three litres of fluid per day and as much cellulose from fruit and vegetables as possible should be given to provide bulk in the diet. Regular habits must be encouraged, mild aperients, such as bulk-producing laxatives, may be given, and an occasional enema administered when necessary.

Bed sores — splint sores

Bed and splint sores have already been discussed and should need no emphasis.

Frame sickness

Frame sickness is a violent form of vomiting, not unlike the vomiting that occurs with an acute intestinal obstruction, and must be reported to the ward sister without delay. It happens when the patient is put on a frame or plaster bed, or even in plaster spica, without the preparation of lying flat for a few days previously. It is more liable to occur when the patient is fixed suddenly with the spine in hyperextension, or the legs in wide abduction. The treatment is prevention, which involves preparing the patient by bed rest, light diet, an enema, and the right psychological approach. Should the condition arise, it may be possible to flex the hips to relax the abdominal muscles and so relieve the abdominal tension. The patient may vomit copiously and so continuously that the resulting dehydration necessitates replacement of fluids intravenously. Gastric suction may be necessary. As a rule this condition rapidly settles down.

Hypostatic pneumonia

Hypostatic pneumonia occurs in the elderly, when there is stasis in the bronchial tubes. If the condition permits it, the head and shoulders should be raised. Failing that, the head of the bed may be raised. It is useful to do this for patients in plaster jackets or spicas. The patient should be kept warm and given breathing exercises with emphasis on expiration. Antibiotics may be ordered.

Renal calculi
In prolonged recumbency and immobilization, there is a decalcification of the whole skeleton with an increase of salts in the blood stream, and therefore, in the urine. Calculi from these salts start to form in the pelvis of the kidney. When they pass down the narrow ureter, there is the violent pain of renal colic in the loins, and haematuria. Before this acute stage is reached, there may be a complaint of pain in the loins and abnormal urine. All patients lying flat should be given what seems an excessive amount of fluids to drink. They must have at least 2 to 2.5 litres a day in addition to meals, and a fluid balance chart should be kept in the early stages. This amount must be drunk, especially in hot weather when body fluid is lost through perspiration, and not merely left on the locker. Some authorities advocate tilting the patient and frequent turnings. As well as routine ward tests, the urine should be sent at regular intervals to the laboratory to be tested for red cells and deposits; such abnormalities if present necessitate more frequent turning and increased fluid intake. Thorough daily cleansing of the genitalia is absolutely essential and particularly after defaecation.

Amyloid disease
Amyloid disease is associated with chronic infection of long standing, such as tuberculosis or osteomyelitis. There is degeneration of the solid viscera with enlargement of liver and spleen. There is oedema of the legs, diarrhoea, albuminuria and a parchment-like skin. It is a condition rarely seen these days, because of the successful treatment of infection by modern surgery and antibiotics.

Muscle wasting and deformities
When lying still over a period the muscles gradually waste — disuse atrophy. Until muscles are sufficiently strong enough to hold the spine erect, a spinal brace may be worn. If, for example,

the foot is allowed to stay in plantar flexion, the anterior tibial group that dorsiflex the foot become stretched and weak and the Achilles tendon contracted.

Flexion deformity of the hip
Flexion deformity of the hip occurs when the patient is allowed to stay in the sitting position for so long that the gluteal muscles become stretched and the hip flexors contracted. The condition is aggravated and accompanied by a flexion deformity of knee, when a pillow has been allowed under the knee so that the hamstrings are contracted and the quadriceps stretched.

On a frame, hip flexion can be caused by the frame and saddle sagging beneath the weight of the patient. The hip flexion caused by the psoas muscle in a hip or spinal lesion subsides on immobilization.

Deformities of the knee
Genu recurvatum is caused by insufficient support for the head of the tibia. Folded felt, wool or suitable pads extending below the tibial condyles must be placed to suport the lower leg comfortably and prevent the knee from becoming hyperextended.

Genu valgum and genu varum
Genu valgum and genu varum occur easily in children and are prevented by correct bandaging to the knock-knee bar. There must be sufficient padding to prevent interference with the circulation. Protection must be given to the lateral popliteal nerve (peroneal) or an equinus deformity of the foot will result because this nerve supplies the muscles that dorsiflex the foot.

Foot deformities
Foot deformities are caused by pressure of the bedclothes, insufficient and incorrect exercises and failure to keep the foot plantar grade between exercises. The exercises should be taught and supervised by a physiotherapist with the nursing staff cooperating and encouraging the patient. The mobility of the feet is most important. A calcaneum deformity (long heel) is due to inadequate packing under the head of the tibia and pressure on the gastrocnemius. It can also be caused by exercises that over-emphasize dorsiflexion and leave out other foot movements. On

an abduction frame, there is a tendency for patients to curl their feet under the extension tapes into a varus deformity.

Deformities of pelvis
Tilting of the pelvis occurs when extensions are uneven or if one groin strap is kept habitually too tight. It can also occur if the position is not checked before applying a plaster spica or jacket.

Shortening of one leg
Shortening of one leg may be due to cessation of growth at the epiphysis at the lower end of the femur.

Deformities of spine
Scoliosis can be secondary to a pelvic tilt or can occur if the patient habitually leans over to one side. It may be necessary to alter the position of the locker to prevent this. Flat back may result because prolonged immobilization can obliterate the normal curves. To avoid this, the patient can be nursed in an anterior plaster shell. Early ambulation with a spinal brace usually restores the normal curves. A poking chin is not so apparent until the patient gets up. Pillows should be varied so that the head is not continually in flexion.

LENGTH OF STAY

Fortunately since the advent of antibiotics the period of frame immobilization associated with tuberculosis or other infective lesions has been greatly reduced. Nevertheless boredom can be a problem and consideration should be given to allowing unrestricted visiting and suitable forms of diversional therapy. Modern drug therapy may also be necessary.

The local education authorities provide facilities for children in orthopaedic hospitals to continue with their education.

SPINAL BRACES

Many types of spinal braces have been designed to hold the spine erect and prevent flexion. No form of support can be designed to relieve the strain of weight-bearing that is taken by the spinal column when a person stands erect. That is why active tuberculosis of the spine is treated in recumbency. A supporting brace limits movement and helps the patient to maintain a good posture. A brace is used for tuberculosis of the spine, when the disease is quiescent and the patient ambulatory. It is used for other spinal conditions, such as anterior poliomyelitis, adolescent kyphosis, ankylosing spondylitis and osteo-arthritis of the spine, when the patient is unable to maintain a good posture.

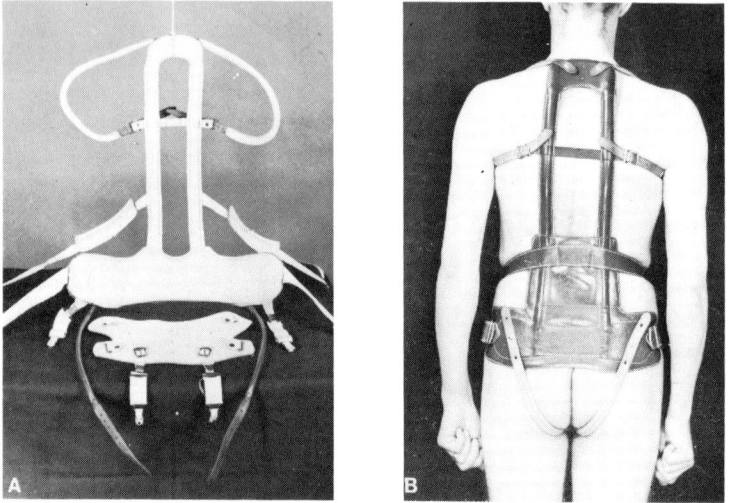

Fig. 42. *Robert Jones brace:* (a) *before application;* (b) *after application.*

THE ROBERT JONES SPINAL BRACE

The Robert Jones spinal brace is comparatively light and comfortable to wear and does not interfere with chest expansion (Fig. 42a and b). It is made of an irregular framework of metal moulded to fit the spinal curves. The brace is covered with felt and soft leather. A strong wide pelvic belt is firmly fixed around the patient between the iliac crests and great trochanters. Padded arm straps are attached to each side and pass around the shoulder and buckle above the middle of the support. Groin straps are buckled to the pelvic belt. They help to keep the support in position. The pelvic belt must take a firm hold of the pelvis. When it has been fully tightened, and the shoulder straps tightened, the back and shoulders are pulled towards the support. This prevents any tendency to flexion. There should be a space of three finger-breadths between the upper part of the support and the patient's spine. This is not liked by the adolescent as it is obvious beneath the clothes, but if the pelvic band is not firm and the support just hangs from the shoulders, it is useless. For high dorsal lesions a supporting collar is attached to the support. An abdominal belt is often added and is essential when the abdomen is protuberant.

To measure for a back support
Place the patient in the prone position.
    Measure the circumference of the chest at the nipple line.
    Measure the circumference of the pelvis between the iliac crests and great tronchanters.
    Measure from the spinous process of the seventh cervical vertebra to the tip of the coccyx, keeping the tape measure in contact with the skin.
    If there is any deformity, a plaster cast of the back must be taken with the patient prone.

Fitting
The pelvic band and groin straps are detached and the pelvic band laid across the pelvis half way between the iliac crest and great trochanters. The patient is then turned and the support laid along the back. It should terminate at the tip of the coccyx. If the part of the brace just over the sacrum is pressed the upper end should stand away from the back. If it fails to do this, and lies flat on the back, the dorso-lumbar curve must be increased. When the fitting is satisfactory, the pelvic band is firmly buckled and the groin and shoulder straps are then secured. The groin straps need not be tight until the patient is ambulant. The patient should then be placed comfortably with pillows under the lumbar spine and knees. Exercises are given and the patient encouraged to move about in bed. The support is more comfortable if it is worn over a thin singlet. After a period of 'kicking free' the patient is allowed to stand. The straps may need adjusting, and an accurate estimate of the fitting can be made. With the patient standing erect, and viewed from the side, no daylight should be visible between the support and the back, and it should be possible to put three fingers between the skin and the upper end.

Daily care

At first the patient may wear the support night and day. There is pressure under the pelvic band and shoulder straps and until the skin hardens these areas should be treated four-hourly and the whole back at least daily. Wash the axillae and areas beneath shoulder and groin straps with soap and water, dry carefully and lightly dust with powder. One advantage of this type of support is that the skin can be treated without altering the position of the spine, provided that the pelvic band is always released last and refastened first. The patient is placed in the prone position with a pillow under the chest and another under the legs so that the feet are comfortable. The shoulder straps and pelvic band are undone and the support is removed. The skin of the back is treated, any points of pressure are observed and the support is cleaned and reapplied. When the pelvic band and shoulder straps have been refastened, the patient is turned into the dorsal position, the groin straps are released, the pelvic band again undone and the skin is treated. Care must be taken not to pinch the skin when replacing the pelvic and shoulder straps, which are rebuckled into the same holes so that the tension on either side is kept equal.

THE FISHER AND ERNST TYPE OF BRACE

The Fisher and Ernst type of brace is made of a metal frame moulded to fit the curves of the body. There are two moulded steel bars supporting the back and fixed to a pelvic bar. A firm grip on the pelvis is obtained by a pelvic bar fitting around the pelvis just below the anterior superior iliac spine, and another bar moulded to the curves of the iliac crest and riveted to the front of the pelvic bar. Also fixed to the pelvic bar are two lateral bars which terminate as axillary crutches. All the metal parts are padded and covered with soft leather. There is a back corset made of white coutil attached to the posterior and lateral bars, with a centre lacing for adjustment. The abdominal corset is attached to the lateral bars and crest piece. It is fastened in front with adjustable buckles and lacing.

Another brace which is sometimes used is the Taylor brace (Fig. 43).

To apply. In this type of brace the strap is undone and the patient placed in the prone position. The support is then put in place, making sure that the pelvic and iliac crest bars fit closely. The axillary crutch should be clear of the shoulder. The patient is then turned over on to a pillow. The pelvic band is first fastened, then the front is laced and finally the shoulder straps are crossed and fastened. The daily care of the patient is the same as that described for the Robert Jones back brace.

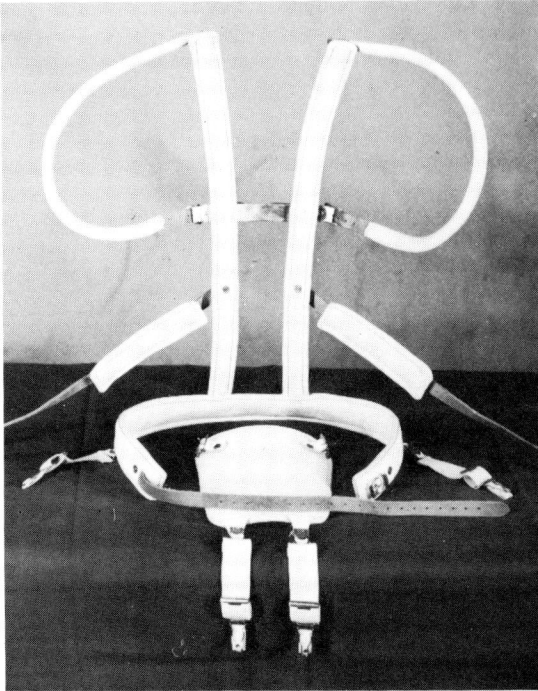

Fig. 43. *The Taylor brace, alternative to the Robert Jones brace used for the same conditions.*

To measure for a spinal brace

Measure the circumference of the pelvis just below the anterior superior iliac spine. Measure the circumference of the waist and of the chest at nipple line. Measure the length from the spinous process of the seventh cervical vertebra to the tip of the coccyx.

This type of support is more satisfactory when a plaster cast is taken, as it is useless and uncomfortable when the moulding of the steel is not accurate.

THE MOULDED LEATHER JACKET

For lesions of the lumbar or lumbo-sacral region, the postural type of support is of little use, nor is relief obtained from a corset support. A moulded leather jacket is made from a plaster cast. The splint-maker moulds wet leather around the cast. When dry and moulded, it is fitted on the patient and marked for trimming. It is then reinforced by strips of Duralumin, lined and polished. It is punctured with holes for ventilation and fastened by laces. It is usual for a plaster jacket to be ordered first and for a moulded block leather jacket to be ordered if that gives relief.

A block leather jacket or spica is used for tuberculosis of the spine in the lumbar region, osteo-arthritis of the spine and paralytic scoliosis and other gross spinal deformities, such as those seen in elderly patients who had rickets when children.

A good cosmetic result can be obtained for these patients by building up the jacket with layers of cork.

LOW BACK SUPPORTS

Surgical corsets, if properly constructed and used under medical direction, can be of great benefit. They are often bought, without medical advice and supervision, by men and women suffering from low back pain and thus are often useless. The correct type of belt can give considerable relief to the patient with chronic low back pain, especially to elderly people with weak abdominal muscles and faulty posture. Before such a belt is ordered by a surgeon, he carries out a full examination to eliminate any of the other causes of backache which might be visceral in origin, or due to referred pain.

As in the case of the spinal brace, there must be a firm grip around the pelvis between the iliac crests and great trochanters. There must be abdominal pressure obliquely upwards and backwards, not just a compression of the abdomen. This, with supporting back steels or a lumbar pad incorporated in the corset, relieves the strain on the lumbar spine and sacro-iliaac joint. The belt is easily adjusted, and the patient is taught to put it on lying down, tightening the lower laces and buckles first (Fig. 44).

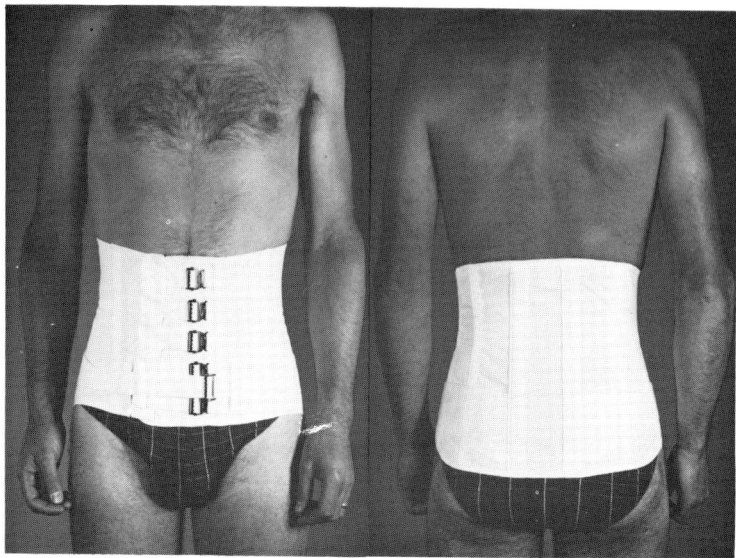

Fig. 44. *Sacro-iliac support* [*Spencer (Banbury) Ltd*].

SPLINTS OF PLASTIC MATERIAL

The term 'plastic' is applied to a synthetic material that can be moulded by the application of heat, pressure or the introduction of a catalyst, into the desired shape. Plastic materiials have many uses in industry and domestic life, and a widening application in orthopaedic work.

Plastic materials make some useful splints. They are light weight, washable and radiotranslucent. They are also non-absorbent and sometimes cause a skin reaction. The following synthetic materials are most commonly used:

Polythene is a solid polymer of gas ethylene, a semi-rigid waxy material prepared for use by heating in an oven, and then held in firm contact with a plaster cast for three-quarters of an hour. It makes useful splints for pool therapy.

Cellular perforated expanded polyethylene is prepared for use by heating in an oven at 140°C and then moulded straight on to the patient and fastened ideally by self-adhesive straps. This type of material is very light, tough, long-lasting and easily washable but some patients find it rather warm to wear. It makes excellent collars and in-soles and if reinforced with polythene strips, jackets can also be made.

CELLULOSE ACETATE AND GLASS FIBRE BANDAGES

The bandages are made of a glass wool fabric and cellulose acetate. When dipped in a setting solution, they become flexible and can be applied in a manner similar to that used for plaster of Paris bandages. Splints can be made by direct application, or over a plaster cast. For direct application, it is advisable to use stockinette or to cover the skin first with French chalk so that the hairs do not adhere.

The glass fibre bandage is dipped into the setting fluid for a few seconds. As it is applied, it is kept partly stretched with each turn overlapping the previous one. The tension should be slacker over bony points in order to avoid pressure. The cast is rigid in about half an hour, but complete evaporation takes over 12 hours with good ventilation. Because of the volatile and inflammable nature of the solvent the patient should not be put under a radiant heat cradle or near a flame.

Splints made of glass fibre are light and strong and not affected by water or excreta. A great advantage to a patient wearing a jacket of this type is the porosity of the material, especially in hot weather.

6 Plaster of Paris

Plaster of Paris or gypsum is obtained by mining. In its natural state the gypsum is composed of 21 per cent by weight of water of crystallization; this forms an important part of the crystalline structure. Its chemical composition is therefore calcium sulphate ($CaSO_4$) plus two molecules of water $CaSO_4 \cdot 2H_2O$. This free gypsum is treated commercially to form the white powder as we know it and is ready for incorporating into the gauze; the excess water is eliminated by the heating process ($2CaSO_4 \cdot H_2O$). The bandages are made ready for use. Water is added once more on immersion of the bandage before use and it is eliminated again after the plaster is applied, gaining its full length when the plaster is completely dry.

Nowadays hospitals use machine-made plaster bandages produced commercially.

Dry slabs for reinforcement can be prepared beforehand with the commercial bandage and a knowledge of the patterns that can be cut out of wide rolls of the gypsum is essential.

REQUISITES FOR APPLICATION OF PLASTER OF PARIS

Plaster bandages and slabs of the required length.

Two or more buckets of water at a temperature comfortable to the hand. The water should be changed frequently or the bandages

will not become soaked. When emptying, allow to stand, pour the
water away and put the plaster that settles at the bottom of the
bucket in the rubbish bin. If it is allowed to go down the drain it
sets in the pipes and causes a blockage.

Padding material which may be stockinette in rolls of various
sizes, splint wool, sheet wadding (also known as dressmakers'
wool), double-faced wool rolls, white adhesive felt, grey felt, or
white felt.

Needle and thread to stitch felt and stockinette.

Plaster knives and shears that are kept sharp.

Indelible pencil for marking.

Protective gowns, gloves, boots, and waterproof aprons.

Tape measures for wet slabs.

Waterproof sheets or newspapers to protect the floor when not
working in theatre or plaster room.

Several pillows with waterproof covers for placing beneath the
wet plaster.

PADDED AND SKIN-TIGHT PLASTERS

Plaster may be applied over felt, wool, stockinette or directly over
the skin. They are usually padded when there will be swelling after
injury or operation. Bony points are protected with felt or sponge
rubber. The padded plaster allows more muscular activity because
the muscles can compress the wool when they contract. The
unpadded plaster gives a better immobilization because it fits more
closely.

APPLICATION OF PLASTER OF PARIS

Before a plaster cast is applied the following points should be quite
clear:

1. From which and to what point the plaster extends
2. The positions of all joints
3. If the plaster case is to be padded or unpadded
4. If it is to be split or unsplit
5. The patient's disability
6. The reason for application.

The patient is placed in the position desired by the surgeon and
any padding fixed in place. Special apparatus, such as a Hawley

table, is often used. The surgeon maintains the position during the whole application. Each bandage is placed in water until the air bubbles cease to rise. It is then lifted out and compressed gently towards the centre. The free end is loosened and the bandage handed to the operator. The next bandage is placed in the bucket to soak. The bandage must be kept in contact with the limb as it is rolled around it. During application, the bandage is moulded to the limb using the palm and never the fingers. Special attention is given to the moulding over bony prominences. Two-thirds of the previous turn is covered. To fit the contours of the limb a small tuck is made at the upper or lower edge of the bandage. Moulding not only prevents pressure on bony prominences but prevents accumulation of air between the layers so that the completed plaster is one solid piece and not weak layers of bandage. Slabs are incorporated between layers of plaster bandages. When the plaster is completed, the edges are trimmed with a sharp knife. They must be smooth and can be finished off by turning the stockinette back and fixing it with a plaster bandage or strapping when dry.

Care of wet plaster

Plaster of Paris does not gain its full strength until completely dry, therefore for the first 24 to 36 hours the recently plastered limb should:

1. Rest on a soft structure, preferably a pillow covered with a rough towel with polythene sheeting on top.
2. The plaster should then be exposed to warm air. The ideal drying conditions are in a warm room or when the weather permits, to sunlight. Owing to the improved drying times of the commercial plaster of Paris bandage it is seldom necessary to use any form of artificial heat.

DANGERS OF PLASTER

Interference with the circulation

Interference with the circulation can be very serious and cause gangrene resulting in loss of part or the whole of the limb.

1. The colour, sensation, movement and temperature of the extremities must be under constant observation, especially after injury or operation. In these cases there will be some swelling of the extremities due to interference of the venous return. It can be

helped by raising the foot of the bed and encouraging movement.

2. Toes should be warm, red and have movement, and if the nurse presses the toe gently with her finger and the blood returns to the part, the circulation is satisfactory. If the toes are unduly white or have the blueish colour of cyanosis it means that there is interference of the arterial blood supply.

3. This sign and loss of sensation or movement should be reported immediately. The surgeon may have the plaster bivalved and the top half removed, or he may split the plaster on one or both sides from top to bottom dividing the padding. Some surgeons do this as routine before the patient leaves the theatre, cutting down both sides in front of the malleoli until the skin is visible. Pressure may be caused by the dried blood of soaked dressings forming hard tight bands around the ankle.

Plaster sores
Plaster sores are due to faulty technique in the application or inefficient handling of the plaster while it is wet, for example:
1. Pulling the bandage into a tight strand during application
2. Roughly trimmed edges
3. Faulty moulding over a bony prominence or inefficient padding
4. Delay in repairing cracks so that the skin is rubbed
5. Moving a joint while the plaster is wet and so causing a ridge
6. Resting a wet plaster on a hard surface.
7. Foreign bodies, such as coins or knitting needles, slipping inside the plaster
8. Plaster applied too loosely and so causing friction.

At first the patient complains of an irritation or burning pain underneath the plaster. This should never be ignored, because the patient loses sensation as the pressure increases and destroys the tissues. There is then an offensive smell — a discharge may appear from beneath the plaster. Children do not complain and the first sign will be restless sleep and fretfulness; constant observation is needed from both day and night nurses.

At the first sign of complaint, a window is cut. If there is no sore the patient must not be taken to task for making unnecessary complaints because this may deter a nearby patient from complaining at a later date. If there is a sore it is treated as an open wound, and when this has been dressed the window is packed with felt or wool held firmly in place by strapping in order to prevent swelling. If the edge of the plaster causes pressure the plaster is split longitudinally and a piece of white felt is inserted and held by strapping. Bits of wool must never be stuffed under the plaster to relieve pressure.

Pressure on peripheral nerves

The nerves most vulnerable to presssure from plaster are the external popliteal (peroneal) nerve as it winds around the head of the fibula and the ulnar nerve as it passes behind the medial epicondyle of the humerus. At first there is tingling and numb-neess of the fingers or toes. This should be reported immediately before loss of movement occurs.

Dermatitis

Dermatitis is rare and occurs when the skin is very dry. It is due to a staphylococcal infection of the hair follicles. There is intense irritation and burning sensation under the plaster. The plaster is bivalved and reapplied over a well-powdered skin and stockinette.

Recumbency

Patients confined to bed in plaster may develop some of the complications of recumbency.

BIVALVING OF THE PLASTER

Bivalving means the splitting of a cast on both sides, the object being to remove the upper half of the cast without interfering with the position of the limb. No plaster is ever cut or removed unless this is ordered to be done by the surgeon. The surgeon may wish to remove the plaster altogether or just the top half for inspection. The bivalved plaster may be retained as a splint. After splitting it is held in position until further orders by bandaging it with a firm calico bandage.

Method of bivalving

The instruments used are plaster shears (Fig. 45), a small saw, and plaster openers.

The patient is placed comfortably on a firm couch with a waterproof sheet under the plaster. An assistant steadies the limb.

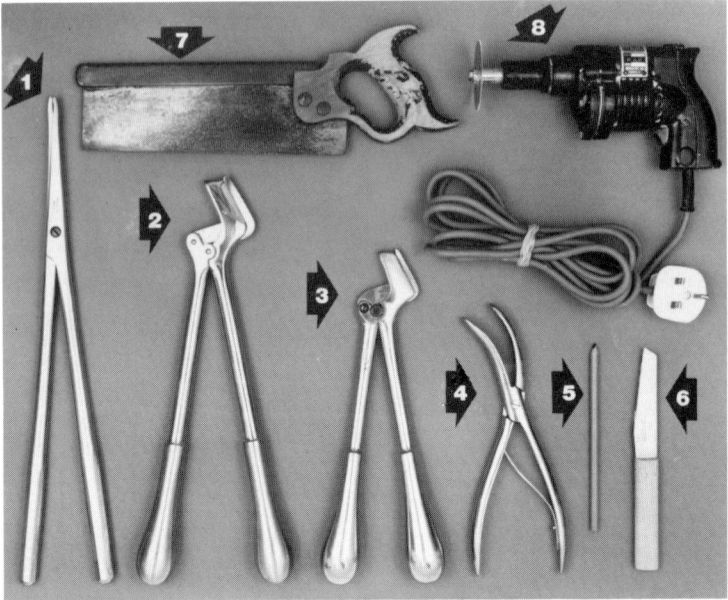

Fig. 45. *Selection of plaster instruments: 1. spreaders; 2. large shears; 3. small shears; 4. benders; 5. indelible pencil; 6. cobbler's knife; 7. saw with wooden handle; 8. electric saw.*

The plaster shears are alarming instruments to look at, so the patient must be reassured by an explanation that it is the plaster which is to be cut, and that it will not hurt. This is true if the nurse is careful and does not rush. The line to be cut is marked in pencil. When the foot is enclosed the cast should be marked with a line behind the internal malleolus and a line in front of the external malleolus. The cutter blade is inserted at right angles to the plaster. The point of the blade should point towards the plaster and not into the patient. The blade must not be pushed too far between the limb and the plaster before cuttting. The plaster is nibbled slowly deviating around bony points. A saw is used for large, heavy casts. The same precautions are necessary if an electric saw is used. This instrument is time-saving but noisy. It is undesirable to use it on a child who is too young to accept a rational explanation of the noise.

SPECIAL POINTS ABOUT CERTAIN PLASTERS

Spicas are applied in a Hawley table or a hip prop. The plaster is taken up to the nipple line. A single above-knee spica is trimmed so that the knee can be fully flexed. If the spica ends below the knee, the head of the fibula is protected. Usually the surgeon fixes the hip in extension neutral rotation, and the degree of abduction he requires depending on the condition. The knee is fixed in 5° to 10° flexion, with the foot plantar grade. In front the sound side is trimmed to allow full hip flexion and behind it is cut around the buttocks at the level of the tip of the coccyx.

Double spicas are joined by a strut or plaster just below the knees. The sacrum and anterior superior iliac spines are protected with felt.

Complete leg plaster

A complete leg plaster extends from the groin to the web of the toes. It is moulded around the patella, the malleoli, and the Achilles tendon. The arches of the foot must be preserved and the plaster is moulded behind the metatarsal heads with the toes

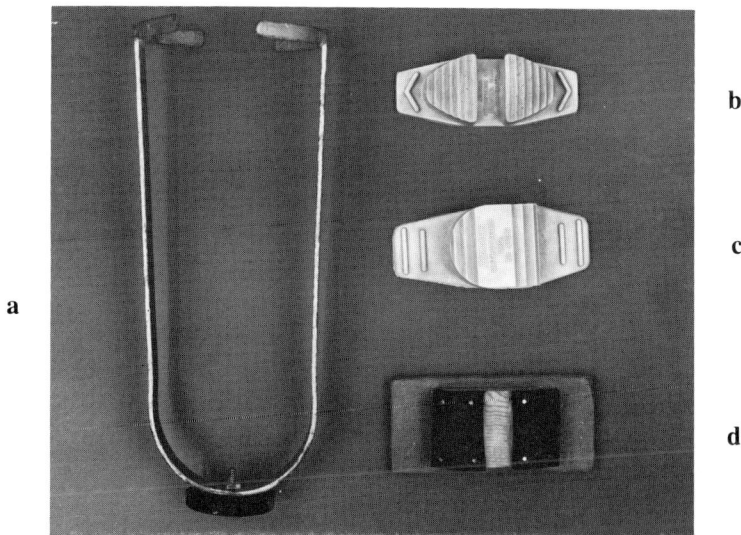

Fig. 46. *Walking heels:* (a) *Böhler iron;* (b) *Zimmer Chinese heel;* (c) *Zimmer walking heel;* (d) *Wooden Chinese heel.*

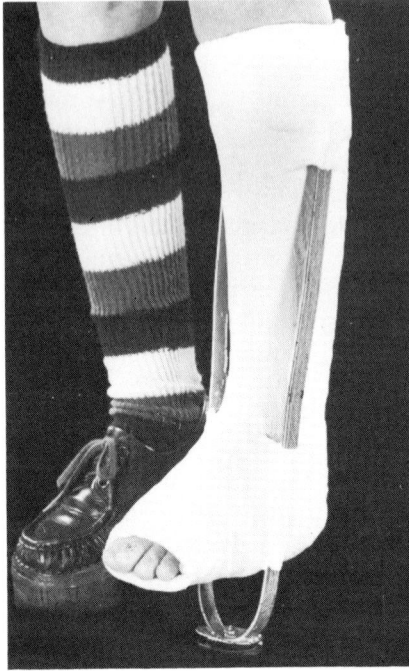

Fig. 47. *Walking in plaster showing a Böhler iron.*

supported. The toes are exercised to prevent a rigid claw foot and the quadriceps can be contracted in the plaster.

Below-knee plasters are trimmed to allow full extension and flexion of the knee.

Walking plasters have the sole reinforced. Sorbo heels or a wooden rocker, are sometimes incorporated. If a Böhler walking iron (Figs 46 and 47) is used, it is applied when the plaster is dry because if it is wet the metal will cause pressure. There should be a space about two fingers' width between the sole and the cross bar. While wearing this iron the patient tends to acquire a faulty gait. A normal gait is easier if a leather boot is worn over the plaster. Plaster boots are specially made in large sizes.

When a leg plaster is finally removed a crêpe bandage or zinc oxide plaster is applied straightaway after washing the leg. The bandage starts at the web of the toes and covers the leg, without any gaps, as far as the knee. This is to prevent oedema.

Knee-guarding plaster

A knee-guarding plaster is applied over stockinette or directly onto the skin, protecting the head of the fibula. It extends from the groin to just above the malleoli. A ring of white felt may be inserted at the lower edge to prevent the plaster from slipping over the malleoli.

Shoulder spica

A shoulder spica must extend over the iliac crests and is trimmed on the free arm side, so that there is no pressure under the axilla. The bony prominences that need protection or careful moulding are the acromion, coracoid and olecranon processes and the internal epicondyle of the humerus. If the patient is not under an anaesthetic he can be seated on a stool while this is applied. The plaster can be dried with the patient sitting and the arm supported.

Forearm plasters

Before forearm plasters are applied rings are removed from the fingers. When applied for Colles' fracture (Fig. 48) the plaster may

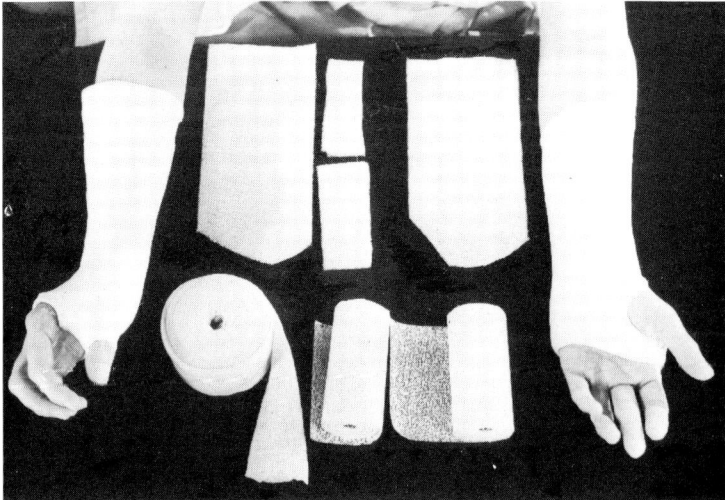

Fig. 48. *A Colles' plaster* (right). *Note freedom of the thumb and fingers. A scaphoid plaster* (left). *Note the position of the thumb. In the centre are shown pattens, bandages and stockinette.*

be started with a slab on the exterior surface of the forearm and extended from the head of the radius to the metacarpal heads. The slab is moulded on the forearm so that it lies on the extensor surface but does not reach far enough round for the edges to meet. It may be held in place by a cotton bandage which can be cut to relieve swelling. A complete forearm plaster is moulded to preserve the arches of the palm. Unless the thumb is included, as for a fractured scaphoid (Fig. 48), the plaster is trimmed to leave the thumb free. The thumb must be able to oppose each finger in a pincer movement. The plaster is trimmed in the palm below the level of the proximal palmar crease to allow full finger movements. An outpatient is allowed to wear a sling while the plaster is wet. This is removed on the following day and the fingers, elbow and shoulder are exercised.

Plaster jackets and corsets
Plaster jackets and corsets are applied over a single or double layer of stockinette with the sacrum and anterior iliac spines protected (Fig. 49). A female patient must have the breasts included or

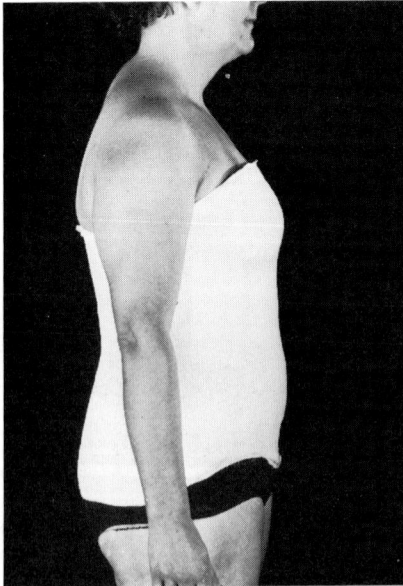

Fig. 49. *A patient in a spinal jacket extending from the upper end of the sternum to the pubis.*

completely free. In front the lower edges are trimmed to allow full flexion of the hip and to the level of the tip of the coccyx behind. A plaster jacket which is applied to keep the spine in extension extends from the interclavicular notch to the symphysis pubis. It is trimmed well away from the axillae. A porthole over the abdomen may be cut when the plaster is dry. Most surgeons do not cut one as a routine, but only in order to relieve abdominal distension.

Plaster for the cervical spine
Before applying the Minerva type of jacket (Fig. 50), the hair must be short and clean. The head is held in extension and an assistant holds the arms with a slight pull to prevent the shoulders hunching up. The occiput is padded to avoid pressure. The chin is included and the plaster extends over the iliac crests.

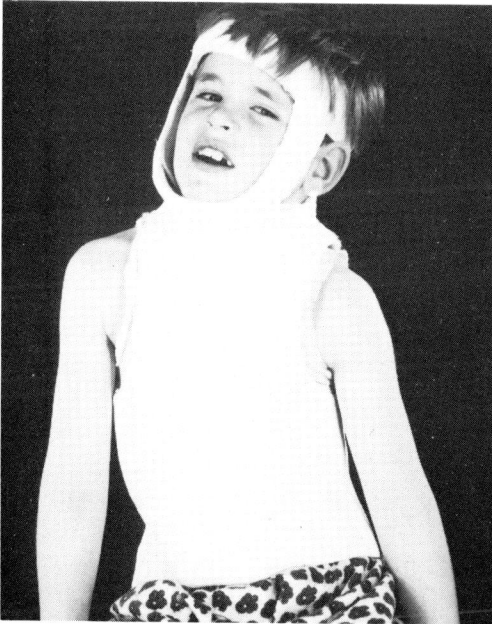

Fig. 50. *Minerva jacket for a patient with right-sided torticollis. Note the rotation towards, and side flexion from the affected side.*

Discharge of patients in plaster
Unless the circulation of the extremities is satisfactory the patient

is not allowed to leave the hospital. All joints not in plaster must be exercised. The patient, unless he lives too far away, usually attends the outpatient department for supervised exercises, until such time as it is obvious that the joints are being mobilized. If there is swelling the exercises must be continued because movement aids the venous return. Between exercises the limb is elevated. The patient is also instructed to keep the plaster dry and to report immediately if there is any cracking or discomfort because this may be due to a plaster sore. A list of instructions is given to the patient.

WEDGING OF PLASTER

A plaster is wedged to improve the alignment of a fracture or correct a deformity such as a flexion of the knee. A well-padded plaster is applied and when set the back of the plaster is split three-quarters of the way around at the level of the knee joint. The split is opened and pieces of cork are wedged in. Larger pieces are gradually wedged in until as much correction as is possible has been obtained.

PLASTER BEDS

If the patient is frightened and apprehensive before the plaster bed is made a sedative may be ordered. The patient lies on the table in the prone position and all details of the position must be checked before starting as alteration is impossible once the bed has been made. The bed extends from the seventh cervical vertebra to the tip of the coccyx. The leg pieces terminate just above the knee or above the malleoli. If the feet need splinting separate plaster shells are made. A head piece may be included. As the patient lies prone the spine must be straight and the head central. The arms are kept to the side and the scapulas level. The hips must be extended and abducted enough for the patient to be easily cleaned after using a bedpan. The knees are held in 5° flexion and the feet hang over the edge of the table. Sometimes the surgeon requires the spine to be in hyperextension and this is obtained by placing a wedge-shaped pillow under the patient's chest. If the patient is emaciated, or there is a sharp kyphos, the bony points can first be covered with felt so that there are grooves fitting these points in the completed

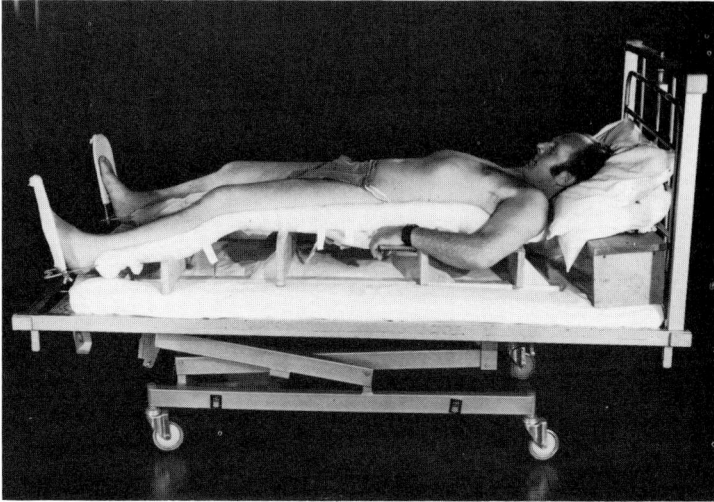

Fig. 51. *A patient in a plaster bed which is supported on a wooden frame.*

bed. The patient's head is protected and the whole skin covered with warm olive oil. Sheets of double plaster muslin are cut beforehand according to the patient's measurements. Plaster cream is made just before starting by mixing thoroughly about 4.5 kg of plaster in a deep bucket of water. Drop the plaster in until some of it floats, then stir thoroughly to form a creamy consistency. A nurse dips a double sheet of muslin into the cream. When it is soaked she hands it to one of the two assistants who stand, one at the foot and one at the head of the table. They open out the sheet, pull it taut and place it over the patient and mould each sheet to the body contour, working away from the midline. There must be no air bubbles between the layers. If it is a long bed, an assistant quickly splits the muslin with a sharp knife between the legs. The sheets must be well moulded over the gluteal fold and upper part of the thigh; this part takes a lot of strain. The sheets must be applied in rapid succession as the cream sets quickly and separate layers make a weak bed. The plaster must be moulded to the sides of the patient but not so far that it cannot be moved. When sufficiently thick it is allowed to set until a ringing noise is heard on tapping. Meanwhile it is marked for trimming. An alternative method of making a bed is by using slabs

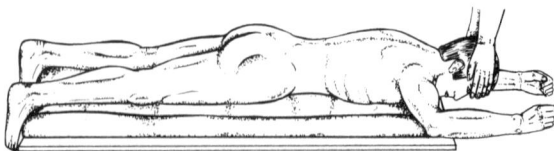

Fig. 52. *Position of a patient for the application of plaster bed. The arms and head must be held or supported on a rest.*

and wide bandages. The patient is prepared as before. A nurse stands at each side of the table and the bandages are rolled over the patient between them, the plaster being moulded and where necessary reinforced with slabs. If a head piece is required it is incorporated when the bed is about half-made and so is the strut of plaster that joins the legs. The completed bed is carefully lifted off the patient. The patient is washed and warmly covered as he will feel chilly on suddenly losing the heat of the plaster. The bed is trimmed so that it is clear of the axillae and malleoli, at the level of the tip of the coccyx and enough around the buttocks for using a bedpan. If too much is cut out the buttocks slip through and become oedematous. If a plaster bed gets continually soiled the

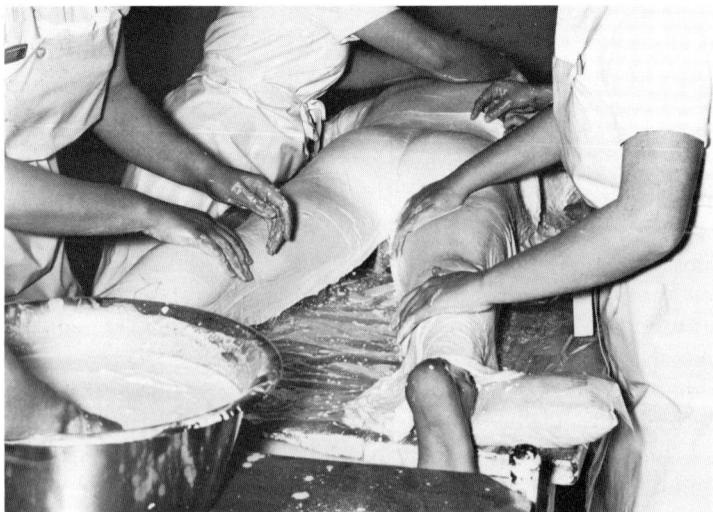

Fig. 53. *Method of making a plaster bed.*

surgeon may give permission for the next bed to be made in slightly wider abduction. Two or three days are needed for drying. A well-made plaster bed should really need no lining and in some hospitals it is smoothed, dusted with French chalk and the patient lies directly in it. A warmer method is to line it either with felt or three layers of splint wool covered with stockinette. Too much felt will alter the shape of the bed and makes the patient feel hot and scratchy. When used the bed is mounted on a wooden stand with three transverse supports. A padded wooden board is fitted at the end which keeps the bedclothes off the feet and provides a support upon which the feet can rest between exercises. Since the support is higher than the bed, blocks are placed on either side for the arm pillows to rest on. The arms can then be rested comfortably in slight abduction and not left to hang. The knees are bandaged. During the daily readjustment of the bandages the position of the patella, which should be straight, is noted. A plaster bed should be quite comfortable, but the patient should be turned if he complains at all.

TURNING CASES

Turning cases are lighter than plaster beds and are maade by the same methods. They are made while the patient is on his frame or plaster bed, the bandages first being undone and the bars bent back. The pubic hair and the face must be protected from the plaster.

PLASTER SPLINTS

Plaster splints are used as night splints for any part; frequently they are used to hold the feet. A complete plaster is made over stockinette, the areas over the bony prominences and the arches of the foot being well moulded. It is bivalved while wet and carefully moved. When dry the posterior half is used as the splint and bandaged over wool to the limb. These will hold the feet in the desired position if correction has already been obtained, and can prevent the feet from acquiring deformities, but a complete plaster is necessary to correct an established deformity.

PLASTER CASTS FOR SPLINT-MAKING

All moulded leather and polythene splints require the taking of a plaster cast. This may also be necessary in the case of severe foot deformity, to give the instrument-maker the correct delineation of the patient's limb or trunk.

Procedure for cast-taking

1. Grease the limb either with oil or petroleum jelly or cover the limb with a well-fitting stockinette.
2. Place a length of fine wire down the side of trunk or limb.
3. Apply the plaster to a sufficient and even thickness to maintain shape of limb or trunk when removed.
4. When the plaster has set, using an indelible pencil make a series of horizontal lines throughout the length of the wire.
5. Take a sharp cobbler's knife in hand and holding the top end of the wire with the other, cut the plaster along the length of the wire as it is being pulled away from the limb.
6. Carefully remove the cast.
7. Join the cast so that the horizontal lines are in opposition.
8. The cast is now ready to be filled with a thick mixture of coarse pink plaster. When this has set the original cast is stripped off, by cutting down the same line as before, and removed thus leaving a complete replica of the limb or trunk, which, having been dried and labelled with the patient's name, is ready for dispatch to the instrument and appliance maker.

Cast bracing

This method of external splintage is often used for fractures of the distal portion of the femur; it allows early ambulation which in turn increases muscular activity and the blood supply, thus stimulating the healing process.

The cast is applied in two parts — the thigh and leg portions. An elastic stocking is applied to the leg and a plastic quadrilateral shell of suitable size is applied to the thigh followed by plaster of Paris bandages. This should fit well up to the ischial tuberosity. The leg portion is applied over a small amount of padding with particular care to protect the head of the fibula. The hinges are applied over the knee; care is taken to see these are parallel. The cast is trimmed to make sure that no flesh impinges when the knee is flexed. A walking heel is usually applied.

X-rays will be taken following application of the cast brace. The patient must be instructed on its care, with particular reference to keeping it dry. If the cast brace has to be changed the operator will take care not to displace the fragments; this can be checked by X-rays on completion.

Other substances used for making coats

Newer materials are available which may be used instead of plaster of Paris. The makers claim special properties such as quicker drying, extra strength and durability. It is right that these should be tried and properly evaluated.

Zorac — Johnson & Johnson. This combines high-quality gypsum with a melamine formaldehyde mixture. Less material is said to be needed to achieve the same result.

Orthoflex — Johnson & Johnson. A stretch rubber elastic gauze fabric combined with plaster of Paris. This the makers claim conforms better and does not constrict.

Scotchcast — 3M. The makers say this is water resistant, light and strong.

Crystona — Smith & Nephew. This is similar to plaster of Paris but less bulky, with a high degree of water resistance.

Baycast — Bayer UK Limited. A cotton bandage impregnated with polymer which reacts with water to give a light strong cast.

The makers of all these materials issue special instructions for their application. These should be read carefully and adhered to, and where appropriate given to the patient.

7 Injuries to bones, joints and soft tissues

Patients with severe injuries are best admitted to an accident and emergency department which has special facilities for treating such patients. The first aid given at the scene of the accident will include measures to establish a clear airway and to give mouth-to-mouth resuscitation if breathing has stopped. External cardiac massage must be started in the case of cardiac arrest, bleeding should be controlled by elevation and direct pressure and the limb splinted if a fracture is suspected.

On admission to the accident and emergency department more efficient methods will be taken to ensure that the airway is clear, which may include the insertion of an endotracheal tube or the performing of a tracheostomy. If bleeding is not controlled, more direct pressure may be applied in the form of a firm bandage or the bleeding vessel may be clamped off with artery forceps. When these emergency measures have been taken which are designed to save life, the doctor will examine the patient carefully, area by area to determine the extent of the injury.

The observations which should be made and recorded will include the temperature, pulse, respiration, blood pressure, pupil reaction and possibly the level of consciousness and girth measurement. The treatment to be given will depend on the extent of the injuries: soft tissue injuries will generally require urgent attention; if there is a wound present it will need to be covered and thereafter closed; fractures will require temporary splintage; administration of intravenous fluids commenced to replace the fluid loss and restore the blood volume and then raise the pressure; antitetanus toxoid may be administered.

Although the team will be involved in urgent life-saving measures for a seriously injured patient, one member should be allocated to give the support and comfort to the relatives and friends which will be needed at this time. This support is just as necessary when the injuries are not so severe. A sympathetic professional approach by one member will help to give the relatives confidence in the whole team.

Having dealt with the general measures which are necessary for the immediate resuscitation of the patient, the surgeon will carry out a more detailed examination of the patient. This is usually done area by area.

When examing the head, fingers are passed gently over the scalp — irregularities can often be felt where they are not easily seen. Bleeding or discharge from the ears or nose is significant. Observation of the chest may reveal diminished or asymmetrical movement, or paroxismal respiration. As well as examination and palpation of the abdomen, measurements of the girth will be taken on admission. Bleeding will cause swelling.

Examination of the limb will be attempting to assess the extent of the damage and its viability. The findings will determine the treatment needed and the nursing care which must be given, keeping in mind the whole patient — not only the limb.

ASSESSMENT

Deformity. The position of the limb will be noted, including angular or rotational deformities.

Skin. Colour is a valuable indication. Pallor or redness suggests decreased or increased blood supply respectively, as does cold or warmth. The extent of skin damage is vital when attempting to close the wound. Failure to be able to close the wound because of skin loss leads to infection, delayed union, and may necessitate amputation, especially of the lower limb.

Blood supply. Colour and temperature have been mentioned as indicators of blood supply. Pressure on the nail causing blanching and observing the reaction, is also helpful. To be able to feel a pulse is the most valuable guide to the blood supply, and therefore the viability of the limb. Nurses should make themselves familiar with the pulses in the leg, the dorsalis pedis artery on the dorsum of the foot, and the posterior tibial behind the medial malleolous.

Sensation. Loss of or altered sensation is an indication of nerve damage. This could lead to pressure or plaster sores or further damage to the limb without the patient being aware of it — this information is very relevant to the nurse. In the case of the hand injury, loss of sensation is a serious disability.

Movement. Loss of movement may be caused by damage to the muscle or its nerve. Extensive muscle damage provides the conditions for infection and will need to be exercised. Injury to a nerve may need to be explored and possibly sutured at a later date.

Swelling. Swelling is produced as a reaction to trauma. It may be due to an excess of fluid in the tissue (oedema), blood in the tissue (haematoma), or blood in the joint (haemarthrosis). It is necessary to compare both limbs to determine the amount of swelling, or by measuring the circumference of limb at the same level each side. Swelling in the tissue leads to loss of function and may further impair thè blood supply. Swelling in the joint may be due to a sympathetic effusion when neighbouring tissues are damaged, or blood in the joint. When the fracture involves the articular surfaces, it is often necessary to aspirate the joint and to do an open reduction in order to get the correct anatomical alignment of the broken fragments.

FRACTURES

A fracture is commonly defined as a break in the continuity of a bone. There may or may not be displacement of the bony fragments.

CAUSES OF FRACTURE

A fracture is caused by some degree of force by:

1. Direct violence which occurs at the point of injury.
2. Indirect violence when the fracture occurs at a point distant
   to the impact.

The amount of damage will depend on the degree of force which caused the injury. It will invariably involve some associated soft tissue which may be more important and require more urgent attention than the broken bone.

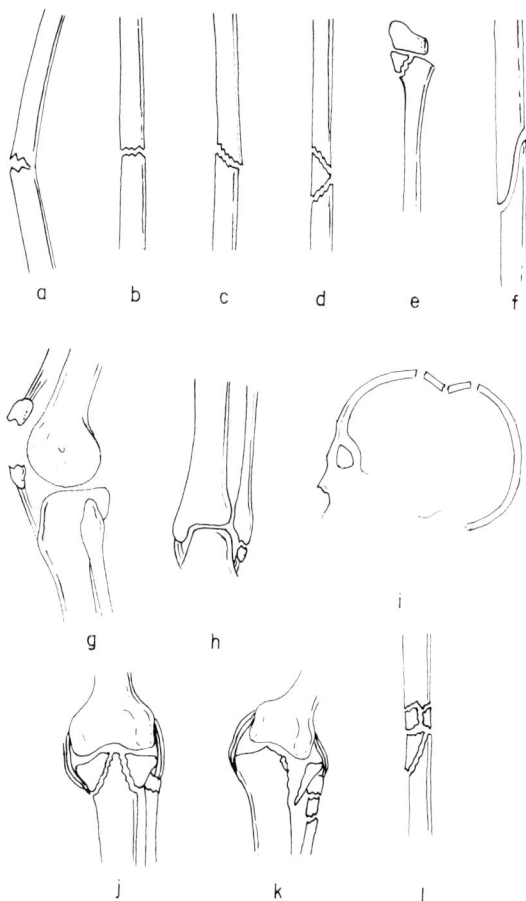

Fig. 54. *Types of fracture:* (a) *Greenstick fracture;* (b), (c) *and* (d) *types of fracture due to bending;* (e) *fracture separation of epiphysis;* (f) *spiral fracture;* (g) *large avulsion fracture;* (h) *small avulsion or sprain fracture;* (i) *and* (j) *depressed fractures;* (k) *splitting;* (l) *comminuted fracture.*

CLASSIFICATION OF FRACTURES

Pathological fractures may be defined as fractures caused by that degree of violence which would not normally produce a break in bone. Conditons which may lead to pathological fractures are:
1. Generalized weakness of bone such as rickets and osteomalacia, fragilitas osseum, Paget's disease.
2. Localized weakness of bone such as infection, e.g. destruction of bone by osteomyelitis, local tumour or bone cyst.

Non-pathological fractures may be defined as fractures where there is no underlying disease of the bone. Fractures may be further classified as:
1. Closed or simple where there is no break in the overlying skin.
2. Open or compound where the overlying skin is broken so that the fracture site is in communication with the outside air; the ends may or may not protrude through the skin.

Open fractures are more serious because of the risk of infection and accompanying damage to blood vessels leading to blood loss.

TYPES OF FRACTURE AND THEIR IMPLICATIONS

Greenstick fractures occur in young children. The periosteum may be torn but remains in contact with the bone. Union is ensured because of the minimal damage to the blood supply.

A transverse fracture is usually stable but may result in delayed or non-union.

An oblique or spiral fracture. The fracture is unstable and may result in shortening but union usually takes place.

A fracture involving a joint is a serious injury which involves bleeding into the joint and may result in irregularity of the joint surface with the risk of osteo-arthritis later in life.

Avulsion fracture. An avulsion fracture occurs when a small piece of bone to which the tendon is attached is pulled off from the bone. It often requires open reduction and fixation.

An impacted fracture. In an impacted fracture the bone ends are crushed together, the fracture is stable, though it may not be in good position.

A depressed fracture applies to bones of the skull; it can cause damage to the underlying brain.

A complicated fracture involves neighbouring structures such as organs, blood vessels, muscles or nerves.

A stress fracture often occurs in the metatarsals (March fracture) or shaft of the tibia in athletes.

SIGNS AND SYMPTOMS

The signs and symptoms of fractures arise from the effects described:
1. Break in continuity of bones causes:
    (a) Tenderness at the site of fracture
    (b) Abnormal mobility and crepitus.
2. Displacement of fragments causes:
    (a) Deformity
    (b) Loss of function.
3. Damage to soft parts causes:
    (a) Pain and tenderness at the fracture
    (b) Bleeding { external and visible; and / internal causing swelling, bruising and shock
    (c) Skin wound
    (d) Paralysis or ischaemia
    (e) Evidence of damage to organs, e.g. brain, spleen, bladder, lungs.

It is necessary to take a careful history of the injury in order to establish the diagnosis. Radiographs are usually taken to confirm the presence of a fracture (anterior, posterior, lateral and sometimes oblique views) and will show the type of fracture, the alignment of the bones and deformity. Radiographs are not infallible as it is sometimes difficult to detect the line of fracture as in a fracture of the scaphoid bone. The other uses of radiographs are to show the presence or absence of callus after a period of immobilization. This together with clinical examination will give the evidence of union; X-ray investigations alone are not reliable enough to determine a satisfactory state of union.

THE PROCESS OF UNION

The process of union depends upon the formation of callus, which can be looked upon as a natural bone cement. The blood shed at the fracture's site clots and then gradually becomes changed into bones as bone-forming cells, or osteoblasts, grow into it both from the periosteum and from the broken bones themselves. Union which is a natural process will restore continuity and rigidity even without treatment but it can be aided by efficient immobilization. Manipulation is necessary to restore alignment and prevent mal-union. Failure of the bone end to unite by bone is called non-union.

TREATMENT

The principles of treatment are:
1. Resuscitation of the patient
2. Reduction
3. Immobilization
4. Re-education or restoration of function
5. The prevention of complications.

Resuscitation
Before considering the treatment of the fracture it is necessary to ensure that adequate resuscitation has been given. This will include the maintenance of a clear airway and satisfactory respiration which may require the patient to be artificially ventilated with a positive-pressure respirator. Blood volume will need to be restored in the case of severe loss which will be accomplished by giving intravenous fluids starting with saline or glucose or similar fluid and followed by blood transfusion when this is available.

If a wound is present it will need to be closed, a dry dressing and firm pad having been applied on admission to the accident and emergency department. The patient will be prepared for theatre and a general anaesthetic, thorough cleaning of the wound, trimming of the skin edges, excision of damaged muscle and suture of the wound will take place. If there is extensive skin damage which prevents suture, a skin graft may be applied to cover the wound.

The bone ends are aligned during the course of the operation. A course of antibiotics is usually commenced and antitetanus toxoid given.

Reduction

If displacement is going to impede function it must be corrected by reduction, which is essentially a matter of pulling to reduce shortening, bending to correct angulation and twisting to correct rotation. This can be effected by manual manipulation by the surgeon, and is usually performed under a general or local anaesthetic. Sometimes the appropriate manoeuvre results in putting the fracture straight in one movement and with little chance of displacement after splintage; this is a stable reduction. In other cases reduction is unstable and can be maintained only by internal fixation or by more or less prolonged traction. Traction may be applied to the skin by strapping or directly to bone by Kirschner's wire or Steinmann's pin in the limbs, or by Blackburn's or Crutchfield's skull traction apparatus for the neck. Some fractures require open reduction which is usually carried out because manipulation has failed or because, as with an avulsion fracture, it could not succeed. It is also used in appropriate cases as a preliminary to internal fixation.

Immobilization

Immobilization must be provided until the callus has gained sufficient firmness to hold the fracture in place against the effects of gravity and muscular action. Immobilization is not carried out for a given period of so many weeks or months, but until union has occurred. This may take anything from less than a month to over a year, depending on the circumstances, but the usual periods are given later when the individual fractures are discussed.

Immobilization is secured by external or internal splintage, but, like reduction, is not always required. Fractures of the ribs and metacarpals, for example, are usually adequately splinted by their surrounding muscles and for some fractures of the humerus a sling suffices but usually some kind of splintage is necessary, most commonly plaster of Paris. Thomas's splint is the only ready-made splint in general use and remains unsurpassed for the treatment of many injuries of the lower limb; it is nearly always combined with traction. An external fixator is a more modern method of providing immobilization. It comprises two Steinmann's pins placed on either side of the fracture site and attached to a rigid bar down one or both sides of the limb. The method has the advantage of resting the soft tissues as well as holding the bone ends in a stable position to allow healing to take place. Inflatable splints are often used to produce temporary immobilization and may be applied by ambulance personnel.

Internal fixation is frequently carried out after open reduction and is achieved by screws, plates or nails of various kinds. These have to be of special metals or they become corroded. Stainless steel and vitallium are most commonly used.

Some fractures fail to unite by bone and are joined by dense fibrous tissue; this is non-union and is not uncommon with some fractures of the tibia, ulna, femur and scaphoid. It is usually treated by a bone graft.

Re-education or restoration of function
The aim of treatment in any fracture is not only to bring about union of the fracture but to maintain or restore the normal function of the limb. Consequently the moment treatment is commenced every effort must be made to encourage full function of the part of the limb which does not require immobilization. The patient must be instructed to use all non-immobilized joints as much as possible. In many cases the patient may carry on with his or her normal occupation. For instance after a Colles' fracture the patient must move the shoulder, the elbow, fingers and thumb as much as possible. After removal of plaster or splint, oedema of the limb is prevented by the application of elastic pressure as by crêpe bandage. This is of especial importance in the lower limb. Joints which have been immobilized will at first be stiff but mobility is regained by active movement. Physiotherapy is directed towards the restoration of function in muscles and joints which involves supervision of active exercises.

GENERAL COMPLICATIONS

Surgical shock
Surgical shock occurs following injury producing changes in the circulation resulting in a fall of blood pressure or feeble pulse. The temperature is subnormal and the skin is cold and moist. The condition is made worse by fluid loss and is treated by fluid replacement.

Fat embolism
Fat embolism occurs almost always as the result of fractures or very occasionally in post-operative bone surgery. The fat from bone marrow enters the circulation and the emboli become systemic or pulmonary. Symptoms can become evident between the first and up to the third day after injury or operation and are characterized by the appearance of skin haemorrhages over the chest and shoulders. General treatment as for respiratory distress is given, but should the embolus settle in the brain the prognosis is very grave.

Hypostatic pneumonia
Hypostatic pneumonia occurs most commonly in the elderly and following head, chest or spinal injuries. Breathing exercises are important to prevent this condition together with the correct positioning of the patient.

Confusion
Confusion is frequent in the aged, who are easily upset by the effects of injury and strange surroundings but because they become noisy at night, interfere with splints and traction and fall or get out of bed, sedatives have to be used on occasion and when ordered should be given early in the evening.

Renal failure
Renal failure is indicated by reduced urinary output leading to anuria and a rise in blood urea. It may need to be treated by renal dialysis.

LOCAL COMPLICATIONS

Local complications occur to neighbouring structures:

Bone

Bone union is produced by callus bridging the gap between the bone ends. When this process takes longer than is expected it is referred to as delayed union. The cause may be damage to blood supply, infection or poor splintage. Non-union describes the condition when the bone ends fail to unite or are joined only by fibrous tissue.

Periosteum

The greater the periosteal damage the greater the risk of delayed or even non-union, periosteum being a bone-forming tissue.

Blood vessels

Complications may involve a particular artery related to a fracture, e.g. the brachial artery which may be associated with a supra-condylar fracture leading to Volkmann's ischaemic contracture or more diffuse damage to blood vessels which accompanies compound fractures. Where there is an increased risk of infection both of soft tissue and sometimes bone there may be delayed or even non-union. Severe damage to blood vessels leading to extensive death of soft tissue may necessitate amputation.

Muscles

Extensive muscle damage requires excision of any muscle which is not viable in order to remove the risk of infection. Apart from this risk, damage to muscle leads to loss of function and may seriously affect the stability of the neighbouring joint.

Nerves

Damage to nerves leads to paralysis and may require a suture of the severed nerve. This is usually carried out at a later date when the risk of infection is reduced and operative conditions more ideal.

Skin

Extensive skin damage can be a serious complication leading to prolonged treatment which may involve skin grafting in order to cover the wound, prevent infection and promote union.

Underlying organs
Damage may occur to underlying organs such as the heart and lungs when the ribs are fractured, to the brain accompanying fracture of the skull and to the bladder or bowel when the pelvis is damaged.

INJURIES TO SPECIAL AREAS OF THE BODY

HEAD INJURIES

Head injuries should never be regarded lightly. They require careful observation and those which are severe will need skilled nursing care; few will require surgery but when surgery is indicated it may have to be carried out urgently in order to prevent the patient's condition from deteriorating. If the patient is unconscious, efficient first aid is needed to save his life: he must be placed in the almost prone position with his head to one side in order to maintain a clear airway; haemorrhage must be controlled by the use of a firm pad and bandage and transfer to hospital as soon as possible is necessary where more advanced treatment can be given.

On admission to the accident and emergency department the most urgent treatment will be directed at maintaining a clear airway to ensure adequate ventilation and oxygenation of the blood. Measures to control haemorrhage and to replace the fluid loss in order to prevent shock will also be performed. A careful history will be taken especially to determine the length of post-traumatic amnesia which is some guide to the severity of the injury. The observations made and recorded in order to establish a base line will be temperature, pulse and respiration, blood pressure, pupil reaction and level of responsiveness. The adverse signs are a rapid, shallow pulse indicating shock, and excessive slowing of the pulse, suggesting rising intracranial pressure.

The pupils may react sluggishly to light and they may be dilated. If the dilation is unequal it is a danger sign which must be reported. A falling blood pressure indicates shock and the need for fluid replacement. Fluid is usually administered intravenously at this stage. A rise in blood pressure indicates intracranial pressure. The temperature may be subnormal as in shock, but there may be hyperthermia indicating damage to the temperature control centre in the base of the brain.

The level of responsiveness can be estimated by the patient's ability to answer simple questions and noting his response to stimuli such as striking the soles of the feet. The maintenance of the chart which records the observations is an essential nursing procedure. A chart showing a rise in blood pressure, slowing of the pulse and a lowering of the level of consciousness indicates intracranial pressure requiring action to be taken.

The nursing care of patients with head injuries

If a patient is unconscious for any length of time and recovers without complications it will be because he has received good nursing care. To ensure adequate ventilation of the lungs it may be necessary to perform a tracheostomy which is not now a routine procedure. On admission the insertion of an endotracheal tube will ensure a satisfactory airway. If a tracheostomy is necessary, a cuffed tube is usually inserted for the first few days and the cuff must be deflated two-hourly; later a Durham's silver tracheostomy tube may be used. Tracheostomy will allow suction to be used to maintain a clear airway.

The patient is placed in the semi-prone position. Care of the skin by turning the patient two-hourly is essential. So too is care of the eyes, especially if they are open. A single stitch may be inserted to retain the eyes closed and protected. Paul's tubing over the penis will ensure that the patient is dry; an in-dwelling catheter will be necessary in the female. It may be necessary to restrain the patient to prevent him pulling tubes out or injuring himself. Sedatives should be avoided because it is impossible to assess the level of responsiveness.

Diet for an unconscious patient will need to be carefully calculated in order to maintain an adequate calorie intake which must include sufficient proteins, mineral salts, vitamins and fluids. Gastric feeding will commence with water, continuing with half-strength milk, then full-strength milk, going on to a powdered complete food. A good diet is a very important factor in the prevention of pressure sores by maintaining healthy tissue although the patient is unconscious. Mobilization is a gradual process, commencing with the addition of a pillow, later sitting up, followed by walking. At this stage if the patient complains of a headache aspirin may be prescribed.

Convalescence is often slow. The family will need counselling to help them give the support which is often needed in order to rehabilitate the patient.

Complications of head injuries

1. The fracture of the skull may not be serious, it is the underlying brain damage which is important. The site of the fracture may be significant because it suggests the part of the brain which might be damaged. A depressed fracture of the skull usually requires surgery to elevate that part of the skull.

2. If there is intracranial haemorrhage causing pressure on the brain, emergency surgery in the form of burr holes in order to relieve this pressure is essential.

3. An intracranial abscess is a serious complication. It may be prevented by giving chemotherapy and antibiotics.

4. Leakage of cerebrospinal fluid from the nose or ear suggests damage to the meninges.

5. Epileptic fits are a serious complication of head injuries.

6. Skull defects may need the insertion of a plate, metal or plastic.

7. Personality changes.

THE SPINE

Fractures of the spine are conveniently divided into the mild and the serious. Mild fractures are caused by twists and wrenches which result in avulsion of the spinous or transverse processes (Fig. 55a) or by forced flexion, which results in simple crush fractures of the vertebral bodies (Fig. 55b). They are treated by rest in a firm bed with sedatives. Exercises can usually be started in bed, after a few days. Many patients can go home in two to four weeks without much stiffness or discomfort although they are not able to resume heavy work for two or three months. The back needs no more support in these cases than is provided by well-developed muscles but the neck often requires a collar of plaster, plastic or leather for six to twelve weeks.

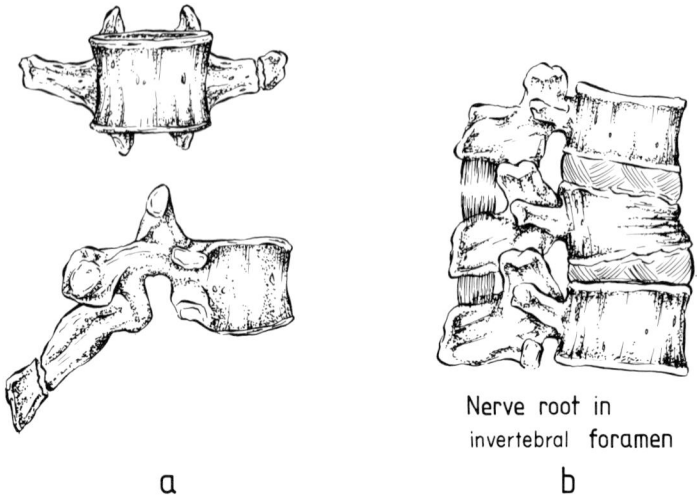

Fig. 55. *Avulsion fractures of vertebral processing* (a); *simple crush fracture of vertebral body* (b).

Major spinal injuries

The serious fractures are produced by great violence and are, in fact, usually fracture-dislocations which owe their seriousness to the fact that they can injure the spinal cord and cause paralysis. Fractures below the first lumbar vertebra damage only the nerve roots in the canda equina and as nerve roots are capable of recovery the initial paralysis may not be permanent. Above this level the spinal cord may be injured and paralysis from this cause is permanent though the accompanying nerve roots may recover (Fig. 56). The higher the injury, the more extensive the paralysis.

First-aid treatment

A person who is lying in a comfortable position immediately after an accident need not be moved until a stretcher arrives, but an awkward sprawl may need to be corrected in order to make sure that the airway is clear and breathing is satisfactory; this is a first priority. A paralysed person can be rolled in safety provided there is enough help to ensure that the spine is moved in one piece, without twisting, flexion or extension. The supine position is satisfactory for all types of spinal injury but a person already prone

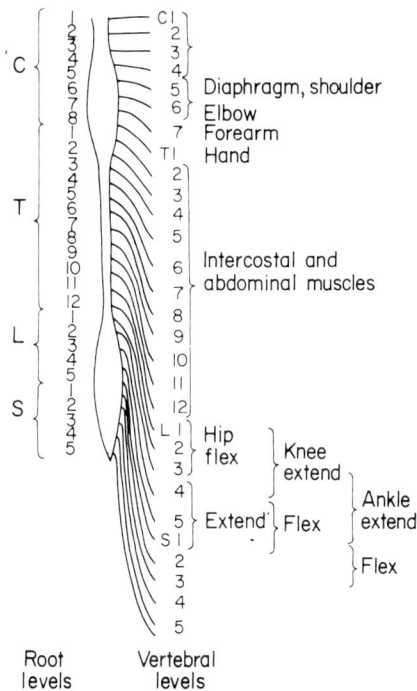

Fig. 56. *Relationships between the levels of origin of spinal nerve roots and vertebral segments and the general localization of functions within the cord.*

may be left so. No time should be lost in padding bony parts. Buckles and hard objects in pockets should be removed to avoid pressure sores. Shock can be reduced by careful handling at this stage and protection from cold.

Examination and investigation

If the patient is unconscious on admission to the accident and emergency department, measures will be taken to ensure that respiration is satisfactory and resuscitation given (page 248). A careful examination will be made to discover the extent of the injury. A patient who has suffered an injury which is of sufficient force to cause fracture or a fracture-dislocation of the spine is likely to have other injuries which may include damage to abdominal or chest organs. Neurological examination will reveal the presence of paralysis and loss of sensation.

Radiography. Radiographs will show the level of the lesion. It is usual for positive recognition to take lateral and posterior projections. Great care must be taken if the patient has to be transferred to the special table, and he may be X-rayed on the stretcher to avoid movement.

Treatment
Multiple injuries accompanying fracture of the spine are not uncommon. Examination will reveal the presence and extent of these injuries. In the light of this knowledge, the programme of treatment will be established.

The treatment of the fracture itself is usually much easier and always much shorter than the treatment of the complications. Fracture-dislocations in the neck are reduced by skull traction, applied under local anaesthesia, and may be continued for a few weeks before a Minerva plaster jacket is applied (see Fig. 50).

Lower down the spine recumbency alone usually suffices but at any level open reduction is sometimes necessary to safeguard the spinal cord. Uncomplicated stable fractures may be immobilized in a plaster jacket after a few days; it is not necessary to hyperextend the spine. The patient should be comfortably erect. Plaster jackets are retained for two to three months and spinal exercises carried out in them. Many surgeons do not immobilize this group of patients at all. Exercises to strengthen the spinal muscles are commenced a few days after the accident. Excellent results are achieved by this active method of treatment.

Unstable fractures where the spinal cord is not damaged are treated by internal fixation, either with some form of plate and screws or a bone graft in order to produce a fusion and restore the stability of the spine. The patient may be nursed on a plaster bed for a few weeks but the period of immobilization is much shorter than it used to be. When the unstable fracture is further complicated by damage to the spinal cord leading to paraplegia, the fracture may be ignored, although some surgeons operate to fuse the spine in order to make nursing care easier.

Re-education. Except for patients where the spinal cord has been damaged, it is important to reassure the patient that complete recovery is usual. Convalescence may be prolonged with patients whose occupations involve lifting, but good results can be expected.

Complications
Paraplegia. Paraplegia is a serious complication of spinal injury and invariably produces further complications which are chest infection, incontinence of bladder and bowel, loss of sensation leading to skin damage and pressure sores, flexor spasm and contracture of joints, especially the hip. The inevitable psychological upset may lead to severe depression.

Management of paraplegic patients in order to prevent further complications
Care of the skin to prevent pressure sores will require careful positioning of the patient on a mattress with a firm base in order to distribute the weight as evenly as possible. Pillows should be placed in position to do this and maintain a good posture in bed, with the hip and knee joints in extension for part of the time. The spine must not be twisted and should not be allowed to sag at the waist when the patient is on his side; a pillow carefully placed will prevent this and keep the spine straight. Pillows will also be needed between the knees to support the leg which is uppermost when the patient is lying on his side and for the head to make the patient comfortable.

The patient's position must be changed two-hourly day and night. Following each turning a careful check must be made to ensure the limbs and the spine are in the correct position, that the patient is comfortable and that everything he needs is at hand.

Care of the bladder. The aim should be to establish an automatic bladder and prevent infection. In the early stage, intermittent catheterization will be performed or alternatively an indwelling catheter may be used. There is controversy as to which of these methods is the best to achieve the aim of preventing infection; with either method strict aseptic precautions must be taken. An adequate fluid intake is important and a fluid balance chart must be maintained. Following the stage of catheterization, manual pressure over the bladder will be carried out in order to train the patient to express his own bladder so that he may become continent. It is important to avoid a residual urine which invariably leads to infection of the bladder and may extend to the kidney with serious consequences.

Treatment
Where there is no disruption, rest in bed until the bruising has subsided and the patient has less pain, followed by gradual mobilization. If necessary support can be given by a well-fitting webbing belt or corset but this is not usually needed; exercise may be given to the lower limbs and the patient should soon regain normal function.

Fractures of the pelvis where the pelvic ring is disrupted with the likelihood of displacement of one side and consequent damage to the weight-bearing mechanism are regarded as serious injuries. The degree of violence which causes this kind of injury will also cause severe haemorrhage; the bladder, urethra or other pelvic organs may be damaged. The injury is accompanied by severe shock and the patient will need urgent treatment to counteract this with transfusion of a large volume of blood. The immobilization which is usually employed for these patients is a pelvic sling, counterbalanced with weights and traction on the affected side, with sufficient pull to reduce the displaced bone. Some traction will need to be applied to the opposite leg in order to provide the degree of abduction needed to stabilize the pelvis.

CHEST INJURIES

Fracture of one or two ribs, though painful, is not a serious injury provided there is no damage to the underlying respiratory organs. The only treatment required is normal activity. Analgesics may be given to relieve pain. Strapping is seldom used. Chest injuries which involve the ribs, pleura, lungs and possibly the heart and pericardium, must be taken seriously. The aim of treatment will be to restore the function of the lungs, which is to oxygenate the blood, as soon as possible and at the same time prevent further complications.

First-aid treatment will be to see that the airway is clear, cover up the wound to seal the abnormal entry from air, turn the patient carefully on to the affected side and arrange for transfer to hospital with the minimum of delay.

On arrival at the accient and emergency unit an examination will reveal the extent of the injury. While one person is observing and recording the pulse, blood pressure and respiration, the nurse will be preparing for the following emergency treatment; an endotracheal tube may be inserted to ensure the airway is clear and may be connected to a positive-pressure respirator. A needle may be inserted if there is evidence of a tension pneumothorax present; drainage of the chest into sealed bottles is carried out. Intravenous fluids are commenced followed by a blood transfusion as soon as possible. If a wound is present it will need to be closed; it may be necessary to aspirate the stomach to prevent vomiting.

Complications of chest injury

A blocked airway may be prevented by efficient first-aid treatment: the insertion of the endotracheal tube and if necessary a tracheostomy tube later. This will make it possible to suck out the respiratory passages if necessary and allow the effective ventilation of the lung with a positive pressure respirator.

Failure of the bellows action of the chest wall is caused by damage to the ribs and loss of stability of the chest wall so that it can no longer move outwards to increase the size of the thorax. The reverse may happen when the chest wall is sucked in, known as paradoxical respiration. The lungs are also prevented from expanding by the blood or air and sometimes by both accumulating in the pleural space. Movement is further reduced because of the pain it causes; a local anaesthetic may be injected into the epidural space to prevent the pain.

Blood loss. The blood collecting in the pleural space which is causing an embarrassment to the lungs is lost to the circulation which means a loss of oxygen-carrying capacity of the blood. The volume of blood lost must be replaced with whole blood as soon as possible.

These complications are serious. If the position is not reversed, death is inevitable but because chest injuries are better understood and treated, the prognosis has improved.

Other complications which may accompany damage to the ribs are injury to the liver, spleen, or kidneys leading to severe internal haemorrhage.

UPPER LIMB INJURIES

Most fractures are caused by falls on the outstretched hand.

The clavicle

Fractures of the clavicle are very common at all ages and usually affect the middle of the bone. They rarely cause any trouble; non-union is exceptional though some irregularity of the bone is common in adults. The subclavian vessels and brachial plexus are close to the bone but are very rarely damaged.

It is customary to try to brace the shoulders back by means of slings or a figure-of-eight bandage round the shoulders. The axillae must be carefully padded and the support should be adjusted every day or two but no matter how carefully this treatment is carried out it is uncomfortable and often causes chafing. Equally good results are achieved by encouraging active movements of the shoulders from the start and providing no more support than a sling for the arm, if required. If irregularity must be avoided the patient should be advised to spend three weeks on the back with a small pillow between the shoulders.

The scapula

Fractures of the scapula are not common; they affect either the body or the neck in most cases and are usually due to direct impact. In fractures of the body the patient may be made more comfortable by a sling but will respond well to active exercises; fractures of the neck commonly leave the shoulder a little stiff. Reduction is usually neither possible nor necessary.

Fracture of the humerus

Fractures of the humerus affect different age groups and present different problems.

Fractures of the upper end. This injury often occurs in the young and in the elderly. It is the latter which is likely to be complicated by stiffness of the shoulder. The patient presents with a painful swollen shoulder and upper arm which she is very reluctant to move. The fracture is often impacted, stable, and seldom requires reduction. The usual treatment is a pad under the axilla, a collar and cuff sling, and sometimes with a body bandage for a few days. This should be removed as soon as possible to allow early movement. Before discharge it will be necessary to ensure that she can cope with dressing, toilet, and feeding at home. Fractures of the shaft of the humerus are treated with a collar and cuff sling. To allow the weight of the arm to maintain the reduction a J-shaped plaster slab is applied to the arm (Fig. 57). Some deformity is quite common but unimportant; fractures occasionally fail to unite. The radial nerve being closely related to the bone is sometimes damaged, leading to radial nerve palsy and drop-wrist which may require splintage but usually recovers spontaneously.

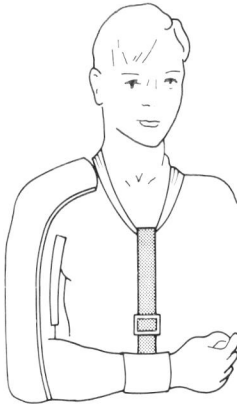

Fig. 57. *J-slab for fracture of the humerus combined with a collar and cuff sling.*

At the lower end of the humerus adults suffer T- or W-shaped fractures. A sling and plaster back-slab give useful though stiff elbows; open reduction and internal fixation is sometimes preferable. In any case movements should be started early.

There are three common varieties of fracture of this region in children. Avulsion of the medial epicondyle, fracture-separation of the lateral condylar epiphysis and, commonest of the three, supracondylar fracture.

The medial epicondyle is often pulled off when the elbow is

dislocated and it is sometimes caught in the joint. Except in these
cases, when open reduction is required, displacement does not
matter and a sling and a plaster slab for two or three weeks suffice.
This fracture also occurs in adults. It occasionally damages the
ulnar nerve, which skirts the epicondyle.

Fractures of the lateral condylar region usually require internal
fixation for they are liable to non-union with much displacement.
The ensuing deformity does not much hamper the use of the
elbows but leads to delayed ulnar palsy, the patient complaining
many years later of numbness and tingling on the ulnar side of the
forearm and hand. The ulnar nerve must then be transplanted.

Supracondylar fracture. Supracondylar fractures occasionally
occur in adults and are common fractures in children. The mother
usually comes with the child who will be crying and in pain. She
should be allowed to stay with her child to comfort him while he is
being examined and X-rayed. X-ray will confirm the presence of a
fracture, and show the position of the bone ends. The lower
fragment is usually displaced backwards and the jagged edge of
the upper fragment causes damage to the brachial artery and
sometimes to the median nerve. These structures run adjacent to
the lower end of the humerus in front of the elbow joint (Fig. 58).

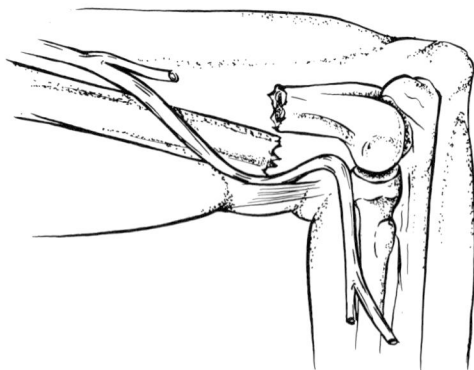

Fig. 58. *Showing how adjacent structures can be injured by a supracondylar fracture
of the humerus.*

The fracture is reduced by manipulation, the limb is immobilized in plaster of Paris with a window cut at the wrist in order to feel the radial pulse, which must be recorded every 15 minutes. Absence of raidial pulse is a warning that the circulation is in danger and may be restored by reducing the degree of flexion at the elbow although sometimes the artery may have to be exposed and the pressure released. Unless circulation is promptly restored, the flexor muscles become hard and tender and any attempt to extend the fingers causes severe pain. Later the muscles are replaced by scar tissue and the hand is crippled by Volkmann's ischaemic contracture. The early signs of this serious complication are the absence of radial pulse, blueness, swelling of the fingers, pallor and pain and must be reported *at once*.

Damage to the median nerve makes the index finger stick out straight and seriously impairs the function of the hand by weakening the power to pinch and to oppose the thumb; it also makes the thumb and forefinger numb. Spontaneous recovery is common. The ulnar and radial nerves are rarely injured.

Sometimes an irregular mass of new bone forms by the elbow which is usually called myositis ossificans but ectopic ossification is a better name.

The forearm
The radius and ulna may be broken separately or together; the latter is more common.

Fractures of the ulna alone usually affect the olecranon, especially of adults. The proximal fragment is nearly always displaced by the pull of the triceps; if comminuted it is removed and the muscle repaired; otherwise it is fixed in place by a screw or stout suture material. Movements are started after two or three weeks in a light plaster and results are good. Direct violence may break the shaft of the ulna and in the rare Monteggia injuries a fracture of the ulna is associated with dislocation of the head of the radius. These are reduced by manipulation and immobilized in plaster for six to ten weeks.

Fractures of the radius alone. Whereas adults break the head of the radius and may have to have it removed children displace the epiphysis, which must be conserved or growth becomes disturbed and delayed ulnar neuritis may ensue. Movements are started after two or three weeks in a sling.

Colles' fracture. Colles' fracture is very common especially in the elderly. It is a fracture of the lowest 2.5 cm of the radius, and often the ulna styloid is avulsed. There is posterior displacement of the distal bone fragment which may be impacted thus giving the classic dinner fork deformity. Smith's fracture has the opposite deformity and is uncommon.

The plaster cast extends from the knuckles to just below the creases of the flexed elbow but where it crosses the palm it must be narrow enough to allow full flexion of the fingers (Fig. 48). The first plaster is often incomplete to allow for swelling and is replaced by a complete one after about a week. Plasters are removed after about five to six weeks. Full use of the limb is encouraged from the very beginning, with particular attention given to exercising the elbow and shoulders.

The main complications are mal-union, which is very common although rarely disabling; rupture of the tendon of extensor pollicis longus, which is rare, and a stiff, painful condition of the wrist and hand known as Sudeck's ostedystrophy. It gradually improves, whether it is treated or not.

Isolated fractures of the shaft of the radius are not common but are apt to be unstable and require internal fixation. Fractures of the styloid process ('chauffeur's fracture') do not usually need any more treatment than a few weeks in plaster.

Fractures of the radius and ulna are very common and vary from the mild greenstick fractures that are easily reduced and give perfect results after three or four weeks in plaster to the badly displaced and overriding fractures that occur in adults and set problems of reduction and immobilization for which even internal fixation is not always a complete solution.

The plaster should extend above the elbow for the first few weeks after both bones have been broken or displacement almost always recurs. The frequency with which children fall makes refracture common unless the plaster is left on for six to nine weeks; adults need longer.

Injury to the wrist

The scaphoid is the commonest site of fracture in the carpus. Sprain-fractures and chip-fractures of other bones, usually the triquetrum, also occur but require no more than strapping or a back-slab for a week or two.

Fractures of the scaphoid have a bad reputation, but provided they are diagnosed early and treated properly they usually unite. When non-union does occur it may cause little trouble but in some cases the fracture cuts off the blood supply to the proximal fragment which undergoes avascular necrosis. Subsequent crumbling of this fragment may cause painful arthritis for which arthrodesis of the wrist is required.

Fractures of the scaphoid may cause such mild symptoms that the patient thinks that the wrist has been merely sprained and does not go to a doctor at all. Nevertheless, if mistakes are to be avoided these wrists should be radiographed from four directions. The typical features are pain, weakness and loss of movement with swelling and tenderness in the anatomical snuff box or over the scaphoid. Manipulation is not required as any displacement is corrected by immobilizing the wrist in slight extension. The plaster is similar to that used for Colles' fracture but includes the thumb as far as the inter-phalangeal joint to allow opposition to the index finger as well (Fig. 48). It is retained for four to twelve weeks according to the speed at which union occurs.

Fractures of the scaphoid are occasionally accompanied by dislocation of the lunate, for which manipulation or sometimes open reduction is required. Otherwise, treatment is the same as for uncomplicated fractures.

Injury to the metacarpals

These bones are quite often the site of spiral or transverse fractures. The spiral fractures are usually so well splinted by the interosseous muscles that treatment is often unnecessary. Transverse fractures are liable to angulation and as external splintage is often unreliable they may need fixation by an intramedullary bone peg.

An uncommon but important injury is Bennett's fracture — dislocation of the base of the first metacarpal. Being unstable it is liable, unless reduced and fixed by operation, to unite with deformity and the risk of later arthritis.

Injury to the phalanges

The fingers are often injured by a crushing force which causes a transverse fracture of the shaft of the phalanx and is often accompanied by a haematoma under the nail and soft tissue damage. Fracture of the phalanx can also be caused by indirect violence displacing one of the articular condyles.

Treatment will include the evacuation of the haematoma. Reduction of the fracture is produced by traction and manipulation. The finger is splinted in flexion (Fig. 59).

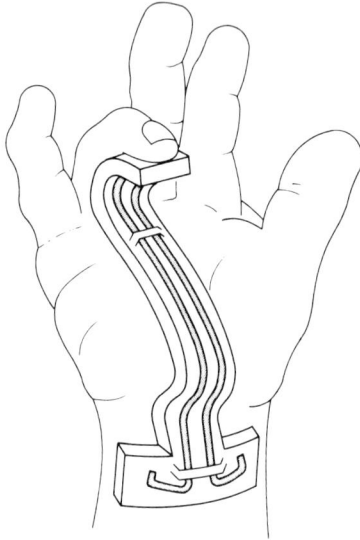

Fig. 59. *Splint for fracture of the phalanx.*

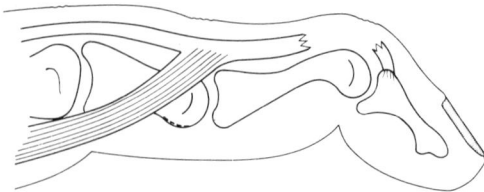

Fig. 60. *Avulsion of the extensor tendon.*

Mallet finger. The extensor tendon is avulsed from its insertion in the terminal phalanx (Fig. 60). In this case the distal interphalanged joint is splinted in extension (Fig. 61).

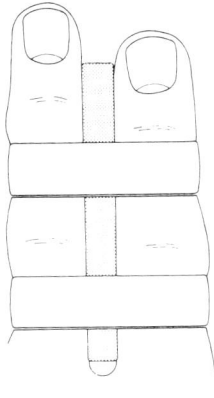

Fig. 61. *Alternative method of splinting an injured finger.*

Some points of general importance

The normal use of the upper limb as a whole and of the hand in particular depends upon the absence of stiffness. Injuries of the shoulder and hand give most trouble of this kind and movements should be started as soon as possible. Those joints which are not immobilized must be exercised from the very beginning and operation is sometimes carried out with the aim of reducing external splintage to a minimum or even avoiding it entirely.

Swelling hampers movement and it also leaves stiffness in its train. Elevation and active movement are the most effective means of prevention and treatment; massage and passive movement are of much less value. It must be remembered that when a triangular or collar and cuff sling is used the elbow, forearm and hand are below the level of the heart and are, therefore, liable to swell. Rings and bracelets must be removed as soon as possible after the injury, before swelling occurs.

Outpatients with plasters must be warned to report *at once* any swelling, pain, discoloration or inability to move the injured limb and it is an advantage to provide them with a printed notice to this effect and to ensure that it is read. Inpatients require careful and repeated observation in this connection.

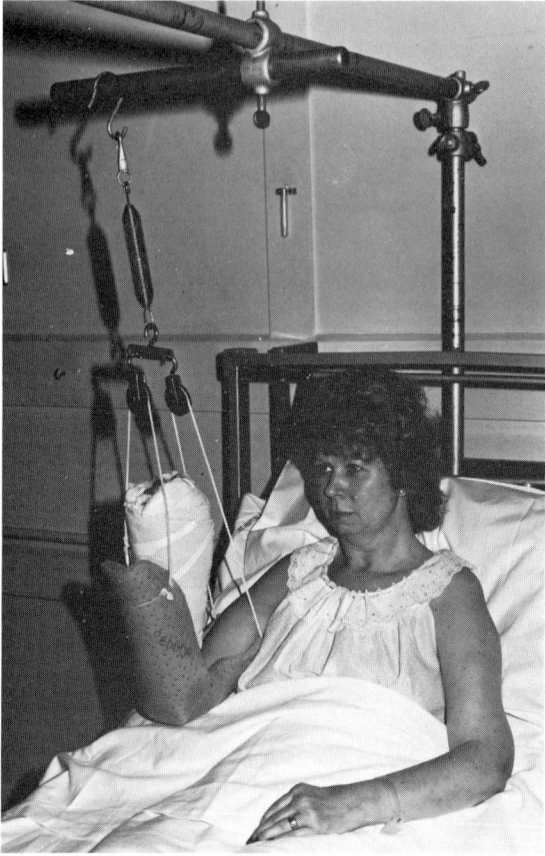

Fig. 62. *A method of elevating the hand to prevent swelling.*

LOWER LIMB INJURIES

The femur

Fractures of the neck and trochanteric region occur characteristically in people of over 65 years of age when the bones have become brittle and unable to withstand the stumbles and falls that are common in the declining years. Fractures of this region carry a serious risk to life for they take up to three months to unite and the aged can develop pressure sores, pneumonia and mental disturbances after only a few days in bed with a broken, painful hip. The aim of treatment, therefore, is early ambulation in an attempt to prevent these complications.

Prior to the operation the immediate treatment is directed towards making the patient comfortable with traction in Thomas's splint or Hamilton Russell's slings while examination and appropriate tests and preparation are carried out.

The object of treatment is to render the hip comfortable so that the patient can move about freely within a matter of days; this cannot be achieved except by internal fixation. With good anaesthesia, prompt, skilful surgery, blood transfusion when necessary, good nursing and determined physiotherapy, it is fair to say in almost every case that a patient who is not fit for operation is not fit to lie in bed and that operation is at times to be regarded as a matter of urgency. Manipulation may be necessary in order to reduce the fracture prior to internal fixation.

Fractures of the neck of the femur (intracapsular). Sub capital fractures carry a high risk of avascular necrosis. Because of the damage to the blood supply, they are usually treated by replacing the head with a prosthesis such as Moore's prosthesis (Fig. 99a) or sometimes by total hip replacement. With a fracture further down the neck, the form of internal fixation is either a three-flange nail, Moore's pin, or sometimes special screws. With intertrochanteric fractures (extra capsular) the risk of non-union is not so high although fixation can be difficult. It is necessary to use a nail which inserts into the neck, combined with a plate which is screwed on to the shaft.

As soon as possible after the immediate post-operative period the patient should be assisted to get up and begin moving again; standing at first, non weight bearing, then walking using such aids as are appropriate.

It is essential to determine whether old people can cope before they are discharged. Old people feel very weak for some time following surgery. They may be managing very well in hospital, where there are good facilities, level floors and plenty of space, but find life more difficult in their own home.

Fracture of the shaft of the femur. The femur is a very strong bone and it takes considerable force to break it unless there is some underlying pathological condition. The degree of violence is likely to damage other structures especially blood vessels causing haemorrhage which leads to shock. The loss of 1 to 1.5 litres of blood into the thigh even with closed fracture is not uncommon. Fat embolism is more common in fractures of the femoral shaft than in other bones and damge to the quadriceps muscle can cause stiffness of the knee.

Sub-trochanteric fracture. The small proximal fragment is difficult to control. It is likely to be flexed and abducted because of the powerful muscles (psoas and glutei) and for this reason open reduction and internal fixation by using a Kuntscher's nail is performed (Fig. 63). Pathological fractures in this area of the bone are not uncommon and are treated in the same way. A Kuntscher's nail may also be used to give internal fixation to any part of the femoral shaft when multiple injuries are present in order to allow the patient greater mobility.

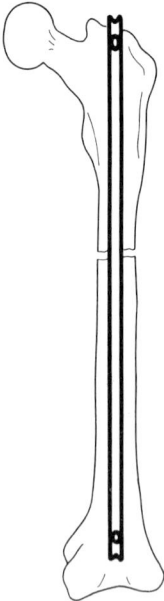

Fig. 63. *Intramedullary (Kuntscher) nailing for internal fixation of femoral shaft fracture.*

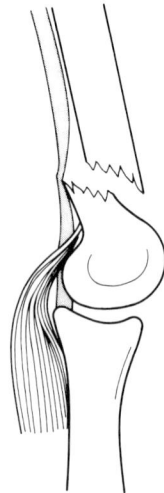

Fig. 64. *Supracondylar fracture of the femur showing displacement of the distal fragment by the pull of the gastrocnemius.*

Fracture of the mid-shaft of the femur. The type of fracture will determine whether it is likely to be stable or not. Reduction is usually by closed manipulation. It is important to get a satisfactory alignment to maintain the natural anterior bowing of the femur and to see that there is no rotational deformity.

Immobilization is achieved by skeletal balanced traction using a Thomas's splint with a Pearson's knee flexion piece on which to rest the limb. The Steinmann's pin is inserted just behind the tibial tubercule; the amount of pull will depend on the strength of the muscles. Carefully placed pads will help to correct angulation and retain the normal contours of the limb rather than using excessive pull.

Fracture of the lower end of the femur — supracondylar fracture. The distal fragment is likely to be displaced backwards because of the pull of the gastrocnemius muscle which has its origin behind the femoral condyles (Fig. 64). Skeletal balanced traction may be used with Thomas's splint and Pearson's knee flexion piece with the angle of splint opposite the site of the fracture. If a pad is used to correct the displacement a careful check must be made to see that the popliteal artery is not being obstructed. The nurse should feel the posterior tibial pulse behind the medial malleolus. Because this fracture is sometimes difficult to control, open reduction and internal fixation is sometimes employed.

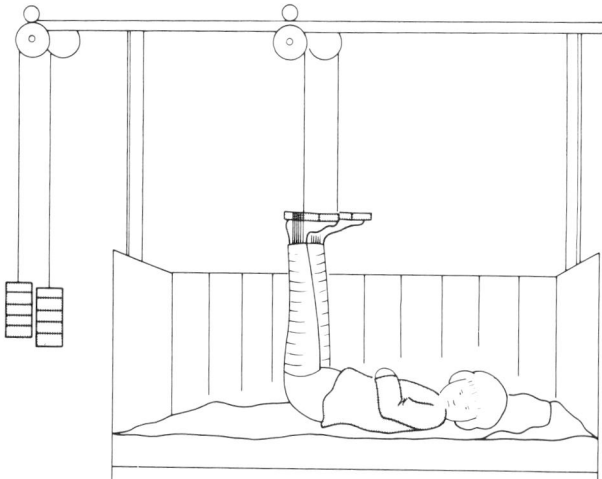

Fig. 65. *Gallows traction.*

Fracture of the femoral shaft in infants. These fractures are treated by gallows traction with the legs suspended from a cross bar so that the buttocks are just clear of the bed (Fig. 65). The contortions in which young children indulge prevent neither union nor perfect recovery in a matter of eight to twelve weeks. This method is suitable for infants up to approximately four years old.

Fracture of the patella

Direct violence causes transverse, occasionally vertical, or stellate fractures with or without displacement; muscular contraction causes transverse fractures with separation. The joint is swollen by an effusion of blood (haemarthrosis) and may require aspiration under strict aseptic conditions.

Fissure fractures require a back splint for two or three weeks but walking and gentle exercises may start after a matter of days in many cases.

Fractures with separation require operation. If accurate reduction can be achieved it is held by a screw or sutures of wire or other strong material, otherwise the patella is removed and the extensor expansion is sewn up. If one of the fragments is small it alone is removed and the gap closed by suture. Quadriceps drill is started at once; walking is allowed when the wound has healed. A plaster tube or well-fitting back splint is worn for six weeks but is removed to allow supervised exercises after three or four weeks. A knee without a patella is often good, but never perfect.

Injury to the tibia

Fracture of the upper end of the tibia. Often the lateral condyle commonly known as a 'bumper fracture' is caused by a force on the outside of the knee and may be accompanied by a tearing of the medial and injury to the cruciate ligaments causing considerable loss of stability. There will be bleeding into the joint and the risk of osteoarthritis if correct anatomical alignment is not achieved. It may be possible to reduce the fracture by closed manipulation followed by immobilization in a long leg plaster, if not it will be necessary to aspirate the knee. Reduction and fixation by screws or bolts may be carried out. The patient is usually not allowed to bear weight on the limb for approximately eight weeks. A fracture of both tibial condyles is likely to need open reduction and internal fixation. If weight-bearing is commenced before there is sound union, the fragments will be depressed causing considerable damage to the knee joint.

Fracture of the mid-shaft of the tibia usually involves the fibula as well. Because the bone is superficial the fracture is likely to be open. It is a typical motor cycle injury caused by direct violence with considerable force involved and there is likely to be extensive soft tissue injury and loss of skin. These factors added together give the risk of infection, delayed union and even non-union is not uncommon; if this is to be avoided prompt emergency treatment in the accident and emergency department is essential. Reduction is usually undertaken when the wound toilet has been carried out. A long leg plaster which not only maintains the alignment but prevents rotation of the fragments achieves immobilization.

In the case of spiral or oblique fractures which are often unstable it may be necessary to apply traction by means of a pin through the calcaneum which is incorporated in the plaster. An alternative method is open reduction and internal fixation using a plate and screw if the fracture is not an open one. Sometimes a single screw is adequate to fix the fragments, but must be accompanied by plaster of Paris. In the post-operative management it is important to elevate the leg to prevent swelling. If there is extensive soft tissue damage an external fixator may be used (see Fig. 66). This form of fixation will hold the bone ends in place and allow reconstructive surgery on the soft tissues such as skin grafting to provide wound cover. If the injury is more severe, amputation may be the treatment of choice to prevent a prolonged series of reconstructive operations over a period of time, as long as two years. Early amputation and the fitting of a prosthesis can be completed in a few weeks.

Fractures and fracture-dislocations of the ankle

These are common at all adult ages and are often referred to loosely as Pott's fractures. Most of them are due to lateral rotation of the foot on the leg and Pott's name is properly applied to these alone. The first degree is a simple spiral fracture of the lateral malleolus (Fig. 67a, b); further violence displaces the foot and lateral malleolus and either pulls off the medial malleolus or tears the medial ligament (second degree) (Fig. 67c, d); yet greater

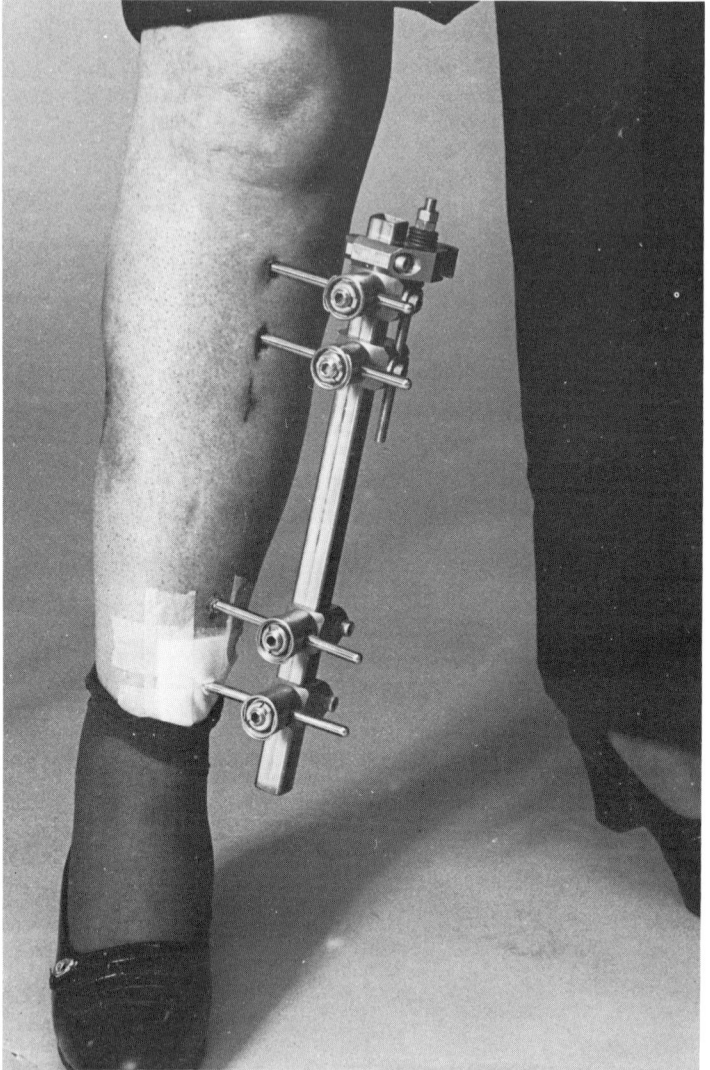

Fig. 66. *The Oxford external fixator (courtesy of Oxford Orthopaedic Engineering Centre).*

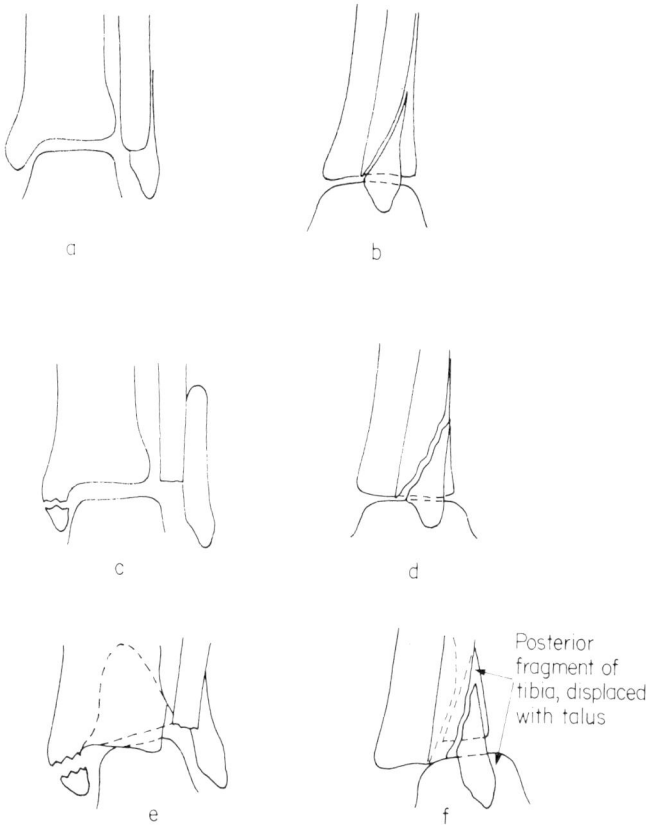

Fig. 67. (a) *and* (b) *first degree Pott's fracture, lateral malleolus only broken;* (c) *and* (d) *secod degree Pott's fracture, both malleoli broken* (*bimalleolar fracture dislocation*) *with talus displaced laterally;* (e) *and* (f) *third degree Pott's fracture* (*'trimalleolar' fracture dislocation*); *the talus is displaced laterally and backwards, taking with it both malleoli and a part of the tibia.*

violence displaces the foot backwards as well, often shearing off part of the back of the tibia (third degree) (Fig. 67e, f). Medial rotation produces inward and backward displacement.

Many of the injuries do well with manipulation and plaster. In the case of second and third degree Pott's fracture this should be extended above the knee. A small incision and a single screw to secure the medial malleolus will help to stabilize the fragments and external splintage using plaster of Paris is also needed. Swelling and stiffness may persist for a long time but good recovery can be expected.

INJURIES TO THE FOOT

The calcaneum. The important injuries are mostly due to falls on the heel; the bone is crushed and the heel becomes broadened and everted. Bruising appears in the sole a day or two later. Even after operative reduction stiffness and aching are common and some surgeons ignore the deformity and prefer to rely upon pressure bandages, elevation and vigorous exercises from the earliest days to reduce swelling and to minimize stiffness. If the fracture has been reduced it must not be walked on for about three months. In non-operative treatment, walking may be commenced earlier. Sorbo padding is incorporated in the sole of the plaster to make a cushion. When the plaster is discarded a similar pad can be placed in the shoe and worn as long as necessary. Pain persists for a long time following fractures of the calcaneum. The force which has been sufficient to fracture the calcaneum will be transmitted to other bones in the body, and may have caused a fracture of the tibia, a crash fracture of the vertebral body, or a fracture at the base of the skull.

The talus. Apart from sprain-fractures this bone is subject to a number of serious injuries which are apt to cause avascular necrosis and severe, permanent stiffness; fractures of the neck with dislocation of the body and dislocation of the entire bone are the chief offenders and usually need open reduction. Simple fractures of the neck unite without trouble and are treated in plaster for ten to twelve weeks, during which time the patient uses crutches.

Fractures of the other bones in the tarsus are not common and not usually serious; they are treated in plaster or strapping and crutches may be ordered.

The metatarsals. Most fractures are caused by weights falling on the foot and causing a crushing injury. This produces much soft tissue damage and swelliing. Treatment consists of elevation to allow the swelling to subside, followed by a below-knee plaster for 4 to 6 weeks. If the injury and swelling is less severe, strapping the foot may be adequate.

Occasionally the neck of the second, third or fourth metatarsal breaks without any known injury. This is a fatigue fracture often called a 'march fracture'. Treatment is a below-knee plaster for 4 to 6 weeks, followed by an insole to maintain the arch, and sometimes a metatarsal bar (Fig. 30) and foot exercises.

The phalanges. Broken toes may be caused by crushing and the patient is wise to go to bed and elevate the foot until the swelling has subsided and the wound is healed.

NURSING CARE

The nursing care of patients following trauma makes special demands on the nurse. She must be able to see the link between the treatment required for the condition and the needs of the person under her care. She must also be able to create the environment in which both treatment and care will produce a satisfactory result. The forms of treatment will vary considerably, from the child with a fractured femur to be treated on gallows traction, to the artisan with a hand injury where the prevention of swelling and retention of movement is so vital, to the patient with a head injury and still unconscious, who has not even begun on the long road back to recovery, or it may be the patient is an old lady with a fracture of the neck of her femur where the risk of complication is great and the mortality rate high.

Each patient whatever his condition will have his own special needs which must be taken into consideration before devising the plan of care for that individual. The needs of the child are different from those of the adolescent and they are different again from the adult patient who may have been involved in an accident. Their special concern may be for their family, their job, or their home — a great number of road traffic accidents come within this category.

The nurse caring for a patient following injury must also be aware of the concern of the family; some of them may have been involved in the same accident; some may have travelled long distances to see their relatives — all will be under great stress at this time.

General remarks

General considerations. All that has been said about the prevention and treatment of swelling and stiffness in the upper limb applies to the lower. Most people told to 'keep the foot up' place it on a stool; it is still dependent and should be at least as high as a chair seat. Swelling responds very well to a pressure bandage (Fig. 68), elevation and exercises and unless slight, is best corrected before plaster is applied. Walking in a well-fitting below-knee plaster does much to reduce swelling and loose plasters should be replaced.

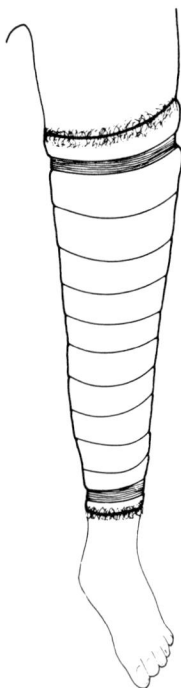

Fig. 68. *Robert Jones pressure bandage.*

The essence of a pressure bandage is a *thick* layer of evenly applied wool secured by a crêpe bandage. The result should be free from ridges and hollows and should be firm to the touch; it should also extend well beyond the swollen part and should be assisted by elevation. The common errors are to use too little wool and to apply the bandage too loosely. An effective pressure dressing is also an effective splint but must be replaced after a day or two.

With unconscious patients especial care is necessary. They must be turned as assiduously as those with paraplegia — often a difficult task with the elderly and semiconscious as they repeatedly adopt a certain position which makes pressure sores very likely. Particular care of pressure areas is necessary and a rising respiratory rate must be reported as it usually means that lung complications are occurring. A good diet is essential and tube-feeding is often necessary; the fortified milk mixture with added vitamins is of great value. Up to 2.5 litres a day can be given. The intake and output of all liquids must be recorded.

Conscious patients may generally be nursed in whatever position they find most comfortable but activity is to be encouraged. Patients just back from the operating theatre should be nursed on the side whenever possible and in all cases the breathing must be watched carefully. Any difficulty must be reported at once. It is also important to make sure that when a patient is on one side there is no pressure on the limb due to the body itself or to plasters. When consciousness has returned the patient should be questioned and examined for evidence of tightness of the plaster or dressings, swelling, discoloration or paralysis. Paralysis may be due to plasters or dressings, the injury itself or to pressure on nerves while the patient is on the operating table.

Care of the bowels is traditionally a nursing preserve but should not be allowed to become a matter of providing aperients simply because a day or two has passed without the bowels having acted. Many patients believe that this is a serious state of affairs. A good diet, activity, especially out of bed, and reassurance may suffice but otherwise aperients should be ordered. A suppository is often effective. Care must be taken to ensure that faecal impaction is not occurring; the patient who has several small motions daily may have a choked rectum and diarrhoea of this type is said to be spurious. Manual evacuation of the rectum is an objectionable task but is much more reliable than any other method in these cases.

INJURIES OF JOINTS

SPRAINS, SUBLUXATIONS AND DISLOCATIONS

The stability of a freely movable synovial joint depends on the shape of the bones taking part. The ligaments which hold the bones together and limit the range of movement may be intracapsular or extracapsular. The muscles which move the joint also provide stability especially those attached close in to the joint, e.g. the short muscles of the shoulder; in large joints are pads of fibrocartilage which also contribute to the stability of the joint. Injury to these structures will affect the stability. The bone ends are covered with articular cartilage which is lubricated by synovial fluid produced by the synovial membrane. Damage to these structures will affect the function of the joint.

Just as the severity of a fracture depends upon the magnitude of the force so does the degree of damage to a joint. A small force stretches or tears a ligament but does not displace the joint — a sprain. A larger force causes more damage to the soft tissues and some displacement of the joint — a subluxation. A larger force still causes the surfaces that normally articulate to lose contact — a dislocation (Fig. 69).

Apart from these, joints may be injured by fractures which extend into them or by disturbance of intra-articular structures.

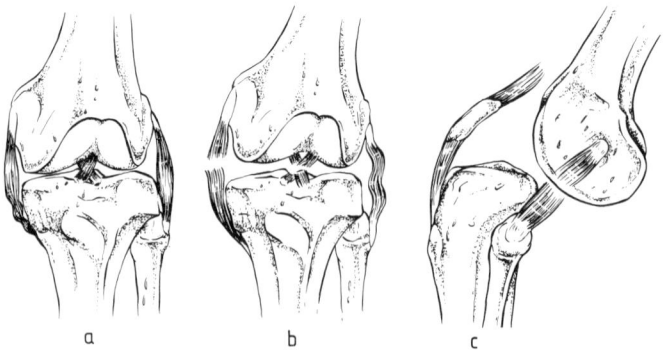

Fig. 69. (a) *Sprain;* (b) *subluxation;* (c) *dislocation.*

SPRAINS

Sprains are very common and are characterized by pain, swelling, bruising and tenderness related to the attachments of capsule or ligaments to bone. The joint is painful to move and often swollen by effusion. As the clinical picture so closely resembles that of a fracture sprains are generally radiographed. In many cases small chips of bone are pulled off as sprain-fractures (Fig. 70).

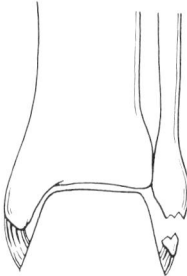

Fig. 70. *Avulsion fracture which may be associated with severe sprains.*

Treatment is by firm support and exercise. For the upper limb a crêpe bandage, strips of zinc oxide plaster or elasto-crêpe bandage is usually adequate but for the lower limb plaster is often a more reliable protection. Sometimes a pad is placed over the sprain before the bandage is applied. Use of the limb prevents swelling and stiffness and the foot should be elevated when not in use. Injecting a sprain with local anaesthetic provides dramatic but usually temporary relief.

Sprains are most common in the ankle and tarsus. Sprains of the wrist are quite common but cannot be distinguished from fractures of the scaphoid without X-ray examination. Sprains and sprain-fractures of the digits can cause troublesome stiffness. Sprains of the hip occur in children and these patients should be admitted to hospital because they closely resemble early tuberculosis.

Sprains of the spine are quite common but are usually labelled lumbago or 'disc lesion' and are treated by various forms of physiotherapy or supports.

SUBLUXATIONS

Subluxations require no separate description.

DISLOCATIONS

Dislocation is a condition where the joint surfaces have been displaced. The force causing the injury damages the ligaments and muscles (Fig. 69c). The clinical features are deformity, swelling, pain and loss of function. The joint is often fixed in an abnormal position. Associated fractures are common.

The jaw
The mouth remains fixed open after a deep yawn or hearty laugh but the dislocation is usually easily reduced by pressing downwards and backwards on the lower molar teeth. No other treatment is necessary.

The spine
For all practical purposes dislocation of the spine does not occur without fracture (see p. 120 for fracture-dislocation of the spine) but an interesting example of subluxation is provided by spondylo-lis-thesis (Fig. 71).

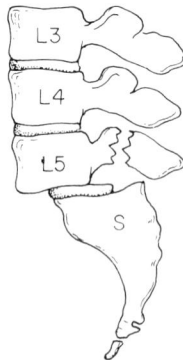

Fig. 71. *Spondylolisthesis. Note forward subluxation of lumbar 5 on the sacrum.*

The clavicular joints
Subluxations are not uncommon and respond well to physiother-

apy. Dislocations (Fig. 72) are rather rare and also respond well to physiotherapy but some deformity remains. This does not usually matter but if it has to be corrected an operation is necessary; pads and strapping are unsuccessful and are liable to cause sores.

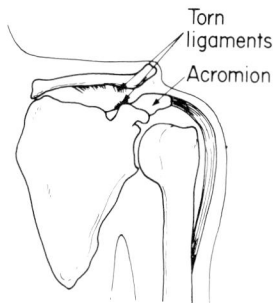

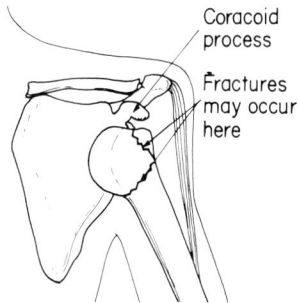

Fig. 72. *Acromioclavicular dislocation.*   Fig. 73. *Subcoracoid dislocation of the shoulder.*

The shoulder

The shoulder is one of the commonest sites of dislocation (Fig. 73) and the commonest site of recurrent dislocation. Displacement is nearly always anterior or subcoracoid, but occasionally posterior or subacromial. There is often injury to the posterior surface of the head of the humerus which may be crushed against the outer rim of the glenoid cavity. There may also be associated fracture of the greater tuberosity of the neck of the humerus. Reduction is by Kocher's or Hippocrates' manipulation. Exercises for the hand and elbow start at once but the shoulder should be immobilized for a minimum period of three weeks to allow the soft tissues to heal. Immobilization is usually with a broad arm sling and body bandage, having placed a pad under the axilla to absorb the moisture. After this period gentle active exercises may commence. Because of the risk of prolonged stiffness of the shoulder in the elderly, the body bandage may be removed earlier to allow movement.

Complications include paralysis of the deltoid and sometimes other muscles due to injury of branches of the brachial plexus. The axillary vessels are rarely injured. The rotator cuff is commonly torn. Recurrrent dislocation is a complication of simple dislocation. The joint dislocates with a minimum of violence; the movement producing it is abduction and external rotation. The patient learns to reduce the dislocation himself but the joint becomes progressively less stable with increasing risk of damage to the articulating surface of the humerus. Treatment is by operation to pleat the front of the capsule and shorten the muscles in front of the joint. Post-operatively the arm is bandaged to the side for three to four weeks to avoid abduction or external rotation. Later active exercises are commenced.

Injuries of the rotator cuff

The rotator cuff is made up of fused tendons that partly enclose the head of the humerus and are attached to the tuberosities. It lies between the head of the humerus and the acromion and is separated from the latter by subdeltoid (subacromial) bursa (Fig. 74). It is readily injured by stretching, as when the arm is

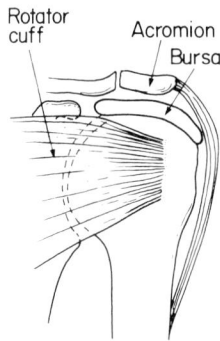

Fig. 74. *The rotator cuff.*

wrenched or the shoulder is dislocated or by crushing between its bony neighbours as a result of a fall on the hand. Young people suffer no more than a painful stiffness that passes off with physiotherapy but over the age of about 40 the cuff has lost resilience and toughness and is liable to be torn, along with the subdeltoid bursa. It is difficult or impossible for the patient to raise his arm and severe, persistent stiffness — 'frozen shoulders' — is liable to follow. Physiotherapy may be enough but surgical repair is sometimes required.

In the past lesions of the rotator cuff have been given numerous names but they all single out mere parts of the whole condition —

subdeltoid (subacromial) bursitis; torn supraspinatus; peri-arthritis, capsulitis or adhesions of the shoulder. As they may cause pain down the arm these injuries have also been labelled 'brachial neuritis'.

The elbow (Fig. 75)

The elbow is commonly dislocated and at any age. Reduction is by manipulation unless, as sometimes happens, the medial epicon-dyle has been caught in the joint (p. 128). A sling is required for two to three weeks and thereafter patience and gentle use; stiffness is common and may be prolonged. Active exercises only are permitted to the elbow joint. Any attempt at stretching is likely to reduce the range of movement and may cause permanent damage to the joint. The nerve and blood vessels are not often damaged.

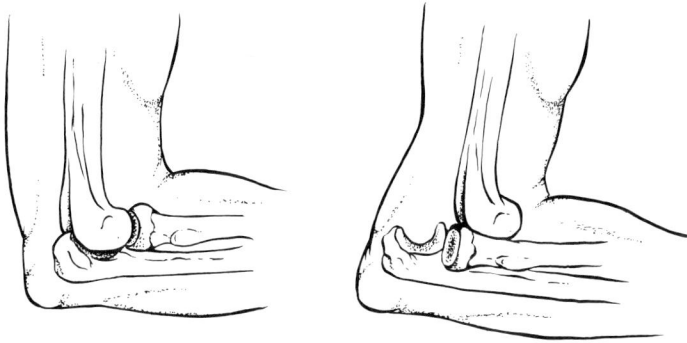

Fig. 75. (a) *Outline of normal elbow;* (b) *outline of dislocated elbow.*

The hip

Great violence is necessary in order to dislocate the hip; the joints may be dislocated in three ways:

1. Anterior dislocation when the head is lying in front of the joint. This is not a common dislocation because of the kind of force needed to produce it.

2. Posterior dislocation is commonly caused by the knee hitting the lower pad of the fascia in a car accident. This violent force on the flexed knee is transmitted via the femur, causing the posterior rim of the acetabulum to be displaced — a fracture-dislocation. Usually it is accompanied by injuries to the knee. Open reduction

and screw fixation may be necessary. There is a risk of damage to
the sciatic nerve in this injury because of its proximity to the
posterior surface of the hip joint.

3. Central dislocation of the hip caused by a direct force to the
side of the hip forcing the head through the acetabulum so that it
protrudes into the pelvis. The shattered pieces of bone caused by
this injury may damage the pelvic organs and the blood vessels in
the area. Traction is often applied to effect a reduction; open
reduction may be necessary. There is a risk of osteo-arthritis
occurring later in life. The traction is applied to both legs, either
skeletal or skin traction, with the legs widely abducted to hold the
pelvis straight. Traction will need to be maintained for 12 weeks.
The nurse must appreciate that this is a major injury often
accompanied by the complications already mentioned.

The wrist
The wrist is not subject to dislocation without fracture (p. 131).

The digits
Open dislocations are less uncommon here than elsewhere.
Manipulation is usually successful but surgical repair of a torn
capsule is sometimes necessary. The injured digit is strapped to a
neighbour (Fig. 61) and early movement is encouraged.

The knee
Dislocations of the knee (Fig. 69c) are rare and carry the serious
risk of damage to the popliteal nerves and vessels. Though it is
astonishing how well strong muscles can compensate for lax
ligaments immediate surgical repair of the badly torn capsule and
ligaments is preferable to mere splintage. In either case a plaster
splint is worn for six weeks, but quadriceps drill, *as with all injuries
of the knee*, must start at once.

The patella
Dislocation of the patella is always lateral and usually recurrent. It
is one of the causes of locking and giving way of the knee and is
treated by transplanting the patellar tendon to a more medial
insertion.

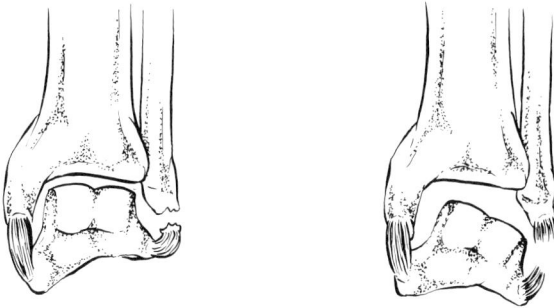

Fig. 76. *Showing the position of the talus following rupture of the lateral ligament of the ankle joint.*

The ankle
Dislocation of the ankle without fracture is rare (see p. 139) but recurrent subluxation may follow severe tears of the lateral ligament (Fig. 76). The torn ligament is replaced by using one of the peroneal tendons and the foot is fixed in plaster for six weeks until the tenodesis has healed soundly.

The tarsus
Dislocations of the tarsus are rare and may be serious (see p. 142) Open reduction may be needed and a walking plaster has to be worn for six to ten weeks.

INTERNAL DERANGEMENTS OF JOINTS

Almost any joint can be affected by sudden episodes of 'locking' or 'giving way' but the knee is by far the commonest. The cause may be either a loose body or some abnormality of an intra-articular fibrocartilage that allows it to interfere with movement of the joint.

A common source of loose bodies is osteochondritis dissecans, a condition in which a piece of articular cartilage comes adrift, most often from the medial condyle of the femur or from the capitulum of the humerus. These loose bodies are sometimes numerous but need not be removed if they are not interfering with the use of the joint.

Injuries of the menisci

Injuries of the menisci are caused by a violent rotational force applied to the knee when it is flexed and bearing weight. It is common in footballers and miners. The medial meniscus is damaged three or four times as often as the lateral. As well as locking and giving way, the knee swells and is painful and there is local tenderness over the affected cartilage; the knee sometimes clicks. Locking is overcome by manipulation, often without anaesthesia, but repeated attacks of internal derangement or irremediable locking are treated by removing the meniscus. This is found either to be torn at one end or to be split in its middle, giving the 'bucket-handle' tear (Fig. 77).

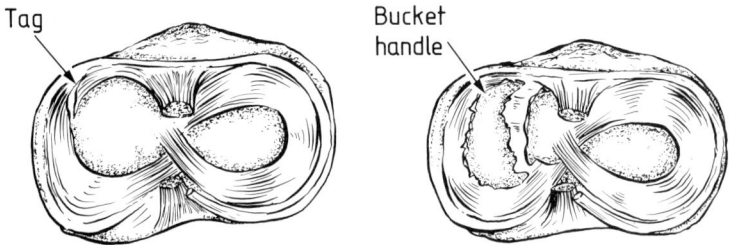

Tag

Bucket handle

Fig. 77. *Torn anterior horn* (left); *bucket-handle tear of meniscus* (right).

After operation it is customary to apply a thick layered dressing of wool and bandage from calf to thigh. Quadriceps drill is started at once. Some surgeons apply a back slab for 48 hours after operation. Walking may be commenced with the bandage still in place. The stitches are removed 10–14 days post operatively. If the wound is healed, there is a good range of flexion and no effusion, the patient may be discharged.

Instructions will be given to continue exercises, either by attending the physiotherapy department or at home. An out-patient appointment will be made, and depending on his occupation the patient should be ready for work about 6 weeks after surgery.

Conditions which resemble torn menisci to a greater or less extent are congenital discoid meniscus, cyst of the lateral meniscus. If these conditions are troublesome, meniscectomy is performed.

Chondromalacia patellae. This condition, not uncommon in adolescents, is a degenerative condition of articular cartilage which becomes soft, roughened and wears away the cartilage on the adjacent femoral condyle which may also be affected. The patient complains of pain especially when going up and down stairs; crepitus can be felt. Treatment is rest in the acute painful stage by wearing either a knee cage (Fig. 78) or cylinder plaster. Surgery to shave off the roughened articular cartilage is sometimes performed, and in rare cases patellectomy.

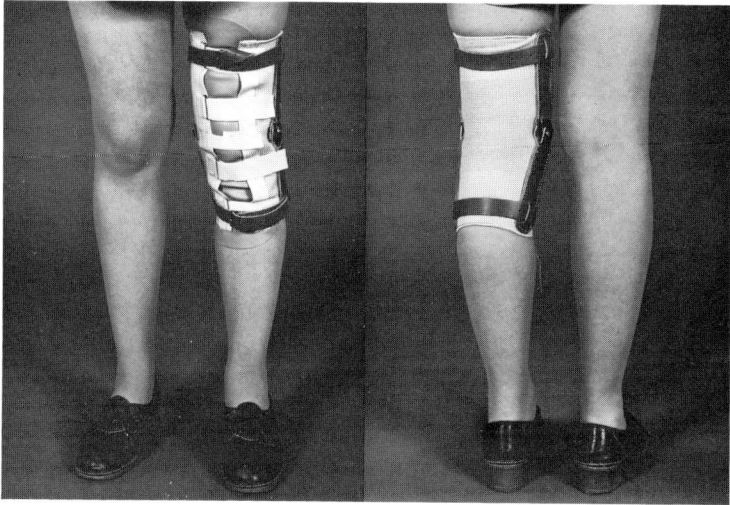

Fig. 78. *A knee cage:* (a) *front view;* (b) *back view.*

Osteochondritis dissecans. A fragment of articular cartilage becomes detached, often with a piece of bone. The commonest site is the medial chondyle of the femur; it then forms a loose body and causes locking. Treatment is removal from the knee joint, or attached back in place with Smillie's pins.

ORTHOPAEDIC BANDAGING

Bandages have been used in the treatment of injuries — for generations they were made usually of linen or cotton. Nowadays bandages and dressings are far more sophisticated; special bandages have been developed for different parts of the body, and for special purposes. The technique of applying them is still an essential skill which should be acquired by the good orthopaedic nurse.

The functions of a bandage are to keep a dressing in place, support an injured limb, and prevent swelling of joints; it may also be used to apply a splint. A correctly applied bandage will give comfort and reassurance to the patient. A bandage incorrectly applied will not carry out the function for which it was applied, and if applied too tightly can cause considerable pain and serious damage, such as impairment of blood supply possibly leading to gangrene.

To bandage a sprained ankle, using a 7.5 cm crêpe bandage, commence the bandaging with two fixing turns at the base of the toes, bandaging from without inwards to keep the foot in eversion. For a lateral ligament injury, carry the bandage over the dorsum of the foot down over the heel, then cover the remainder of the foot with a figure-of-eight bandage, covering at least half of the preceding turn, extending up the leg to just below the knee. Keep the bandage under tension to give the necessary support, but not so tight as to cause discomfort or impairment of the blood supply.

A stirrup may be used in conjunction with this bandage, starting on the inside of the leg below the knee, passing down and under the foot, extending to the same level on the lateral side of the limb. If used, the stirrup should be applied before the encircling turns. Similar bandages can be applied to support an injured wrist or thumb.

8 Diseases of bones and joints

ACUTE HAEMATOGENOUS OSTEOMYELITIS

Acute osteomyelitis is an inflammatory condition occurring most commonly in children under the age of 16. Inadequate nutrition, a low standard of hygiene, and injury are predisposing factors. Any pyogenic organism may cause the infection but usually it is a *Staphylococcus aureus* or a streptococcus. The infecting bacteria reach the bone by the blood stream and settle in the bone where there may have been some slight trauma giving rise to mild inflammation from a primary focus of infection elsewhere in the body. There may be a history of some minor skin lesion, such as a boil or septic abrasion, or there may have been a mild infection of the nasopharynx. Any bone may be involved but the commonest sites are the upper end of the tibia, the lower end of the femur, fibula, radius and humerus. In children the focus of infection is at the metaphysis of a long bone. It may occur in any part of the bone in the case of an adult but usually it starts in the shaft of a long bone where the nutrient artery enters. The highly vascular area of the metaphysis has narrow capillaries that slow the rate of the flow of blood and is an ideal site for bacteria to multiply and produce their toxins. The changes of inflammation take place, i.e. vascular engorgement, exudation of lymph and escape of white corpuscles into the part. When pus is formed, there is an increase of tension and the pus tracks down the medullary canal or under the periosteum forming a subperiosteal abscess that separates the periosteum from the bone and deprives it of its blood supply (Fig. 79). The abscess will eventually break through into the soft tissues. The vessels in the Haversian canals of compact tissue become thrombosed by pressure and infection, so that the blood supply is cut off and the bone dies. If treatment is begun at an early stage the necrosis of bone may be negligible but it is possible for the entire disphysis to become necrotic.

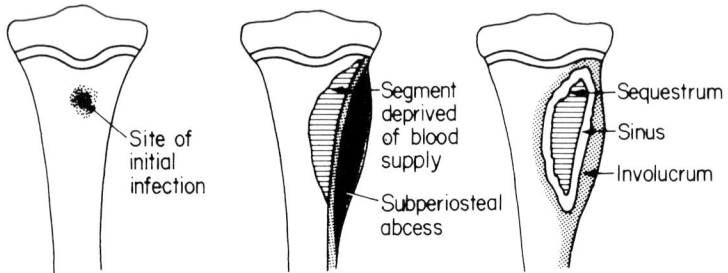

Fig. 79. *The inflammatory process of osteomyelitis.*

Signs and symptoms

General. The onset is sudden and there may be a rigor. There is always some degree of bacteraemia (bacteria multiplying in the blood stream), and toxaemia if the bacteria are of a virulent type. The face is flushed, the pulse rapid, the tongue furred, and the temperature raised to 40°C (104°F). The child may be dull and apathetic or restless and delirious. There is scanty urine which may contain albumen.

Local. There is a definite area of pain increased heat and localized tenderness near a joint. As the pain increases in intensity the child is unwilling to move the limb and holds the joint in flexion. Handling is resented. Radiographs show up no abnormality until the tenth day.

NURSING CARE

This very sick child must be received into a ward. Preferably his mother should be with him to help him settle down and allay his fears. She will be able to give some history of the condition, and supply the necessary background information which will enable the nurse to get to know the child, and to be able to assess his needs and plan his care accordingly. The child is put to bed with a bed cradle to support the bedclothes and must be kept quiet. Fresh air and warmth are essential. The diet should be light and nourishing with plenty of bland fluids. Attention must be given to the mouth and pressure areas, and the bowels regulated. The temperature, pulse and respiration are recorded four-hourly. Tepid sponging will make a hot, restless child comfortable.

INVESTIGATIONS

Blood is taken for culture in order to identify the organism and determine its sensitivity to antibiotics; the blood is put into a bottle containing a culture medium and sent to the laboratory at once. Blood is also taken to estimate the haemoglobin level (these children are often anaemic), the white cell count and a deferential count — the leucocytosis may reach as high as 25 000. The blood sedimentation rate will be raised. It should be taken on admission and repeated later — a lower rate is an indication that the infection is subsiding.

Although no changes will be visible for the first 10–12 days, X-rays are usually taken to exclude other conditions of bone.

TREATMENT

General treatment will include the administration of antibiotics, either by the intra-muscular or sometimes by the intravenous route. Penicillin, which is the usual antibiotic, is given in large doses, three or four-hourly, commencing as soon as possible after the blood culture has been taken, the usual dose being 250 000 units daily, continuously for a fortnight. Alternatively daily or twice-daily injections of antibiotics may be ordered. It is essential to keep constant the level of penicillin in the blood. If sufficient fluids are not being taken by mouth, an intravenous transfusion is started.

Local rest. The limb is immobilized in a splint, such as a plaster shell, gutter splint, a Thomas's knee splint for the femur or a shoulder abduction splint for the humerus which is kept open for inspection. After the acute symptoms have subsided a complete plaster may be used. Ths is especially important when a weight-bearing bone is involved, in order to prevent a fracture occurring.

Operative treatment. If treatment is started early and the disease is of short duration changes may occur to bring about healing of the bone without surgery. However, surgery may be needed because there is poor penetration of the antibiotic into the diseased bone owing to reduction of the circulation due to the disease. Operations are performed to relieve tension and to remove pus which produces substances that are a barrier against penicillin. The subperiosteal abscess is opened and drained. The bone may be drilled to let out the pus. When the general condition is good and healing has occurred, the use of the limb is resumed.

OSTEOMYELITIS OF THE SPINE

The onset may be acute or insidious. The pain is not severe and it is difficult to distinguish it from a tuberculous spine. The treatment is the same as that for a tuberculous spine with the appropriate chemotherapy. In this case the spinal fusion is performed by nature.

CHRONIC OSTEOMYELITIS

The chronic type of osteomyelitis may be a sequel to acute osteomyelitis or may be due to an organism of low virulence so that there is no early acute illness. The infection may be the result of a penetrating wound. Because the blood supply is deficient sequestra are formed. These are found in cavities of dense bone laid down under the periosteum. From these cavities an opening leads to a discharging skin sinus. The condition may seem quiescent for a long period, following which there may be recurring attacks of subacute inflammation with abscess formation. These are accompanied by local swelling and tenderness with a dull, aching pain. There is some rise of temperature but the constitutional upset is not severe.

Treatment

Rest and care of general health are essential. Chemotherapy is ordered if possible. Often the bacteria are low-grade and resistant.

Operative treatment

Sequestrectomy. The surgical treatment of this condition is performed to: (1) establish the causative organism, and consequently provide the appropriate antibiotic cover; (2) to open the bone abscess by a wide saucer-shaped incision which permits easier removal of dead and sclerotic bone; and (3) to transfer healthy tissue, muscle or skin pedicle grafts, into the bone defect. After the operation the wound may be packed and a padded plaster applied. This is left on even when discharges seep through it. It can be encased in deodorant felt to overcome the smell. It is changed only when necessary so that the newly formed granulation tissue is undisturbed.

BRODIE'S DISEASE

In Brodie's disease there is a small abscess localized at the end of a long bone and caused by an organism of low virulence. Often it remains quiescent and symptomless for years, but later there is pain and tenderness with reddening of the overlying skin. Radiographs reveal the abscess walled off by a ring of dense bone.

Treatment

The abscess and dense bone are excised and the space filled with bone chips.

ACUTE INFECTIVE ARTHRITIS

Acute infective arthritis is an infection of a joint caused by pyogenic organisms. Infection can enter the joint: (1) directly from a penetrating wound; (2) from a neighbouring focus of infection, usually bone; (3) through the blood stream, as in acute osteomyelitis; and (4) as the complication of an acute specific infection.

Pathology

The synovial membrane becomes inflamed and there is an effusion into the joint. At first this is serous fluid; later there is a serofibrinous exudate and, unless the condition is treated, pus forms. If suppuration continues the articular cartilage is eroded and the infection spreads to the epiphysis causing an osteomyelitis, or it may perforate the joint capsule and spread to surrounding soft tissues. Destruction of bone and soft tissue may be followed by a pathological dislocation. If treatment starts early resolution can take place leaving a normal joint, but when there has been gross bone destruction the fibrous tissue ossifies leaving a bony ankylosis.

Signs and symptoms
There is general toxaemia with a high swinging temperature. The joint is hot, tender and swollen. The pain is severe and is increased by any movement, however slight. Even bumping the bed causes intense pain. There is muscle spasm and the limb is quite rigid; the patient holds the joint in semiflexion — the position of greatest ease.

Treatment
The general nursing care is that already described for acute osteomyelitis. The joint is aspirated and the fluid investigated in the laboratory. Antibiotics may be introduced into the joint and also given systemically. If the pus is too thick to be aspirated an operation is necessary. The joint is opened, the pus evacuated, the joint washed out and an antibiotic introduced. Drainage may be needed. The joint is immobilized, as in acute osteomyelitis, in the optimum position in a splint that allows for inspection. The hip joint requires skin extension and traction and a Thomas's bed knee splint with skin extensions is used for the knee.

Later treatment. If there has been no bone destruction bed exercises and graduated weight-bearing are started under the supervision of the physiotherapist. If there has been bone destruction followed by ankylosis, a protective splint, such as a caliper, is worn. Any surgery to consolidate the joint is delayed until there is no possibility of the infection becoming active.

Acute infective arthritis occasionally occurs in children under one year. Provision must be made to admit the mother who may be breast feeding the child. Although the condition is not common it may have serious consequences to life, and the future function of the limb. The infection is spread either by the blood stream or from a neighbouring matephysis. Pus from an osteomyelitic lesion of the upper end of the femur can cause septic arthritis of the hip joint because the metaphysis is intracapsular. Skilled surgical and nursing care is essential for the child, together with reassurance and support for the parents.

NEUROPATHIC ARTHRITIS (CHARCOT'S JOINT)

Charcot's joint (Fig. 80) occurs when there is a disorder of the nervous system such as tabes dorsalis, syringomelia, peripheral neuritis or transverse myelitis. When the sensory nerve supply to a joint is impaired the joint is insensitive and the rapid tendon reflexes that normally protect the joint against sudden strains do not function. Following a minor injury there is a quickly increasing, painless effusion into one of the larger joints, such as the knee, shoulder or elbow. In a short time the joint structures are destroyed and the joint easily dislocates.

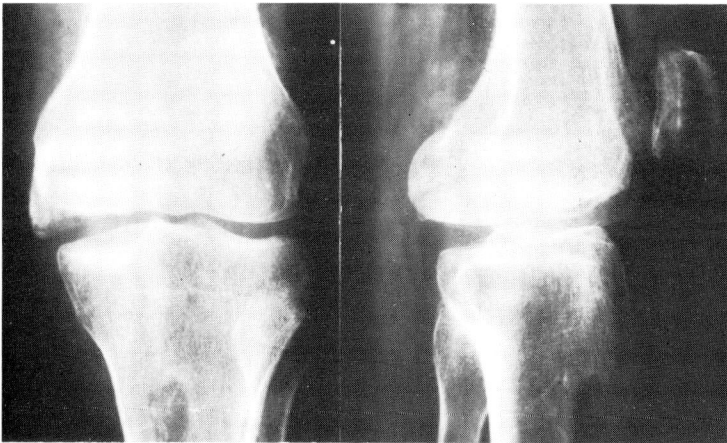

Fig. 80. *X-ray showing Charcot's disease of knee joint.*

Treatment
Protective splinting such as a caliper or elbow cage is ordered to prevent further joint damage. The fluid is aspirated and a pressure bandage applied.

SYPHILIS OF JOINTS

A syphilitic epiphysitis occurs in infants with congenital syphilis. A Wassermann reaction of mother and child is taken. General antisyphilitic treatment is given while the limb is immobilized until the epiphysitis has subsided so that there is no risk of the epiphysis separating from the diaphysis. A more chronic form of arthritis due to congenital syphilis (Clutton's joints) is occasionally seen in adolescents. There is painless effusion into both knees. Clutton's joints and joints affected by acquired syphilis respond to anti-syphilitic treatment.

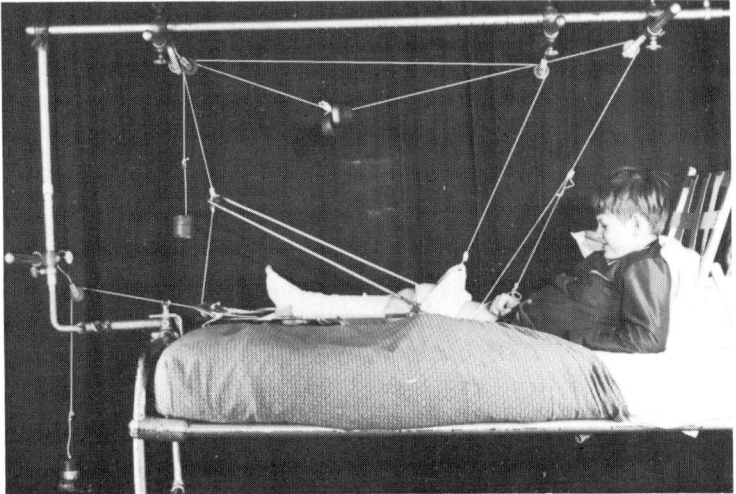

Fig. 81. *Reverse dynamic splintage.*

GONOCOCCAL ARTHRITIS

Gonococcal arthritis is a form of suppurative arthritis following gonococcal urethritis unless the infection has been controlled by antibiotics. It may be polyarticular or may affect only one joint, such as the knee or ankle.

The orthopaedic treatment is the same as that for any acute suppurative arthritis with treatment of the disease by antibiotics given systemically. They may also be injected into the joint following aspiration.

HAEMOPHILIA

Haemophilia is a hereditary sex-linked condition in which the clotting of blood is delayed due to the absence of a blood protein necessary for coagulation, AHG (antehaemophilic globulin) Factor VIII. There are approximately 4000 haemophiliacs in the United Kingdom. It is transmitted from females to their sons, occurring very rarely in females. Although present at birth it may not be evident until the child is a little older, more active and more prone to injury.

Inheritance

All daughters of a haemophiliac are carriers, but all his sons are normal. The sons of carriers have a 50:50 chance of being haemophilic. The daughters of a carrier have a 50:50 chance of being carriers. In approximately one-quarter of cases a family history of haemophilia is not known. Severe haemophilia — the man with no Factor VIII — bleeds for little or no apparent reason. His life is disrupted and he may become crippled unless bleeds are treated early. In severe haemophilia it is mostly joints and muscles that are affected. With less severe haemophilia there is more than 1–2% of Factor VIII in the blood; these men may lead near-normal lives unless injured or subjected to surgery, then they should be managed as severe haemophiliacs. Superficial cuts are not usually troublesome.

Management of persons with haemophilia

All should be registered with a centre for haemophilia, they will then carry a card identifying them with the centre. The centre is usually linked with an orthopaedic department where bleeding into the joint can be treated effectively in order to prevent joint damage and deformity. The haemophilia centre is responsible for the treatment of the blood disorder. The staff at the centre will also give valuable advice to the family regarding treatment and the ways that disabilities can be prevented. This advice can be extended to those who have contact with haemophiliacs, such as the school teacher and, later, the employer. Persons with this condition can now have a near-normal life expectancy and the quality of their life has been greatly improved.

Treatment
The aim is to control bleeding, to relieve pain and restore function. Bleeding is controlled by giving sufficient Factor VIII concentrate, and it will be continued in order to prevent further bleeding and to allow healing to occur.

Administration
Sterile water is added to the concentrate, the solution is drawn up with a plastic disposable syringe through a filter needle. The phial is then gently rotated — not shaken — and the filter needle is discarded and replaced with a suitable intravenous needle. The solution is then slowly injected into the vein (20 ml in about 5 min). Factor VIII may also be administered by continuous intravenous infusion. Tranexamic acid may be given for up to 14 days to control bleeding following such operations as total hip replacement.

Analgesic drugs used for patients with haemophilia include Palfium, given orally, or pethidine, orally or intravenously. Buprenorphine is given sublingually or intravenously.

Bleeding into the joint is treated by rest and the application of a pressure bandage. Aspiration is less commonly carried out now. Later, gentle exercises will be commenced under Factor VIII cover. Recent advances in treatment allow the patient to have home therapy. This gives the haemophiliac much greater freedom to travel and live a more normal life. Careful assessment will be made by the staff of the haemophilia centre in order to determine the suitability of the patient and his environment. Training on administration and advice on storage and maintenance of a continuous supply of Factor VIII will be given.

CHRISTMAS DISEASE

Christmas disease is much less common than haemophilia. It presents the same signs and symptoms and is a genetic defect of the X chromosomes, producing a deficiency of Factor IX. The aims of treatment are similar to those previously mentioned. Factor IX therapy is given to arrest bleeding.

RHEUMATOID ARTHRITIS

Although orthopaedic nurses will be meeting patients with

affected joints it must be remembered that rheumatoid disease is a systemic disease involving connective tisssue. Parts of the body which may also be affected are the skin, lungs, eyes, arteries, kidneys and blood-forming tissues; some degree of anaemia is almost always present.

Rheumatoid arthritis affects about 1 000 500 people in this country. If properly treated in the first year, 70 per cent can go into complete remission; untreated, 40 per cent heal with little or no deformity; the remainder will suffer disablement — some severe. The disease, affecting as it does women in the active period of life, has many social implications. They usually have heavy family or career commitments which add to the stress.

Aetiology
The cause of rheumatoid disease is unknown. It affects women much more often than men; it can occur at all ages but is more common in the first half of life and middle age. The course of the disease is affected by various factors such as environmental and emotional balance. It is a generalized disease with local manifestations.

Pathology
The disease process begins in the synovial membrane which thickens and becomes fringed in appearance. The joint capsule becomes fibrous so that the joint movement is restricted. A layer of granulation tissue, a 'pannus', spreads over the articular cartilage and destroys it in patches. The granulation tissue becomes fibrous and a fibrous ankylosis is produced. Occasionally the ankylosis is bony. The joints are easily subluxated. There is gross and rapid wasting of the muscles with fibrous tissue between the muscle fibres. In the later stage X-rays will reveal porosis of bone and cyst formation.

Signs and symptoms
The patient complains of general malaise, tiredness and presents symptoms of anaemia, joint pains and swelling with crippling early morning stiffness.

The general malaise is due both to moderately accompanying anaemia and also a raised erythrocyte sedimentation rate. There is nearly always fatigue due to battling with the progressive debilitation caused by the illness. Joint pain can be so severe as to cause flexion deformities, but in most cases of early onset the deformities are more likely due to swelling with effusion and accompanying tenderness. Even in the early stages of the disease there can be early morning stiffness, which may last anything up to three hours after waking.

Investigations
The investigations will include a full clinical examination and social history. Blood will be taken for erythrocyte sedimentation rate (ESR), haemoglobin, white cell count. It will also be tested for the presence of the rheumatoid factor by carrying out a sheep cell or latex fixation text. Radiography will show changes in the structure of bone.

Principles of management
The overall general health of the patient can best be undertaken in hospital, preferably in a unit dealing with patients with rheumatoid disease. These units will have the specialized knowledge of the condition and be aware of the problems which it presents. They will be able to provide the right atmosphere for treatment and care which is so essential, especially in the acute phase of the illness.

Treatment
The aims of treatment will be:

1. Relief of inflammation and pain (Mowat 1970)
2. Correction and control of systemic manifestations
3. Prevention of deformity
4. Correction of existing deformity
5. Improvement of functional capacity

Following admission to hospital the patient will be investigated and the treatment ordered. This will be carried out by members of the team. The nurse will need to make a detailed assessment of the patient's needs, and be able to plan the nursing care accordingly; she will also need to be aware of the part played by other members of the team so that treatment and care can be co-ordinated. The family must also be aware of the plan — they too have their part to play in encouraging the patient. Many of the principles initiated in hospital will need to be continued after discharge.

The problems which the patient is likely to experience are those of constantly feeling unwell and in pain. Limited mobility makes it impossible to play a full part in family life. Sexual problems may exist because of pain and stiffness. Breakdown of the marriage is not uncommon. An awareness of the patient's problems and the ability to communicate with them effectively, is essential when nursing patients suffering from this disease.

The overall general health of the patient can best be undertaken in hospital where the necessary rest can be enforced and radiography and other investigations carried out. The diet should be attractive and well balanced. Overweight can be an added burden to inflamed and damaged joints and a programme of weight reduction can be supervised. Rest in bed during the active disease relieves the symptoms of pain and muscle spasm and improves the general well-being of the patient. During this period care must be taken to secure adequate support and correct positioning of painful joints. Accordingly splints for arms and legs are provided. A fixed bed-cage with a padded foot rest to keep the weight of the bedclothes off the inflamed joints prevents foot-drop when leg splints are not worn. Slipping down the bed is also avoided by this method (Fig. 82).

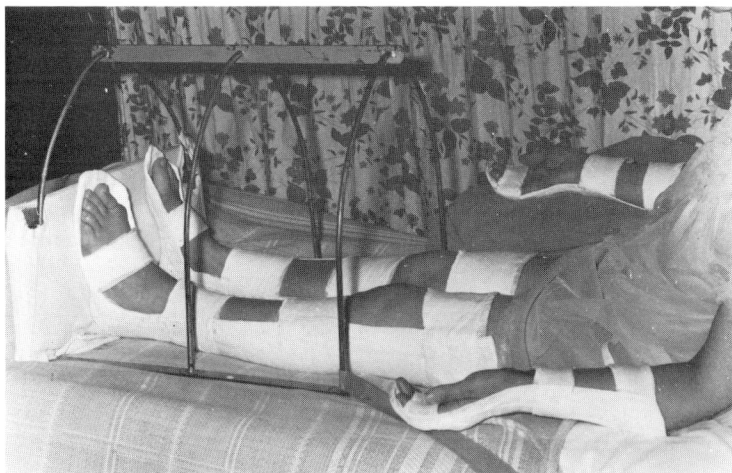

Fig. 82. *A patient 'cuffed' into hand and leg splints. Note:* (a) *the 5° flexion of the knees;* (b) *the good position of the feet;* (c) *the cuffing allowing inspection of the joints and coolness of the limbs;* (d) *the freedom of the limbs;* (e) *the slight finger flexion for comfort; and* (f) *the padded bed cradle with foot rest tied to the bed to enable the patients to sit upright if they wish.*

Only one pillow should be allowed at night and the patient taught to lie prone for a period of at least one hour each day.

Local treatment of joints. On completion of the tests, the process of treating joint manifestations of the disease can commence. Joint effusions, particularly of the knee are removed by aspiration and local injection of hydrocortisone cuts down joint pain and prevents the formation of further effusions due to inflammation. Such procedures require the use of careful aseptic technique.

Leg rests. Leg rests are made with the patient lying in the prone position on a plinth with the knee flexed at about 5° by placing a sandbag under the ankle. The plaster of Paris slabs should extend from the gluteal fold to the end of the toes over a well-oiled skin which has no other covering. The patient is lightly bandaged into the leg splints for 24 hours before 'cuffing'. The cuffs are merely bands of plaster over a layer of felt and are placed above and below the knee joint, above the ankle and across the foot. This method of immobilization allows observation of the joints.

Skin-tight unpadded plaster of Paris splints which hold the limb in the correct position are bandaged on at night and for rest periods during the day. Night splints are effective in relieving morning stiffness and reducing the inflammatory process (Fig. 83).

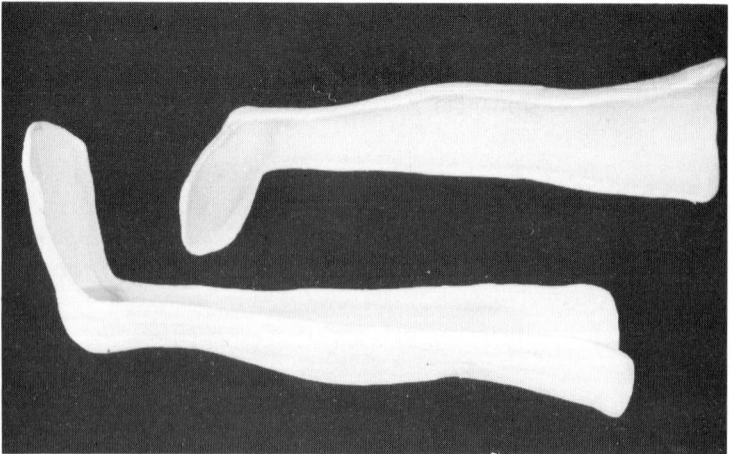

Fig. 83. *Long leg plaster night splints, unpadded.*

Sedatives to ensure restful sleeping in splints for the first few nights can be helpful. These unpadded skin-tight splints, properly made, are very comfortable and will last for many weeks. Later the patient should live a regulated life with balanced rest and exercises and local treatment to the joints. Measures are taken to improve the general health. Septic foci, such as decayed teeth, are removed because these always have an ill effect on the general health. The diet should be mixed and must contain all vitamins and minerals and plenty of fluids. If the patient is in bed the calories should be lowered by cutting down carbohydrates. Anaemia is treated by intramuscular or intravenous injection of iron.

Corrective splints

Correction of deformity before contractures have occurred can be achieved at any joint but especially the knee, with the use of serial plaster of Paris splints. Flexion deformities of the knees are common in the early phases of the disease and must be corrected to prevent serious disability in the later stages. A posterior shell is applied in the position of the deformity and no force, traction or manipulation is used. The shell is fixed to the limb by a circular plaster of Paris cuff above and below the knee. Pain, muscle spasm and joint swelling settle rapidly. After a week the lower cuffs are removed and any gain in extension is maintained by application of new splints (Fig. 84).

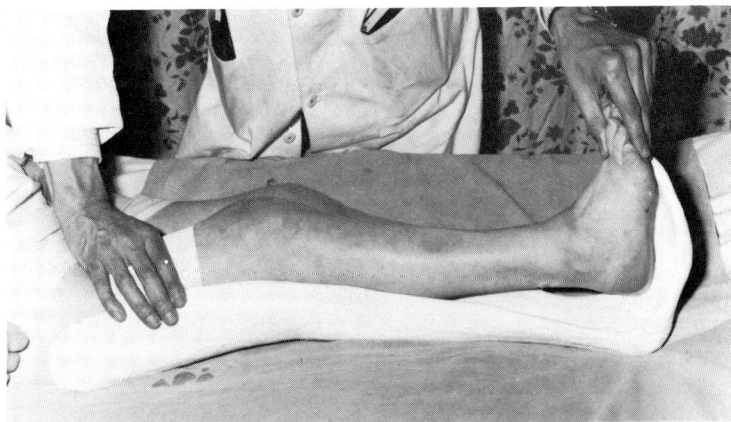

Fig. 84. *Knee flexion deformity straightened by serial splinting. Note the degree of extension obtained following one week in plaster. A new splint is then made to contain further extension.*

Fixation splints

Support for painful, unstable or permanently deformed joints is provided by a removable splint which is used to hold the joint in a position of function and so improve the everyday activities. These splints can be made in materials such as polythene, leather and fibre glass, all of which combine lightness, strength and durability. Simple fastenings should be used and care taken to ensure that they are placed so that the patient can use them.

Splints of this sort besides permitting the activity in a single joint or limb to settle without the need for complete rest can be used to reassure the patient that any surgical fixation of a joint will not produce the disability they fear. They are also particularly useful long-term aids for patients who may not be considered suitable for surgical fixation (Fig. 85).

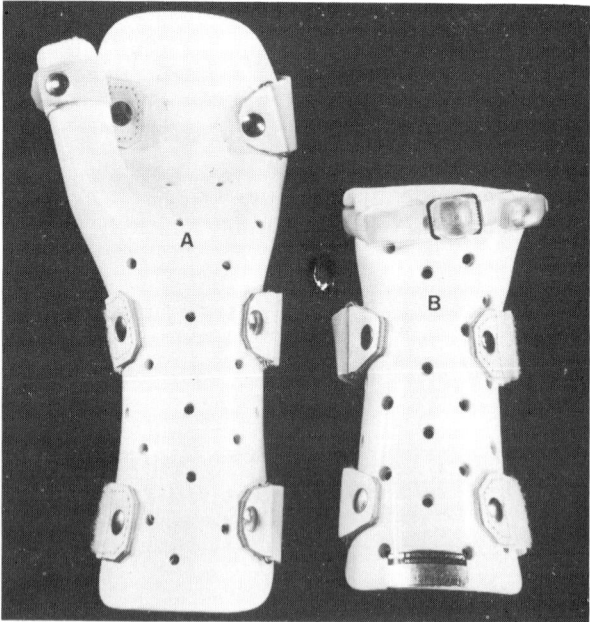

Fig. 85. *Fixation splints:* (a) *resting splint;* (b) *splint for daily use.*

Footwear

Severe deformity requires surgical footwear in which alterations providing support can be effected. A variety of new materials and methods are now in use which provide seamless shoes for these patients, i.e. the 'space' shoe (Fig. 86).

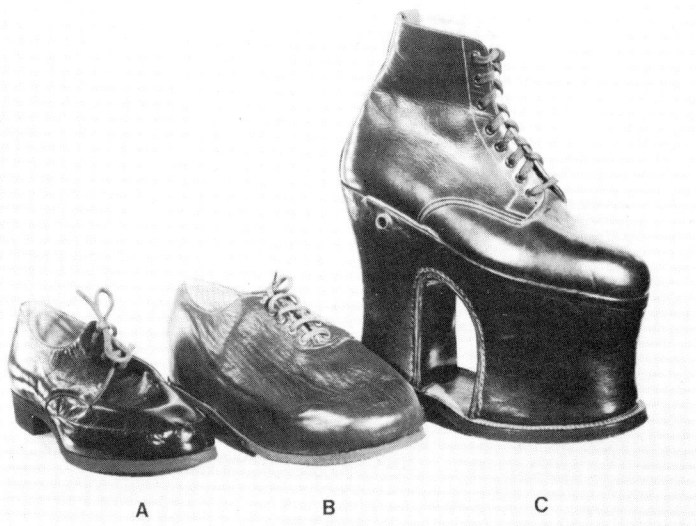

Fig. 86. (a) *Ski-front surgical shoe;* (b) *space shoe;* (c) *shoe with deep cork raise sometimes known as a bridge cork.*

Management of rheumatoid knee

Serial splinting is a method of straightening the joint without force. The patient is cuffed into a plaster splint as previously described with the knee in the degree of flexion deformity present; two weeks later, the cuffs are removed and the leg gently removed from the plaster and a new set of plasters made to accommodate the improved degree of extension of the knee joint; this procedure is repeated until a position of maximum extension is obtained. After a period of rest, active physiotherapy is given and the patient re-educated in walking.

Instability of the knee may be treated with other forms of splintage such as calipers, glass fibre splints or light plaster shells.

SURGERY IN RHEUMATOID ARTHRITIS

Surgical procedures are carried out in order to relieve pain, improve function and to stabilize joints.

The hip
Total hip replacement is the commonest surgical procedure for the
hip joint. Surgical difficulty is sometimes experienced due to the
poor quality of the bone and the fact that the patient's general
health is not as good as the patient who undergoes this procedure
for osteo-arthritis, but the management will be similar (see p.
185).

The knee
Synovectomy is designed to inhibit the diseased process of the
synovium from destroying the joint and may be either chemically
or surgically performed.

Chemical synovectomy. Radioactive gold is injected into the joint
and the patient is confined to bed, in a non-weight-bearing
position for a period of 24 hours.

Surgical synovectomy. This is performed by excision of the
inflamed synovium. A Robert Jones pressure bandage is applied
post-operatively.

Mackintosh prosthesis. A metal wedge is used to correct valgus or
varus deformity (Fig. 87). It rests on the tibial plateau either
laterally or medially on both sides and articulates with the femoral
condyles. The post-operative care is the same as that which follows
synovectomy.

Total knee replacement. Total knee replacement is used when
there is extensive damage to the joint by the diseased process.
There are many different types in use. They can be grouped under
two kinds, the hinge variety which have a spike extending up the
shaft of the femur and down the shaft of the tibia and the kind
where a small amount of bone is removed from the femoral and
tibial condyles to be replaced by a component made of metal and
one of the high density polyethylenes. The later type of total knee
replacement is more commonly used now; the cruciate ligaments
are preserved in order to maintain stability. In the Oxford total
knee replacement a disc is placed between the femoral and tibial
components. This acts as a 'spacer' similar to the meniscus; it
creates a compression force on the bone ends, and a tension on the

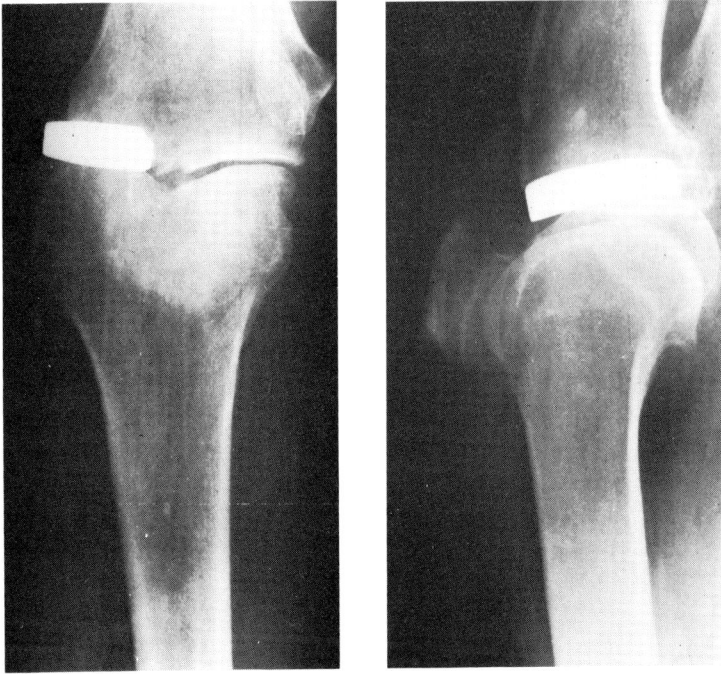

Fig. 87. *Mackintosh's arthroplasty of knee showing prostheses in place; anterior position* (left); *lateral view* (right).

ligaments and tendons, thus restoring the function these structures have in a normal joint, that of maintaining stability.

Preparation for operation. The patient will be admitted a few days prior to operation — this will allow time for the patient to get used to her surroundings, and for the staff to assess her needs, to give breathing exercises, and to explain to the patient what is to be done and what is expected of her — this will allay her fears. Investigations prior to surgery will include taking blood for haemoglobin estimation, grouping and cross matching, and electrolyte balance. The drug therapy may need modifying at the time of surgery.

Post-operative care. On return from theatre the temperature,

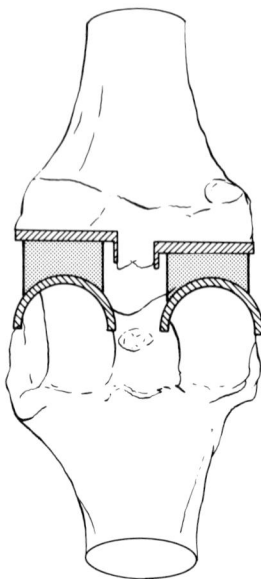

Fig. 88. *Diagram of the Oxford Knee in situ.*

pulse, respiration and blood pressure will be recorded, and the circulation of the limb checked; the foot of the bed may be elevated. Intravenous therapy will be continued and a fluid balance chart maintained. The Redivac drain is removed after 48 hours which willl necessitate removing the outer dressing and the firm bandage applied in theatre. Analgesic will be needed and antibiotics are usually given for approximately one week or until there is no evidence of infection.

The patient is usually confined to bed for the first 5 or 6 days during which time she will need help to carry out normal activities. Static quadriceps exercises are commenced early. The back slab applied in theatre is removed after 6 days and knee flexion commenced gradually. If there is good quadriceps control the patient may start walking. Stitches are removed after 12 days, and if the knee is satisfactory the patient can be discharged home with instruction as to what she is able to do and what must be avoided. An out-patient appointment is given.

In an alternative regime the knee is held in flexion, the bandage

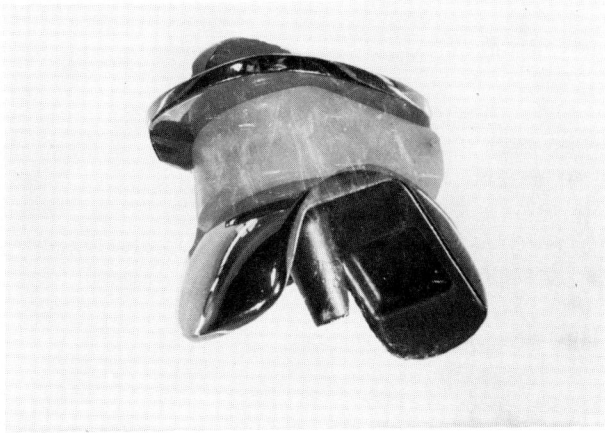

Fig. 89. *The Oxford total knee prosthesis.*

is removed daily after the third day for a short period when the knee is held in extension and then in flexion, the time and range increased each day. When full extension and 90° of flexion is achieved the patient is allowed up in a plaster back slab, after stitches have been removed on the twelfth day. If the patient can cope with stairs, etc. she is allowed home.

Arthrodesis. Arthrodesis may be performed to give stability to one knee when both are involved with the disease and it can also be used when arthroplasty has failed. The compression method is usually adopted and the limb is encased in plaster of Paris.

The ankle
Stiffness of the ankle can often be freed by simple manipulation under general anaesthetic. If necessary an arthrodesis can be performed because there are neighbouring joints allowing compensatory movements so that the results of arthrodesis are good. Plaster of Paris is applied to the limb until fusion has taken place.

The elbow
Synovectomy and excision of the head of radius is aimed at relieving pain and increasing the range of movement. A pressure bandage is applied. The arm must be elevated on return from the

theatre and it is essential to check the circulation of the hand and encourage finger movement in order to prevent swelling. Sutures are removed on the fourth post-operative day.

The wrist

1. *Synovectomy* and removal of the ulna styloid increases movement and relieves pain; the post-operative regimen is similar to the elbow operation.

2. *Arthrodesis* will stabilize the wrist joint and should relieve the pain. A pressure bandage is applied, usually reinforced with plaster of Paris. Elevation and finger movement are essential to ensure success of the operation.

Hand operations

Synovectomies, repair of ruptured tendons, prosthetic replacements and arthrodesis are operations which may be performed on the hand. Following surgery, a boxing glove type of dressing is usually applied and gently active exercises are commenced as soon as possible within the limits of the pain.

Post-operative management. The limb is placed on a pillow for comfort, the foot of the bed is elevated and the limb is observed for swelling and circulation. Movement of the toes is encouraged. Physiotherapy is commenced the following day and will include quadriceps exercises, straight leg raising, ankle movement and the hip joint will be put through a range of movement within the limits of pain. Analgesics will be necessary during this period. The pressure bandage must be checked to see that it not too tight. The pressure bandage is removed on the fifth post-operative day, flexion exercises commenced and gradual weight-bearing resumed; walking aids will be necessary at this stage but will gradually be discarded, possibly retaining one walking stick (Fig. 90). Sutures are removed on the fourteenth day.

The ambulatory patient. When the patient starts to walk he must wear well-fitting laced shoes and not loosely fitting slippers. Metatarsal domes or arch supports may be needed. Walking may start either unaided or with a walking machine, sticks or crutches. Special attention is given to posture.

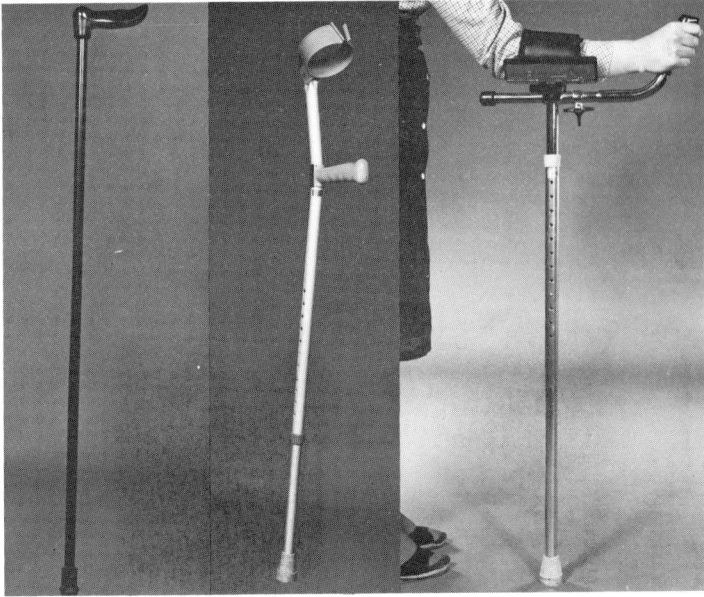

Fig. 90. *Walking aids:* (a) *Stick with moulded hand grip;* (b) *forearm trough crutch;* (c) *elbow crutch.*

Discharge. When the patient goes home definite instructions regarding the splints and the positions he must avoid are given. It must be stressed that independence through self-help must never be carried to the point of fatigue. Patients should also be told of gadgets that help, such as long-handled combs, lipstick holders, shoe horns and specially designed cups (see Fig. 91).

DRUG THERAPY IN RHEUMATOID ARTHRITIS

Drugs used in the management of rheumatoid disease will aim at relieving the pain, reducing the inflammatory process and preventing or alleviating joint stiffness.

Groups of drugs
Non-steroidal anti-inflammatory drugs
    Aspirin
    Ibuprofen (Brufen)

Indomethacin
Naproxen
Steroidal anti-inflammatory drugs
  Adrenocorticotrophic hormone
  Hydrocortisone injected into joints
  Prednisone
Other anti-inflammatory drugs
  Gold (Myocrisin)
  Chloroquine
  Penicillamine

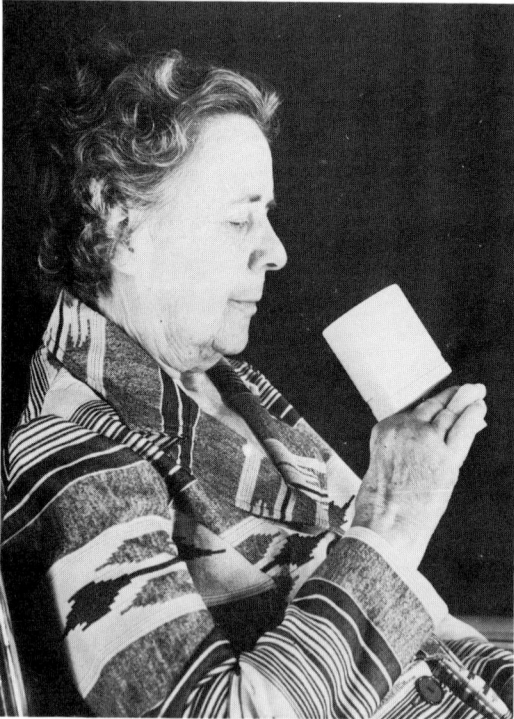

Fig. 91. *The Mandy cup, specially designed for rheumatoid hands.*

STILL'S DISEASE

Still's disease is a very acute form of rheumatoid arthritis that occurs in children (Fig. 92). The symptoms and signs at the onset

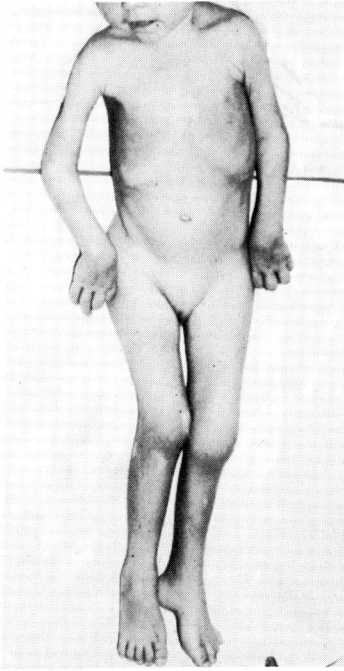

Fig. 92. *Still's disease.*

are far more severe than in the case of an adult with extensive joint involvement. The general treatment is the same with rest in the functional position for the joints. Rest in bed with separate splints for the limbs with the child spending some time in lying flat on his face is often not as satisfactory as a full-length plaster bed. With almost every joint involved this is an effective method of preventing contracture deformities and the relief of pain it affords is followed by an improvement in general health. These children need years of skilled and knowledgeable care.

OSTEO-ARTHRITIS (DEGENERATIVE ARTHRITIS)

Osteo-arthritis is essentially a disorder of the joints and not part of a general disease of the body as in rheumatoid arthritis. Since there is no infection present the term 'arthritis' taken from the

Greek 'Arthron' meaning a joint and 'itis' meaning inflammation, is not a correct description of the condition. For this reason the term osteo-arthrosis is considered more descriptive.

Aetiology
The cause of primary osteo-arthritis is unknown. The weight-bearing joints are most often affected, e.g. hips, knees, spine. Age, obesity and occupational stress appear to have some contributory relation.

Secondary osteo-arthritis
Certain well-known orthopaedic conditions can predispose osteo-arthritis, e.g. Perthes's disease; inter-articular fractures; infection of a joint affecting the articular cartilage; and untreated congenital dislocation of hip.

Pathology
The earliest changes are in the articular cartilage which becomes soft and eroded. Small bony growths, osteophytes or lipping, occur at the margins of the articulating surfaces. Gradually the whole cartilage is destroyed. The underlying bone becomes dense and the surface glistens like ivory, known as eburnation. Cyst-like spaces surrounded by local sclerosis are formed.

Signs and symptoms
The patient may be overweight but the general health is usually good. The clinical features are:

Pain. At first there is an aching of the joints after exercise and weight-bearing movement. This is relieved by rest but during rest the joint becomes stiff and pain is again felt when movement is started. Sleep may be disturbed because during sleep muscles relax and cause involuntary movement.

Stiffness and deformity. Movement of the joint becomes more restricted so that the patient becomes unable to perform certain movements such as taking a step up. As the disease progresses the limitation of movement causes deformity. Muscle wasting is due to disuse rather than to the disease itself. Radiographs show osteophytic lipping and loss of joint space.

Treatment

Conservative. In the early stages physiotherapy in the form of heat and exercises may be of value. Reduction of weight in obese patients should be advised. The use of a stick in the opposite hand may relieve mechanical stress. Analgesic drugs give the main relief.

Operative. Overall assessment of the patient's general condition, together with age, occupation and home environment are important considerations prior to surgery, together with the routine physical examination given to all patients. It is important for the patient to be admitted a few days before operation, not only to complete presurgical investigations but also to be taught breathing exercises by the physiotherapist.

OSTEO-ARTHRITIS OF THE SPINE

Osteo-arthritis of the spine is one of the many causes of chronic back pain. As the pain and stiffness increase the deformity of kyphosis develops. The typical radiograph changes of irregularity of joint outline and lipping are present in the spine of many people over middle age. They may give rise to practically no symptoms and are discovered only when a radiograph is taken for some other quite unrelated condition. It will alarm a patient considerably to hear the word 'arthritis' spoken in an unguarded manner without qualification.

Treatment

General treatment as described is given. A spinal brace or corset support may be ordered. In advanced osteo-arthritis of the cervical spine there may be root pain due to pressure on the spinal nerves as they pass through the intervertebral foraminae; the pain radiates into the occiput or down the arms. A snugly fitting Thomas's collar may relieve symptoms.

OSTEO-ARTHRITIS OF THE KNEES

Osteo-arthritis of the knees is often caused by repeated minor injuries such as kneeling on a hard floor or follows a fracture in the region of the joint. Loose bodies of bone or fibrous tissue such as a torn semilunar cartilage damage the articular cartilage as they get caught between the joint surfaces.

General treatment
As osteo-arthritis of the knees is frequently seen in women at the menopause, the predisposing causes of obesity and flat feet are treated. Physiotherapy in the form of graduated exercises especially for the quadriceps is given.

A supporting bandage, knee cage or caliper may be used for protection by restricting movement.

Operative treatment
Removal of loose bodies. Patellectomy, for relief of patella femoral arthritis. Upper tibial osteotomy, correction of valgus or varus deformity and relief of pain. Total knee replacement may be the operation of choice where there is severe joint destruction (see earlier in this chapter the treatment of rheumatoid knee). Arthrodesis may still be performed if only one knee if affected, or if an arthroplasty has been carried out on the opposite knee. To arthrodise two knees is severely disabling.

OSTEO-ARTHRITIS OF THE EXTREMITIES

In elderly people, usually in women, small swellings occur at the terminal interphalangeal joints of the fingers, known as Heberden's nodes. Osteo-arthritis of the carpo-metacarpal joint of the thumb interferes with the use of the thumb and therefore with the use of the whole hand. There is a great deal of pain and discomfort and the hands look unsightly. The patient needs reassurance. There is usually a response to remedial measures. An arthrodesis of the carpo-metacarpal joint is sometimes performed.

OSTEO-ARTHRITIS OF THE ANKLE

Usually as a result of injury, e.g. fracture or infection. Conservative treatment may relieve this condition in the early stages. A firm double below-knee iron with either flat ends to prevent plantar flexion or normal ends with back check stops is used.

Operative treatment
Arthrodesis of the ankle joint providing there is a good range of movement of the neighbouring joints of the foot.

ARTHRITIS OF THE FOOT

Usually follows injury, rheumatoid arthritis or infection. Conservative treatment as for the ankle.

Operative treatment
Subtalar arthrodesis or triple arthrodesis.

OSTEO-ARTHRITIS OF THE HIP

Osteo-arthritis of the hip is the most disabling form of degenerative arthritis. The characteristic pain that becomes worse after exercise and is relieved by rest may be in the region of the hip joint itself or referred to the knee on the same side. There may be pain in bed during the night. As movement becomes more limited the patient complains of inability to stride out, cross his legs or take a wide stance. He nearly always complains of difficulty in putting on his socks and shoes as he cannot flex the hip enough to get at the foot. The hip becomes fixed in flexion adduction and external rotation. The flexion may be compensated by a lordosis. Adduc-

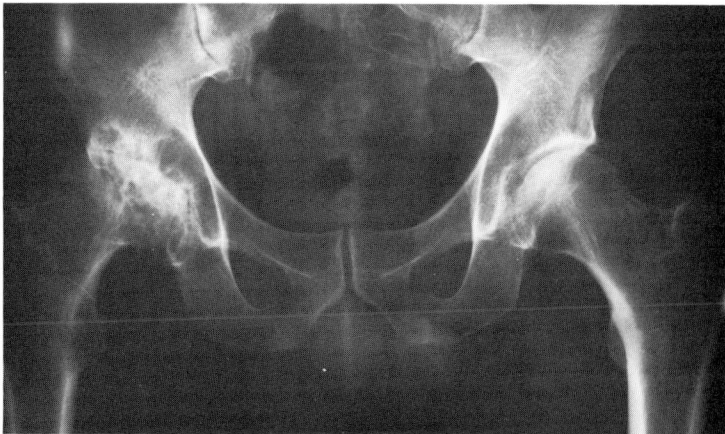

Fig. 93. *Osteo-arthritis of the hip joint showing joint destruction.*

tion causes apparent shortening which prevents the foot touching the ground. There may be severe backache which may be due to the strain put on the lumbar spine when sitting down with a stiff hip or possibly to arthritic changes in the spine itself.

The restrictions to daily activity caused by increasing stiffness and the pain which may keep the patient awake at night, are indications for surgery. This not only relieves the pain but greatly improves the quality of life for these elderly patients, thus enabling them to maintain a higher degree of independence.

Treatment
Conservative treatment is carried out on the principles already described.

Operative treatment

Arthrodesis is the fixation of the joint using a nail (Watson-Jones). All movements of the joint and pain are eliminated. It is not indicated when both hips are involved.

Osteotomy (Fig. 94) is the division of the bone between the trochanters and medial displacement of the shaft. This operation is usually combined with internal fixation which allows earlier mobilization. Hamilton-Russell traction is applied for three weeks

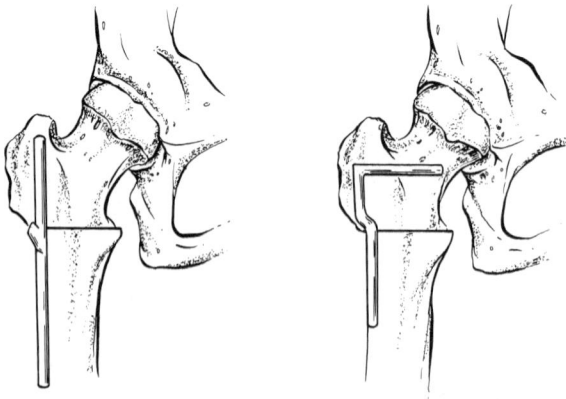

Fig. 94. *Osteotomy combined with Wainright's spline fixator* (left); *and a Muller-Harris compression plate* (right).

post-operatively followed by partial weight-bearing on crutches for six weeks. Full weight-bearing in twelve weeks.

Arthroplasty. The aim of this operation is to obtain a good range of movement and a stable joint. The results are not certain. When selecting a patient for arthroplasty of the hip the surgeon is guided by the temperament of the patient, because cooperation and concentration during the post-operative period is essential.

1. *Girdlestone's operation (pseudarthrosis)* (Fig. 95). Excision of the head and neck of the femur forms a fibrous joint, pain free but with a resulting shortening which varies between 1 and 2 inches. It is useful when all else fails.

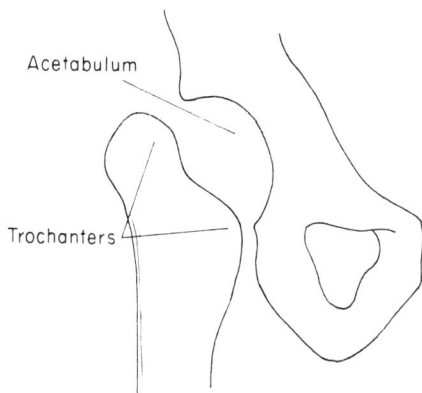

Fig. 95. *Girdlestone's arthroplasty. Fibrous tissue forms in the gap between the acetabulum and the trochanters thus allowing movement.*

2. *Smith–Petersen's operation*, using a vitallium cup (Fig. 96). The hip joint is exposed and the femoral head and acetabulum are reshaped to correspond to the vitallium mould.

3. *Total hip replacements.* Replacement of the upper end of the femur and the acetabulum with an articulated prosthesis which is cemented to the bone by acrylic cement (Figs 97, 98 and 99). The patient is nursed free in bed. Alternatively traction may be applied to the limb, either Tulloch–Brown or Russell traction; or the limb may rest on a splint such as the Cockin splint (Chapter 5, Fig. 39)

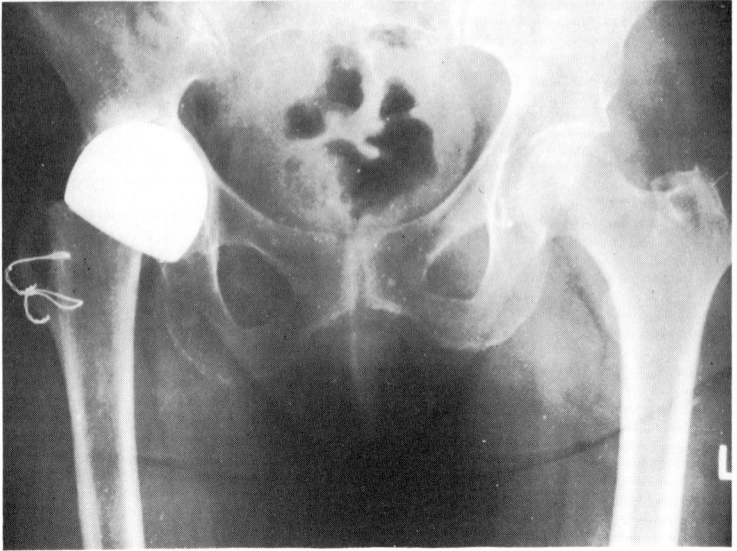

Fig. 96. *Smith–Petersen cup arthroplasty in a young person.*

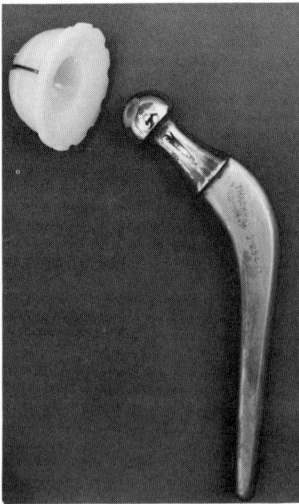

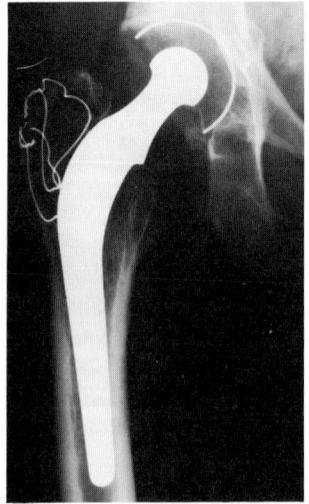

Fig. 97. *Charnley total hip replacement: Charnley prosthesis* (left); *Charnley prosthesis in situ* (right).

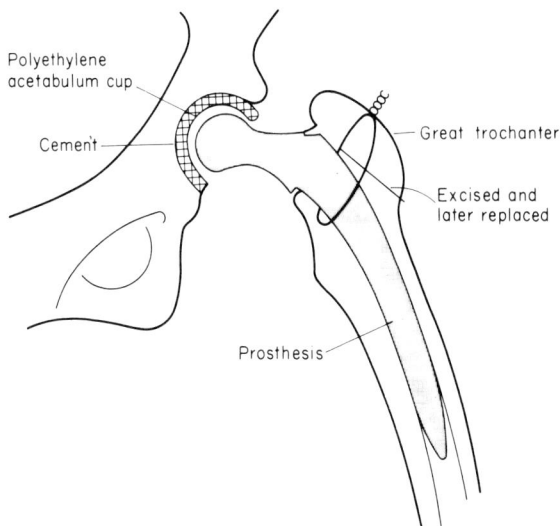

Fig. 98. *Charnley total hip replacement. The great trochanter is removed at operation then replaced and held in position by wires when the prosthesis is in situ.*

or Thomas's splint (Chapter 5 Fig. 16). The advantages of traction are that the limb is held in a comfortable position, thus enabling exercises to commence early; these will be directed at strengthening the abductor and extensor muscles and increasing the range of movement. The stay in hospital is usually 2–3 weeks, during which time the patient will gradually be mobilized and prepared for discharge.

Pre-operative care. The patient will be admitted a few days before his operation, to allow time for him to adjust to the ward, and for the necessary pre-operative care and investigations to be carried out. An assessment will be made in order to plan the care needed. The investigations will include taking blood for grouping and cross-matching, and haemoglobin and electrolyte estimation. An enema or suppositories may be given. The skin area is shaved. The type of skin preparation will depend on the surgeon – it will include a bath and antiseptics may be used.

Post-operative care. In the immediate post-operative period the

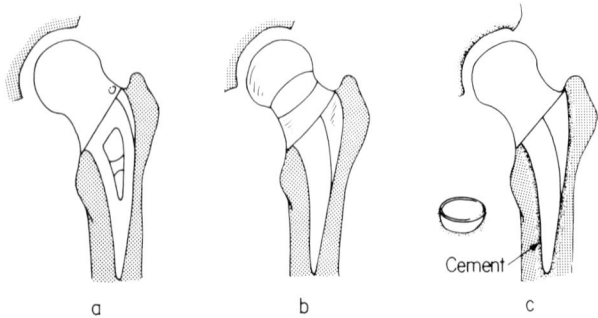

Fig. 99. (a) *Moore's prosthesis, with intramedullary stem in which consolidation of the bone occurs;* (b) *Thompson's prosthesis, similar to Moore's in that post-operatively Hamilton-Russell traction may be ordered for two to three weeks followed by partial weight-bearing with elbow crutches;* (c) *McKee-Farrer total hip replacement, replacement of the upper end of the femur and the acetabulum with articulated prostheses which are cemented to the bone by acrylic cement.*

patient may have a Charnley wedge pillow placed between the legs to reduce the risk of dislocation following surgery. Observation of temperature, pulse, respiration and blood pressure will be recorded. The wound will be observed to see that the Redivac drain is functioning and that there is no oozing from the wound. Care must be taken that the limb is in a good position and the circulation adequate. The physiotherapist will commence exercises to the chest, ankle and foot quite early, the patient having been shown how to do these before operation. The nurse must check the intravenous equipment frequently. Blood transfusion started in the theatre is followed by saline or a similar solution. Antibiotics which are often commenced intravenously may be continued for about five days. Some surgeons advocate the use of anti-emboli stockings or placing the limb in a foam trough to reduce the risk of thrombosis. An x-ray may be taken next day to check that the prosthesis is in position.

Twenty-four hours later the intravenous infusion will be discontinued if the patient is taking fluids well; the aim should be 2½ litres per day. At this time the patient may be blanket bathed with particular care to see that the area of the groin is clean and dry. With the removal of the intravenous infusion he will be better able to help to move himself, using the monkey pole; this will be good for him and will reduce the risk to the nurse's back. The patient must lie flat, with two pillows for 1–1½ hours twice daily. The Redivac drain is removed after 48 hours and the wound redressed. Abduction exercises are commenced and activity is gradually increased. If the condition is satisfactory the patient may get up and begin walking on the 4th or 5th day with a Zimmer frame or elbow crutches. At this stage he will go to the gymnasium each day to be taught walking and climbing stairs. About the 7th day the Occupational Therapist will assess his ability to cope with dressing and the activities of daily living, which will gradually be increased. Stitches are removed on the 12th day, and if his condition is satisfactory he may be discharged on the 14th day. It is essential to check the home conditions prior to discharge, and to instruct him on how to sit, get up from a chair, and how to lie in bed; also how to get in and out of the bath.

The nurse must be aware that most of these patients are elderly, and that they may have problems in passing urine, having their bowels open, etc. and that these conditions can be exacerbated by being in bed and in hospital. If traction is used she must see that it is functioning correctly.

Other joint replacements

Other joints of the body are being replaced in the case of disease or injury, such as the shoulder, elbow and small joints of the hand. Research continues on design, materials, method of fixation and the general management of patients with replacements. The reader should refer to a more detailed text for further information.

ANKYLOSING SPONDYLITIS (SPONDYLITIS ANKYLO-POIETICA)

In ankylosing spondylitis the joints and ligaments of the spine become ossified. It is classically a disease of the young male adult but now cases are being seen in older patients and females, possibly on account of better diagnosis. The cause is unknown. There is a tendency for the disease to progress with remissions and exacerbations of symptoms to a final state of rigid kyphosis.

Signs and symptoms

The onset is insidious starting with pain in the lumbosacral region which radiates down the buttocks and thighs. At this phase there may be complications of secondary anaemia and iritis. The back muscles tend to go into spasm. The patient is easily fatigued and complains of malaise. The blood sedimentation rate is raised. The stiffness of the back is due first to spasm and later to a fibrous ankylosis which becomes osseous, involving the sacro-iliac joints, the intervertebral joints throughout the spine, hips, and shoulder joint. The tempero-mandibular joint is sometimes affected, the extremities are not usually involved. The ankylosing of the intercostal joints limits chest expansion. The lumbar curve becomes obliterated and the dorsal curve greatly increased so that the patient cannot extend his head and struggles along usually with two sticks unable to look beyond three feet in front of him without stopping, straining and flexing his knees (Fig. 100).

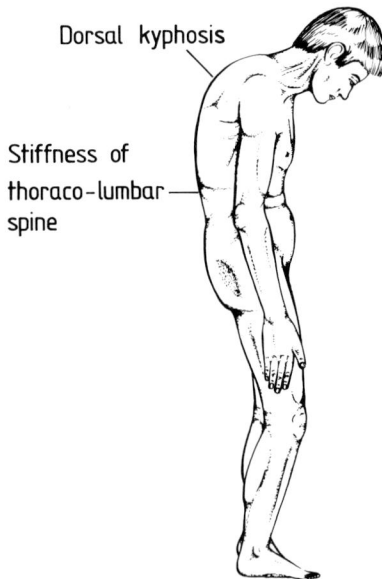

Dorsal kyphosis

Stiffness of
thoraco-lumbar
spine

Fig. 100. *Posture in ankylosing spondylitis.*

Radiographs
The first changes shown by radiograph are seen in the sacro-iliac joints. Later radiographs show a type of fusion between the intervertebral bodies. The most characteristic change is due to

calcification of the longitudinal ligaments so that the spine resembles a bamboo rod.

Treatment

The aims of treatment are:

  (a) to maintain and restore spinal and thoracic mobility
  (b) prevention and correction of deformity
  (c) the relief of pain

A period of intensive physical rehabilitation is needed in order to maintain the mobility of the spine, together with breathing exercises to retain or improve chest expansion. These exercises must be simple and properly taught because the patient may have to carry them out for the rest of his life. Exercises will be needed for other joints to retain their mobility. Hydrotherapy is helpful.

Prevention of spinal deformity

The patient should have a firm bed with only one pillow under the head; a small pillow may be allowed for the natural lumbar curve. If the patient cannot tolerate the flat position, more pillows may be allowed at first, then gradually decreased in order to prevent or correct kyphosis. A period of lying prone will also help to prevent flexion deformity of the hips when these joints are involved. The patient should be encouraged to maintain a good posture at work and at home. All spondylitic patients should sleep flat and should develop this sleeping position as a habit even when the disease is quiescent. By standing with his heels, buttocks, shoulders and occiput against a wall the patient can assess his progress; any deterioration indicates exercises should be increased.

Correction of spinal deformity

For more advanced cases with pain, spasm and rapidly increasing kyphosis, a plaster bed may be ordered. The plaster bed must be well moulded, with the spine extended as much as possible. A turning case is also made.

These patients are often emaciated and the skin requires careful attention. As pain and muscle spasm subside a fresh plaster bed may be necessary to fit the improved dorsal curve. While the condition is acute, physiotherapy is confined to breathing exercises. These exercises are most important for maintenance of the mobility of the thorax. Chest expansion also helps to counteract the spinal deformity. Progress can be checked by recording chest expansion at regular intervals. The patient can follow this record with interest and is encouraged to maintain, if he cannot increase, the expansion. Breathing exercises must be continued throughout the course of the disease even when the patient is at home.

Corrective and protective splintage may be:

1. A plaster jacket applied in head suspension or in hyperextension in the prone position, extending from the interclavicular notch to the symphysis pubis.
2. A Minerva type of jacket if a cervico–dorsal flexion deformity is occurring (Fig. 50).
3. A plaster jacket of the Doll's type which may be replaced later by a removable one of leather or plastic. This is worn for a period of about one year and gradually discarded when the disease is quiescent.
4. A spinal brace with a Thomas's collar or brow band may be used as an alternative.

Operative correction
Spinal osteotomy may be performed in the quiescent stage. It carries considerable risk and is only performed after a careful assessment of the deformity and the patient's disability. The operation consists of a V-shaped osteotomy across the articular processes in the lumbar region at one or more levels and then hyperextending to provide a compensatory lumbar lordosis for the rigid dorsal kyphosis. It may be performed in two or more stages for severe cases. The pre-operative and post-operative nursing care is the same as that described for a spinal graft. Following the operation the patient may be nursed in a plaster bed with a turning case or the surgeon may apply a plaster jacket in the theatre. A plaster jacket is worn until fusion is complete. This is an operation that may cause profound shock. Among the post-operative complications are:

1. Respiratory infection which may be prevented by breathing exercises. Postural drainage may be required.
2. Injury to the cauda equina causing a transient and partial paralysis of one or both lower limbs. Conservative treatment for the paralysed muscles is given while recovery is awaited.

Arthroplasty of hip

A patient with an ankylosed hip and a rigid spine is practically bed-ridden. Restoration of joint movement will give the patient greater ability to walk, sit and stand. Pre-operative and post-operative nursing care is the same as that described when the operation is performed for osteo-arthritis (see p. 185).

Relief of pain and stiffness

Medication for patients with ankylosing spondylitis is similar to that of rheumatoid arthritis — Aspirin, phenylbutazone, indomethacin and naproxen. For severe cases corticosteroids may be required. A short course of these drugs or ACTH may reduce pain, stiffness and muscle spasm. The nurse must be aware of the possible side effects.

Radiotherapy, once the most popular method of treatment, is now seldom used because of the increased incidence of leukaemia. It may still be used in some cases which do not respond to other drugs.

General consideration

The natural progress of this disease often led to a gross deformity of the spine and stiffness of other joints. With modern management the patient can look forward to a full and active life, and in most cases is able to carry on with his normal occupation. He will, however, need a great deal of encouragement from all concerned, which means that members of the team must be aware of the treatment and plan of care — all have their part to play, including the relatives. The plan may have to be modified in the light of progress and experience.

AFFECTIONS OF THE EPIPHYSES

Osteochondritis is a non-inflammatory affection of the epiphyses which disturbs normal growth. Each epiphysis is liable to be affected at a definite age period. The cause is obscure but it is thought to be due to an impaired blood supply, mild trauma being a possible factor. The commoner conditions affecting small bones and epiphyses are:
  1. Osgood-Schlatter's disease of the tubercle of the tibia occurring between ten and fifteen years.

2. Köhler's disease of the tarsal scaphoid occurring between five and ten years.
3. Sever's disease of the os calcis occurring between five and ten years.
4. Freiberg's disease of the head of the second metatarsal occurring during adolescence.
5. Kienböck's disease of the carpal semilunar bone, occurring during adolescence.

They are all treated by rest, which is usually enforced by plaster fixation and non-weight bearing, followed by muscle re-education.

PERTHES'S DISEASE (LEGG-CALVE-PERTHES'S DISEASE, PSEUDOCOXALGIA)

In Perthes's disease the upper femoral epiphysis is affected between the ages of five and ten years (Fig. 101). It is more common in boys than girls and is usually, but not always, unilateral.

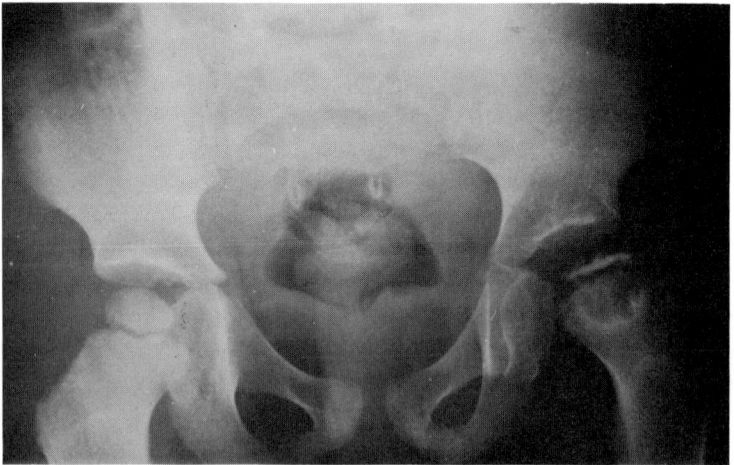

Fig. 101. *Perthes's disease showing abnormality of right femoral head.*

Signs and symptoms
The general health is good. At first the child walks with an intermittent limp; pain is slight and if present is often referred to the knee.

Sometimes after the early pain and limping the child appears to recover but on examination there is found to be a limitation of hip movements chiefly abduction and internal rotation. Muscle spasm and pain are not severe and disappear with rest. A radiograph shows an abnormality of the femoral epiphysis which goes through the phases of increased density, fragmentation and finally regeneration.

The earliest changes are an increase of joint space and density of the epiphysis. Later fragmentation is seen and the femoral head appears broader and flatter so that it is mushroom-like in shape. The femoral neck becomes thicker and there may be changes in the acetabulum.

Healing is spontaneous. The bone structure regenerates so that the femoral head is reformed in shape. There may be residual changes in the head and neck of the femur in spite of efficient treatment, leaving some restriction of movement. The prognosis is better in the younger age group.

Treatment

The aim of treatment is to minimize the secondary changes which can take place. The length of time needed for the stages of recovery to take place is 2 to 3 years. That the child should be confined to bed non-weight-bearing for this length of time is not now acceptable — it causes too much disturbance of the child's life. Whatever method of treatment is used the child is usually given a bed rest in the early stage, with traction applied keeping the leg in abduction. This will relieve the pain and overcome the muscle spasm. A double abduction frame with the legs in internal rotation may be used.

Splints designed to relieve weight and so prevent deformity of the femoral head are employed while recovery is taking place. Thomas's patten-ended caliper is described on page 53 (Fig. 21). The Birmingham splint (Harrison's) (Fig. 103) can be worn as an alternative to a caliper. It allows the affected leg to be off weight-bearing and maintains slight flexion and abduction with full internal rotation. The child mobilizes on crutches.

Alternative methods include the containment of the head within the acetabulum. If weight bearing is then allowed there is an overall force applied to the femoral head which does not deform as would pressure applied to a partly sublaxed head. This can be

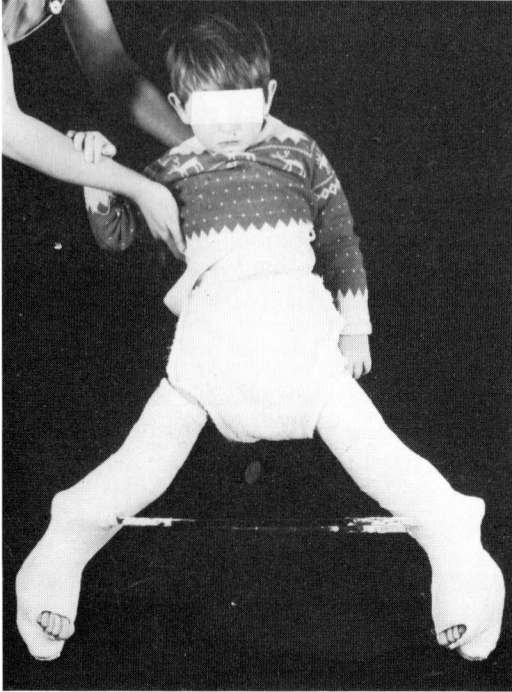

Fig. 102. *Petrie plaster. Note the abduction and internal rotation of the hips and the angle of the walking heels.*

achieved either by:

(a) *Application of Petrie plasters.* The legs are fixed in full abduction and internal rotation by applying plaster of Paris to each leg and incorporating a broomstick between (Fig. 102). The position of the limbs is of great importance as it maintains the head of the femur within the acetabulum. The patient can stay at home and with help can move around. He should attend the hospital at three-monthly intervals in order to have a check radiograph, mobilization and a re-application of the plaster.

(b) *By surgery.* A hip spica is applied for a short period with the affected leg abducted and internally rotated. A subtrochanteric external rotation and varus osteotomy is performed. A double hip spica is applied for 6–8 weeks to allow the osteotomy to

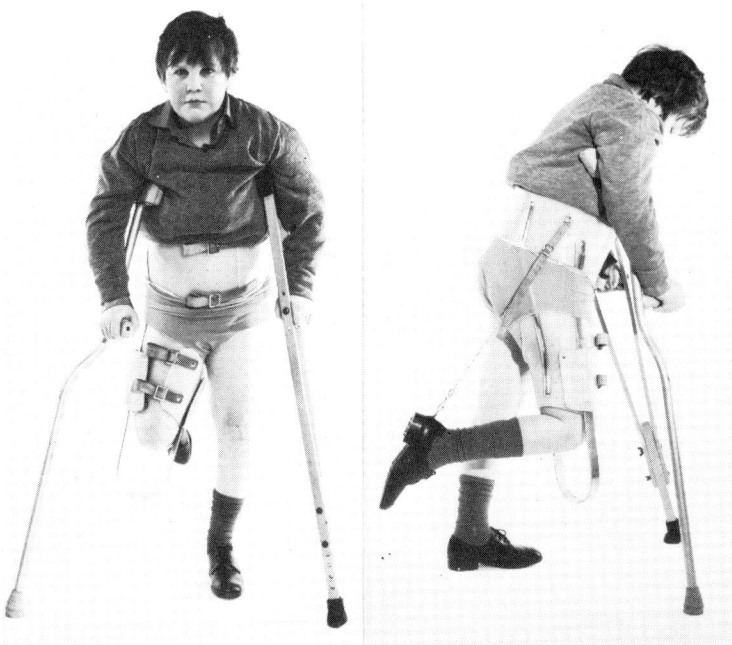

Fig. 103. *Harrison's splints for Perthes's disease of the hips to maintain weight-relieving and internal rotation and movement of the hip. Note use of staggered crutch.*

unite. Following removal of the hip spica, full weight bearing and normal activity is resumed. By this method there is a minimal disturbance of the child's activity and life style.

Posture and gait are expressions of an attitude of mind and personality and depend on the physical and mental make up of the individual. Since the variation is so wide normal posture cannot be defined. It is only possible to describe certain features that make up what we call a good carriage, such as the erect head, level shoulders and pelvis, the spine with normal curves and flat abdomen. If the erect position is assumed and the body is properly balanced and a plumb line is hung from the ear, it should pass through the centre of the shoulder and hip and in front of the ankle joint (see Fig. 104). This is achieved by a complicated neuro-muscular mechanism. The position of the hips is a vital factor

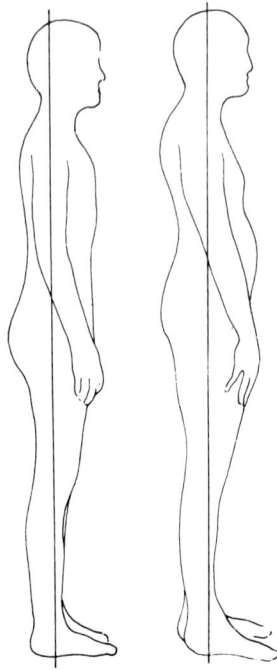

Fig. 104. *Posture: good* (left); *bad* (right).

because this determines the tilt of the pelvis on which the spinal column rests, also the position of legs and feet. The position is maintained by a balanced contraction of the muscles on each side of the weight-bearing joints. The muscles are controlled by the central nervous system which receives and controls afferent (sensory) impulses from muscles, skin, eyes and ears. At the same time it sends out a continual stream of efferent (motor) impulses to the muscles. Ligaments play an important role in preventing execessive bending but the amount of strain they can take is limited. When overstretched they become painful and sensory impulses pass to the spinal cord and reflex motor impulses to the muscles in front of the hip (psoas), behind the knee (hamstrings) and to the calf muscles so that they contract and move the line of weight. This is seen by watching the constant change of position adopted by a line of people standing in a queue.

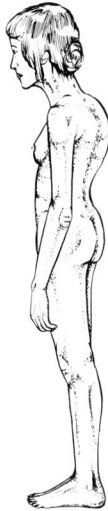

Fig. 105. *Adolescent kyphosis.*

OSTEOCHONDRITIS OF SPINE (VERTEBRAL EPIPHYSITIS, ADOLESCENT KYPHOSIS, SCHEUERMANN'S DISEASE,** Fig. 105)

Vertebral epiphysitis occurs between the ages of 12 and 18 years. It produces a deformity which is not attractive in young people; they are aware of it and will be looking for help to correct it. The patient should be admitted to an adolescent unit of a children's ward (see chapter 12) to provide the right atmosphere for treatment and nursing care.

Signs and symptoms
Pathological changes of the vertebrae cause the gradual develop-ment of a dorsal or dorsolumbar kyphosis. There is a smooth kyphos in the mid-dorsal region. In compensation the cervical and lumbar curves are increased. Pain comes on after the deformity. It is never severe but the child complains of an aching back at the end of the day or after playing games. The round shoulders, flat chest and poking chin of poor posture are to be seen. The hamstrings are often tight. The signs and symptoms are slight and not very incapacitating so that there is a tendency for them to be

disregarded. Treatment, however, is essential in order to prevent deformity of the spine and pain from osteo-arthritic changes later in life.

Radiographs show irregularity of the vertebral epiphyseal plates and wedging of the vertebrae in the affected area.

Treatment

In the early stages, while the spine is still mobile, rest and postural exercises may be sufficient. Usually it is necessary to immobilize the spine in hyperextension to correct the deformity.

A straight frame or a straight frame with a sunken head piece may be used. The hyperextension is gradual. After the patient has settled on the frame he is turned in the turning case. The frame is marked at the peak of the kyphos so the instrument maker can hyperextend it to the degree ordered (5° to 10°). After a short period the frame is again hyperextended and this is repeated until maximum correction has been attained. General care is described in Chapter 3.

A plaster bed which is made with as much correction as possible without exaggerating the lumbar curve may also be used. Extension of the spine can be increased gradually by: (1) renewing the plaster bed; and (2) gradually filling the hollow in the bed that fits the kyphos with white felt cut to fit exactly and with bevelled edges.

The patient is taken off the frame or bed for remedial exercises. These are given in both prone and supine positions and include abdominal, leg, arm and breathing exercises as well as back raisings to strengthen the erector spinae and exercises for the glutei.

Later treatment. The patient is allowed up when there is freedom from pain and no further correction is possible. Remedial exercises are continued. If the back muscles are strong the surgeon may not order a support but desire the patient to sleep in the plaster bed. A plaster jacket or a spinal brace may be ordered. The fitting of a brace is described in Chapter 5 (see p. 81). It is more satisfactory if made from a plaster cast. It must be fitted so that the dorsal spine is extended without exaggerating the lumbar curve.

Since the shoulder straps will be fairly tight careful and frequent treatment of the skin is needed. Several readjustments may be required. The support is discarded gradually and exercises must be continued at home. Supervision is needed until final growth is completed. Throughout the whole period of treatment a positive attitude should be encouraged by the nursing staff. The aim should be to see the young adult less deformed and taking part in all the activities of a person of his age group.

ADOLESCENT COXA VARA (SLIPPED FEMORAL EPI-PHYSIS)

This occurs between the ages of 12 and 15 and is more frequent in boys than in girls. The upper femoral epiphysis becomes displaced and if untreated causes the deformity of coxa vara. The cause is obscure, but an endocrine disorder is considered to be a factor because many cases, especially when the condition is bilateral, are found in the heavy type of child with under-developed genital organs, showing evidence of the Fröhlich's syndrome.

Signs and symptoms

In an acute slip the history resembles that of a fracture with a sudden onset of pain and inability to bear weight on the affected limb, which lies in external rotation. In the insidious type the onset of pain is more gradual; it may be in the hip, down the front of the thigh or in the knee. It is accompanied by a limp, and in some cases the Trendelenburg sign is positive. Examination shows the hip to be held in external rotation and adduction with limitation of abduction and internal rotation.

Radiography. In the early stage it is not apparent in the anteroposterior view, but a lateral view will show external rotation of the neck in relation to the head. Later when a definite deformity develops the neck is shortened and the great trochanter displaced upwards. It is important to remember that the epiphysis is in normal relation to the acetabulum; it is the shaft which has moved so that the epiphysis is now displaced backwards and downwards in relationship to it.

Both views of both hips are taken for initial and check X-ray examination as a later slipping may occur in the sound hip.

Treatment
Treatment depends on the degree of slipping and the length of time between the displacement and commencement of treatment. For the acute slip reduction is usually attempted either by traction or by gentle manipulation. Skeletal traction with a Kirschner wire through the femoral condyles allows for a pull on the femur and a pull to correct external rotation. Skin traction may be used but it may not be adequate to bring about a reduction.

Manipulation carries with it the risk of damage to the epiphyseal vessels which supply the head of the femur, resulting in avascular necrosis of the femoral head.

When reduction has been achieved Moore's pins are inserted through the neck into the head to keep it in place; alternatively a single screw may be used.

In the treatment of a gradual, less severe slip it is usual to accept the position and insert Moore's pins to prevent further slipping.

When the slip is severe and the epiphysis has fused and the position is unacceptable because of the degree of coxa vara, a subtrochanteric osteotomy is performed to correct the alignmennt of the shaft with the neck of femur.

Complications
Avascular necrosis leading to osteoarthritis presents a major problem in a person of this age. A Smith-Petersen cup arthroplasty, a Thompson prosthesis, or in some cases a total hip replacement may be performed.

Nursing care
In the early stage of treating an adolescent with this condition the nursing care will be directed at maintaining the traction, together with his other needs. After operation to insert the Moore's pins he will be confined to bed for some weeks. Later when fusion is obtained he can be allowed up non-weight-bearing. This degree of inactivity is very boring for a person of this age group. Visits from his peers will be a welcome diversion, along with other measures to keep him occupied.

After treatment
When fusion in a good position is obtained, gradual exercises and weight-bearing start.

9 Tuberculosis of bones and joints

In the last 50 years there has been a concerted medical and social effort to eradicate tuberculosis. Because of this, the mortality rate has reached a much lower level, nevertheless it is still a serious medicosocial problem in spite of the improved social services and all the advances made in diagnosis and treatment.

Tuberculosis is an infection of the blood and lymphatic streams, caused by invasion by the *Mycobacterium tuberculosis*, or Koch's bacillus. Two types of bacillus affecting man are: (1) human type which is acquired by inhalation or droplet infection from someone suffering from tuberculosis; (2) bovine type, which is ingested in milk from infected cows.

Methods of spread
Tuberculous infection spreads from the bronchial glands or from the gastrointestinal tract into the lymph vessels and blood stream. The reaction of the body to both types of the bacillus is identical and tuberculous lesions are liable to occur in almost all the organs of the body. The degree of natural resistance, susceptibility to the disease and ability to overcome the infection differ in individuals and races. These variations cannot be fully explained. People who live in a civilized community have usually become infected with tuberculosis some time or other in their lives. Infection does not necessarily mean progressive infection, because it may remain

sub-clinical and not be recognized. There is evidence that the natural resistance is raised from one generation to another and that races suddenly brought into contact with tuberculosis succumb quickly. The role of climatic and racial factors is small in comparison with those played by economic and social conditions. The incidence is high among people living in overcrowded conditions and having a low standard of nutrition, especially when first-class proteins are deficient. Children are more prone to bone and joint tuberculosis than are adults.

The bacilli reach bones and joints via the blood stream from a primary focus. This may be an infection in a lymphatic gland that does not itself cause symptoms or it may be severe enough to be detected. There is often a history of slight injury. When the tissues are devitalized and there is stagnation of the circulation, an ideal medium is produced for the growth and multiplication of the bacilli.

Localization usually begins at the ends of long bones. A focus near a joint is seldom restricted to the bone; almost invariably it spreads to the joint, causing a specific arthritis. Rarely, a lesion occurs in the shaft of a long bone, flat or irregular bones, causing a tuberculosis osteitis and not a typical tuberculous arthritis. At the site of infection the changes caused by inflammation take place. There is increased vascularity and exudation of lumph. Lymphocytes surround the bacilli with a formation of characteristic giant cells. Normal tissue is destroyed with the formation of the typical tuberculous nodule or granuloma (tumour of granulation tissue). One characteristic of the tubercle is that it is avascular, having no blood supply. In this it differs from an acute inflammatory focus, which is hot, tender and causes throbbing pain due to a local increase of blood.

The tuberculous nodule becomes necrotic at the centre from lack of a blood supply and the protective cells are destroyed by toxins liberated by the bacilli. The production of tuberculous material is known as caseation. Tuberculous granulation tissue covers the synovial membrane, which becomes thickened, and the cartilage erodes. The destruction of articular cartilage gives the radiographic appearance of a narrowing joint space. The bones become delcalcified and appear on an X-ray plate less dense than normal bone. In the advanced stage there is destruction of bone and formation of sequestra.

When the caseous material perforates the surface of a bone or joint capsule, it forms an abscess. The tuberculous abscess forms slowly and is known as a 'cold' abscess because there is no heat or pain. It may remain localized near the site of the disease, e.g. para-vertebral abscess, or it may track a considerable distance, diverted by muscles, muscle sheaths, blood vessels or nerves, and appear as a subcutaneous fluctuant swelling, e.g. a psoas abscess that results from a lesion of the lumbar spine. The wall of the abscess is composed of fibrous tissue and the contents are broken down tissues and tubercle bacilli. The abscess may perforate the skin spontaneously and form a channel between the deeper tissues and the skin; this is called a sinus. Pus is discharged in varying quantities.

If the resistance of the individual is good and the conditions favourable, tubercle formation ceases. The bone recalcifies and the tuberculous granular tissue is converted into fibrous tissue. The fibrous tissue walls off the disease but it is possible for tubercle bacilli to remain dormant in a healed lesion and cause trouble in later life. There is a fibrous ankylosis or union of the joint; bony ankylosis, which is sound, seldom occurs unless there has been secondary infection. A joint with fibrous ankylosis is unsound and unable to take any great strain. The operation of arthrodesis is performed which fixes the joint in the optimum position. The articular surfaces are excised and the bones unite. The joint is immobilized until there is sound union.

If resistance is poor, tubercle formation is followed by caseation, abscess formation and possibly sinus formation, unless treatment is carried out to check the disease.

In establishing diagnosis the Mantoux skin test is commonly used.

Mantoux skin test

Tuberculin is an emulsion containing dead tubercle bacilli. When injected into the skin of a person who has not been infected by tubercle bacilli no reaction takes place at the site of inoculation. If the body has been infected at some time there is localized redness and swelling. If the reaction is negative the intradermal injection is repeated using tuberculin of a higher concentration. A positive reaction does not establish the presence of active tuberculosis at the time but is of diagnostic value.

BCG vaccination

The vaccine is prepared from a cultivated strain of the Bacillus Calmette Guérin. It was introduced into Great Britain in 1949 and given to negative Mantoux reactors of school-leaving age with the object of preparing these youngsters to meet the tuberculosis of early adult life.

Diagnosis

The surgeon bases his diagnosis on general and local signs and symptoms confirmed by radiography and laboratory tests.

General signs and symptoms

There is a history of loss of appetite, decreased weight and the patient complains of being easily tired. There may be a rise of temperature 1° to 2° in the afternoon or evening. Sleep may be restless with night sweats.

Local signs and symptoms

Pain. If pain is present it is of an aching character which is worse after exercise and relieved by rest. It may be referred to a point away from the lesion which has the same nerve supply. A lesion of the hip joint may cause pain in the knee owing to the distribution of the obturator nerve. The muscles that control the joint go into spasm which is protective and limits movements in *all* directions.

A limp is often the first symptom noticed in lesions of lower limb and spine.

Muscle atrophy. There is definite wasting of the muscles controlling the joint due to disuse.

Deformity may be due to the pull of stronger muscle groups in spasm, or in the later stages may be due to bone destruction.

Swelling. On palpation there is swelling and tenderness. Joints that can be easily palpated, like the knee, have a 'doughy' feeling. There may be abscess formation with sinuses. X-ray examination may show general decalcification of bone, loss of joint space and irregularity due to destruction and loss of joint space. In early cases when the synovial membrane only is affected, there is little or no X-ray evidence especially in young children. These children are often referred to as an 'observation hip' or 'observation knee'. The nurse should remember that they are admitted to be observed. The child is put to bed and kept at rest until the signs and symptoms of an 'irritable' joint disappear or become definite. An accurate report of sleep and appetite must be given and instructions may be given to record the temperature at hourly intervals for several successive days.

Pathological investigations

In order to confirm diagnosis the following tests are carried out:

The Mantoux skin test

Aspiration of an abscess or any joint effusion is performed so that the fluid or pus can be examined microscopically for tubercle bacilli or the suspected material injected into a guinea-pig. Six weeks later the guinea-pig is killed and examined for the presence of tuberculous glands.

Biopsies. A small piece of lymph gland or synovial membrane may be removed for microscopic or guinea-pig examination.

Joint biopsy carried out on children and adults under antibiotic cover.

Treatment

The infection may appear to be localized in one joint only, but nevertheless it is a general infection and tubercle bacilli are present in other parts of the body. Recovery depends on the ability of the normal defence mechanism of the body to check and overcome the bacilli. While the affected joint is immobilized, the patient must be in surroundings that assist his own natural forces to overcome the infection. The treatment for all cases of joint or bone tuberculosis is rest. The patient is rested and the affected joint is rested in the best functional position until healing has occurred. The general and local treatment are interdependent and are best carried out in the regimen of an open-air orthopaedic hospital. Any condition that lowers the general health, such as decayed teeth or septic tonsils, should be detected and treated, and a radiograph of the chest taken. It is possible in lesions of the upper limb to give adequate splintage and allow the patient to exercise the rest of the body before the local lesion is healed. All means available must be used to keep the patient happy and occupied. There should be freedom from worry and emotional stress because these have an indirect but far-reaching effect on the physical condition.

Other important factors are:

1. *Fresh air*. The patient is nursed continuously in the open air or in a well-ventilated room.

2. *Diet*. The diet should be varied and contain the necessary vitamins and mineral ssalts, have a high protein content and include 2–3 litres of fluids per day. It should be served in such a way that the patient will eat and enjoy it. Casilan added to sweetened milk is valuable to raise the protein content of the diet in an easily digested and economical way.

3. *Exposure to sunlight and fresh air*, when available, is beneficial in stimulating metabolism and in giving a sense of well-being. Excessive exposure is dangerous as it causes dehydration and too much sun can 'flare up' a lesion. Exposure should be graduated as to period and the area of body exposed, so that an erythema is never produced, but the skin is gradually pigmented. The best time of day at first is early morning before the sun becomes too hot.

Chemotherapy

Treatment of tuberculosis has been revolutionized by the advent of antibiotics. The combined use of chemotherapy and the local measures described in the following pages have served to reduce the period of hospitalization.

Streptomycin may be given by intramuscular injection for a period of three months, average adult dose being 0.5 g twice daily. It can also be given by local injection into joint cavities.

Para-aminosalicylic acid (PAS) is given in conjunction with streptomycin and acts by preventing the bacilli from becoming resistant to streptomycin. Twelve to 20 g given daily either twice or six-hourly.

Isonicotinic acid hydrazide (isoniazid) (INH) is given by mouth and is thought to have a lethal effect on the tubercle bacilli. The average dose is 50 mg twice daily or four-hourly.

A combination of these drugs may be used in treatment. Streptomycin may be given with PAS or INH or both.

Rifampicin (Rifadin) is one of the new antituberculous drugs. The average daily adult dose is 600 mg given once daily before meals.

Ethambutol-isoniazid (Mynah) The dosage of this combined drug for an adult (72 kg) is INH 300 mg and ethambutol 1895 mg administered once daily.

Complications

Streptomycin can produce damage to the eighth cranial nerve resulting in headaches, giddiness and ringing in the ears, deafness and gastrointestinal upsets. These symptoms must be reported and will probably necessitate stopping the administration of the drug for a short time, or if the symptoms persist in producing an intolerance, then stopped altogether.

After-care

The treatment does not end when the patient is discharged from hospital. He should be examined thereafter at regular intervals. Any splints worn are overhauled and checked by X-ray examination. A watch is kept on general health and home circumstances because once a person has had clinical tuberculosis there is always the possibility of a fresh lesion. Suitable work should be followed. This may mean retraining in a similar occupation. For instance, a motor mechanic with tuberculosis of the spine can be trained to work with precision instruments.

When caring for any tuberculous lesion, it should be remembered that the principles of general treatment, and possibly the complications of recumbency, described in Chapter 3, apply to all patients with surgical tuberculosis.

It is quite common for the bacilli which are in the blood stream to attack another part of the body. Variation in temperature, cough, gastrointestinal disturbances and complaints of pain in

ORTHOPAEDIC NURSING

another joint should be reported. Loss of weight or appetite and increasing lethargy are unfavourable signs. The disease may appear in the pulmonary form or in another joint, or as tuberculous meningitis or peritonitis, or it may affect the kidney.

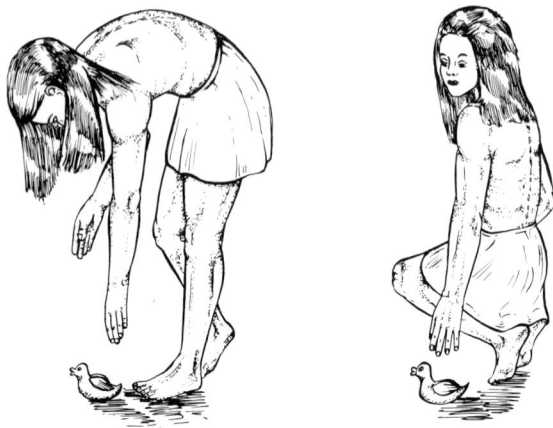

Fig. 106. *Pott's disease:* (a) *a normal child picking up a toy from the floor;* (b) *a child with Pott's disease keeping the spine rigid but flexing the knees.*

TUBERCULOSIS OF THE SPINE

The spine is the commonest site of bone tuberculosis (Pott's disease, Fig. 106) especially in children. The dorsolumbar region is most frequently affected, since this region is the most mobile part of the spine and takes the stress of weight-bearing. Infection usually starts in the anterior part of the vertebral bodies and rarely in the transverse spinous processes of laminae. The blood supply to the intervertebral discs is cut off and they break up. There is loss of joint space. The infection spreads to the body above and below. It may be present in other bodies not necessarily those that are adjacent. The vertebral bodies are eventually destroyed and collapse, causing the spinous processes to angulate sharply to form a bony knuckle under the skin known as kyphos or gibbus. It is sometimes the first sign noticed and is more marked if the lesion is in the dorsal region.

Signs and symptoms

The general signs and symptoms have been outlined. It is an

insidious disease and the early signs and symptoms are easily overlooked. The pain is not usually severe and the patient complains of a dull ache that is increased by sudden movement such as jumping, or the slight continuous jarring of riding in a bus. The pain is often referred up the back of the head in a cervical lesion, around the chest wall if the lesion is in the dorsal region, or down the legs if it is in the lumbar region. The back muscles go into spasm to keep the spine rigid and movement is limited in all directions. The patient acquires the gait and posture that will guard the painful areas. Walking is done gingerly and stooping avoided. An object is picked up from the floor by flexing the hips and knees to keep the spine rigid. If there is a cervical lesion the patient will support his head with his hands with the elbows on the table.

There may be a slight alteration in the normal spine curves or a very definite kyphos. The skin over the kyphos may be tender on palpation. Abscesses are not so obvious in lesions of the dorsal region, but in a lumbar lesion an abscess may appear as a large swelling in the groin.

Complications

An abscess commonly occurs with a tuberculosis of the spine (Fig. 107). Some abscesses may remain deep-seated and are revealed as a shadow on an X-ray plate. The cold abscess is often without symptoms and the patient may be quite unaware of it. The nurse should know where abscesses are liable to occur. It has happened that they have been detected during the toilet routine of a patient. The results of abscess formation may be:

1. If the general condition is good, the abscess may calcify, be absorbed and leave behind harmless fibrous tissue.
2. It may perforate the skin or lining membrane and enter an adjacent cavity, e.g. the retropharyngeal abscess of a cervical lesion.
3. It may press on another structure, e.g. an abscess in the upper or middle dorsal region passing backward and pressing on the spinal cord resulting in paraplegia.
4. A cold abscess may be found a considerable distance from the site of the disease as the pus has tracked away, diverted by nerves, blood vessels or a muscle sheath.

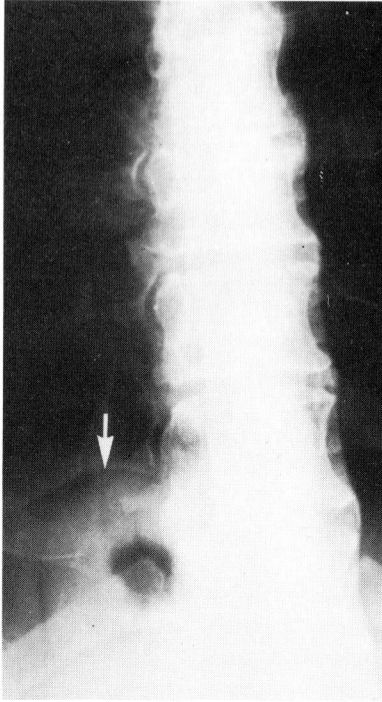

Fig. 107. *Tuberculosis of the spine showing abscess.*

Where cold abscesses occur. In the cervical region an abscess may form in front of the vertebral bodies behind the prevertebral fascia which it may perforate and enter the pharynx and mouth. This is called the retropharyngeal abscess. It may track between the lateral surfaces of the vertebrae and the posterior neck muscles and be seen at the posterior edge of sternomastoid muscle.

In the thoracic region an abscess may pass back and press on the spinal cord. It may remain localized in front of the vertebrae. It may perforate the anterior common ligament and enter the posterior mediastinum. It may track around the sides of the vertebrae and appear on the dorsum, or follow the course of the intercostal nerves and appear in the mid-axillary line.

In the lumbar region the commonest cold abscess is that which tracks down the sheath of the iliopsoas muscle and is seen below the inguinal ligament (Poupart's) on one or other side of the femoral vessels. Or the pus may: (1) track down the psoas to pass outward under the fascia of the iliacus and appear close to the anterior superior iliac spine; (2) follow the great vessels into the pelvis or inner side of the thigh; (3) extend laterally along the sheath of the quadratus lumborum and become superficial above the iliac crest; or (4) follow the posterior primary nerve division and appear under the skin of the lumbar region.

Treatment

If the general condition is good, the abscess may absorb and the surgeon may not consider it necessary to aspirate. Aspiration is performed to prevent the abscess from breaking and the formation of sinuses. A wide-bored needle is used at a point below the abscess on healthy skin and the point of puncture sealed. The abscess may refill by the next day and should in any case be observed, because the surgeon, if necessary, will repeat the aspiration. If the contents are too thick for aspiration, an incision is made and the pus evacuated.

Secondary infection is a danger and the strictest asepsis is observed. The pus may be copious so it is necessary to provide both a sterile test-tube for laboratory purposes and a receiver for the excess pus. After use, the syringe, needle and anything else that has been in contact with this highly infective pus must be conscientiously sterilized.

Since the contents of the abscess are largely composed of the broken down cells and tissue fluids of the patient, the value of a high protein diet and fluid needs no emphasis.

Sinuses. If a sinus forms, it provides a means by which other bacteria can enter. It may look small and unimportant but should be dressed and kept covered with the same aseptic technique given to a more spectacular dressing, as sepsis added to tuberculous infection greatly increases the trouble.

Sinuses will heal if the general condition is good and if secondary infection is avoided.

Paraplegia is a serious complication and occurs most frequently in lesions of the dorsal spine (see p. 222).

Local treatment of tuberculosis of spine
When the disease is active, all weight-bearing must be removed from the vertebrae and any movement of the spine prevented. The aims of treatment are: (1) to limit bone destruction; (2) to prevent deformity; and (3) if deformity is already present, to produce compensatory curves.

Children usually need a more rigid form of immobilization than do adults. Immobilization methods are described below.

Plaster bed. The nursing is comparatively easy providing the bed is well made. It is used especially for patients with a marked deformity because the plaster can be moulded over the kyphos. It is a good method when the patient is either very fat or frail. If well made, lateral movement of the spine is prevented and the legs are held in a good physiological position.

Frame. When a frame is used the Thomas's straight frame is the one of choice.

Cervical and high dorsal lesions. In the case of lesions at these levels, the head must be immobilized and kept hyperextended. A sunken head piece with a collar is used with a frame or a head piece incorporated in the plaster bed. Some form of head traction such as a halter may be ordered. Washing and feeding must be done with care, because moisture inside the collar or in the head piece, will be very uncomfortable. The possibility of a retropharyngeal abscess must be remembered and any difficulty in swallowing, or pain in the neck or throat, must be reported. Pressure sores may occur on the occiput, mandible or ears. Any signs of spasm or muscle weakness should be reported. Tilting mirrors are essential if the patient is to see anything of his surroundings and keep mentally alert. With correctly placed mirrors, these patients can watch films and television, the head end of the bed being placed nearer the screen.

Dorsal lesions. For these the frame may be hyperextended 5° to 10° at the level of the lesion. The frame is marked at the point of the kyphos for the guidance of the instrument maker, and the patient turned while the frame is altered. Hyperextension is held in the active stage in order to protect the diseased bone from pressure

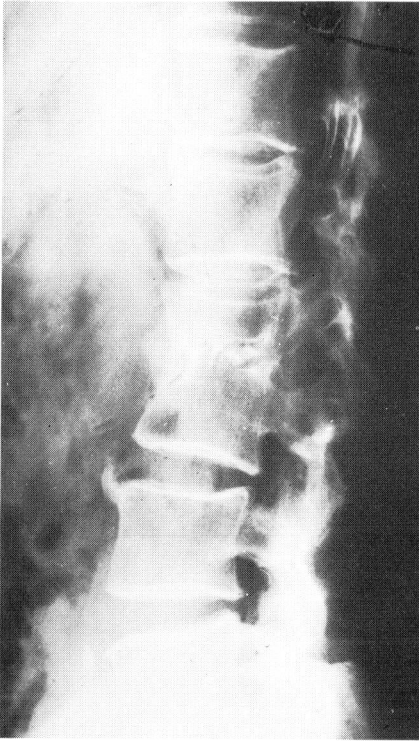

Fig. 108. *Tuberculosis lesion of the lumbar spine showing affection of the disc and vertebral bodies.*

and not with the intention of preventing the vertebrae from collapsing, which is nature's method of healing. Compensatory curves are produced by padding above and below the kyphos, while the kyphos itself is protected by graduated pieces of felt. When the patient is up and dressed, the compensatory curves are not very obvious. Some surgeons prefer an anterior plaster shell which is made like a plaster bed, the posterior turning case being the shallower half (Fig. 110). In this, the erector spinae muscles can be exercised and the knees mobilized and if the treatment is of long duration it gives the patient a change of view and position which is very welcome.

Lumbar lesions. The head piece can be dispensed with and pillows

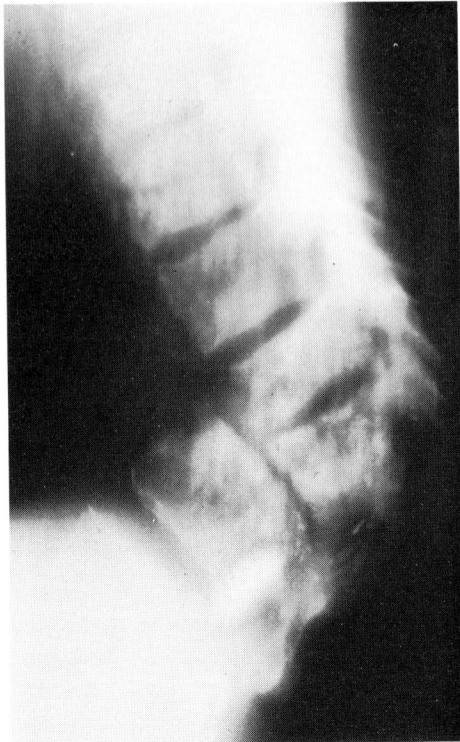

Fig. 109. *Tuberculosis of the spine showing collapse of the vertebrae and the formation of a kyphos.*

used. Immobilization is increased by means of groin straps or a pelvic band.

Later treatment

It is considered safe for the patient to assume the erect position when: (1) the radiographs which have been taken at regular intervals show that bone destruction has ceased and that recalcification has taken place; (2) the blood sedimentation rate is satisfactory and there is no pyrexia; and (3) the patient eats and sleeps well and looks happy. Some form of protective splinting is used to prevent spinal flexion. The patient is turned and measured and, while waiting, a pelvic band may be ordered and the legs mobilized and exercised. This has a very good effect on the

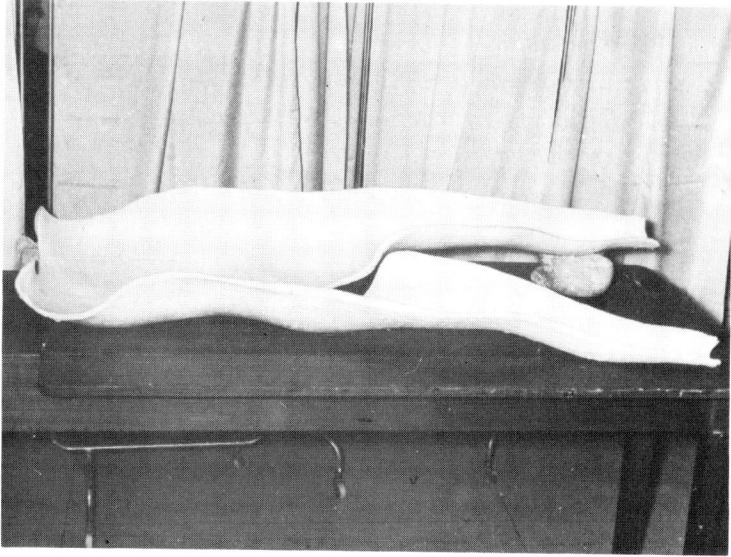

Fig. 110. *Anterior shell for turning the patient.*

patient's morale but care must be taken so that the patient does not move the spine.

Protective splints for different regions may be provided as described below.

For cervical lesions. The surgeon may use a back brace with a brow band; Minerva plaster jacket; Doll's collar of plaster of Paris; leather, celluloid or plastic material.

For high dorsal lesions. The surgeon may use either a plaster jacket which includes the neck or a spinal brace with a collar.

For lower dorsal lesions. The surgeon may use a spinal brace or a jacket made from plaster of Paris, leather, celluloid or plastic material.

For lumbar lesions. The surgeon uses a spica, including one leg above the knee, made of leather or plaster of Paris. At first the

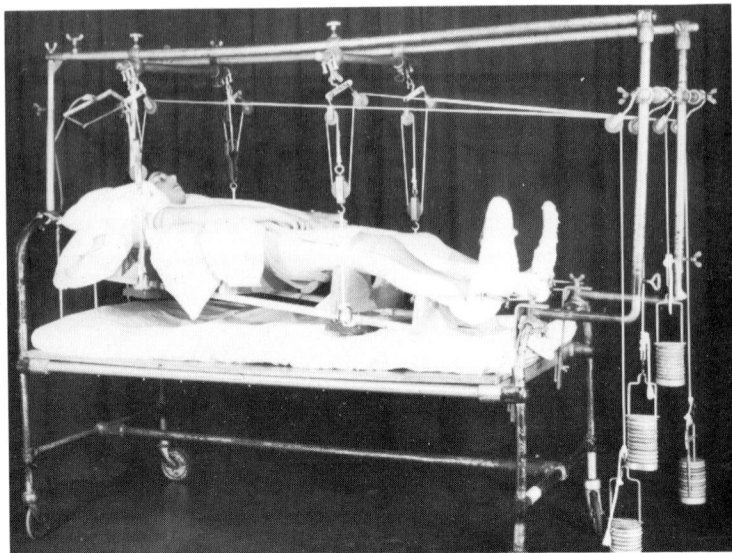

Fig. 111. *A triple pulley attached to a plaster bed allows the patient to change position while retaining full immobilization of the spine.*

patient wears the splint in bed and is then allowed to get up for gradually increasing periods each day. Supervision of walking at this stage is essential. When the patient has been up all day for a period he is discharged. Instructions are given regarding the care of the support, and this is possibly demonstrated to the patients. The support is not to be left off without the surgeon's permission. The patient reports at the after-care clinic after three months. The supports are usually discarded gradually when consolidation has occurred.

Operative treatment
The vertebrae affected are fused together — sometimes the vertebrae above and below are included. This part of the vertebral column is then without movement. The Albee type of operation consists of fusing the spine with a bone graft taken from the tibia, ribs, iliac crest or a piece from the bone bank. An anterior fusion may be done for a lumbar spine lesion or it may be anterior and posterior. In the Hibb's type the spinous processes are fused together. The operation is performed when the disease is quies-

cent either before the patient gets up or after the patient has been up in a brace living a fairly active life without any signs of reactivation. The operation does not shorten the period of recumbency, but does shorten the period during which a patient must wear a brace. The graft acts as an internal splint that protects the diseased area from trauma, maintains the compensatory curves and prevents any increase of deformity.

General preparation. The nature of the operation is explained to the patient or parents. Usually the patient wants the operation and feels hopeful. The general health, blood sedimentation rate, blood pressure and state of the kidneys must be satisfactory. Prior to the operation the patient is turned for the general treatment of the skin of the back as frequently as it is necessary. The knees are mobilized so that one knee can be flexed to 90° if the graft is being taken from the tibia. The frame or plaster bed is overhauled. The turning case in which the operation is often performed must be in good condition. If the patient is ambulatory a plaster bed is made and the patient allowed to lie in it for at least a week. A sample of blood is taken to ascertain the patient's blood group for blood transfusion. The patient is turned and the whole of the skin of the back is prepared for operation, the chest and axillae being shaved if the patient is adult. The area from which the graft is taken is also prepared. On the day before operation the patient is given a light diet with glucose drinks and a cleansing enema. A sedative is ordered the night before.

Post-operative care. Shock may be severe and a transfusion may be ordered. The patient must be kept warm and quiet, the pulse recorded half-hourly at first and any vomiting or restlessness reported. A sedative will be ordered. The area from which the graft has been taken must be watched for any undue haemorrhage and any loss of toe movement must be reported if the graft has been tibial. After three weeks the patient is turned and the back stitches removed. If a tibial graft has been taken a firm bandage will be applied over the dressing to prevent oozing. A back slab supporting the foot at a right angle with a few encircling turns may be added. The stitches are removed after 10 days and the wound redressed if necessary. Plaster of Paris may be applied to protect the weakened bone. Healthy bone bleeds profusely and because layers of blood-soaked gauze are uncomfortable, the dressing may be changed before taking the stitches out. When the graft is consolidated a brace is fitted and the patient allowed up.

POTT'S PARAPLEGIA

Pott's paraplegia is a spastic paralysis of the lower limbs caused by pressure on the spinal cord. It occurs in disease of the cervical and dorsal spine. It is practically unknown in the lower lumbar region as the spinal cord terminates at the level of the second lumbar vertebra. Pressure on the cord is caused by an abscess, thickening of the cord coverings, interference with the blood supply, tuberculous granulation tissue or sequestra. It is broadly classified into three types.

1. The onset may be early with the symptoms increasing as the disease becomes more active and decreasing when the disease becomes quiescent.

2. The onset may be early and the paraplegia does not improve when the bony lesion heals.

3. It may be of late onset when the disease has apparently been healed for years and is reactivated. It may be the first sign in an adult. The onset is insidious and may occur during fixation, so that a careful watch must be kept for early signs and symptoms. Efficient early treatment affects the prognosis. When there is pressure on the spinal cord the pathway that transmits nerve impulses is broken. The cortex of the brain cannot control voluntary muscle movement below the level of the lesion and reflexes are uncontrolled. At first the patient complains that his legs feel weak and that he seems to be walking on cotton wool. The gait is unsteady. Voluntary movement at first is weak and later completely lost and spasm increases. Examination shows an increase of the knee jerks, the presence of ankle clonus and a positive Babinski sign. Both legs are affected but the paralysis may be more marked in one leg. As the condition progresses skin sensation is lost. Voluntary control of bladder and rectum are lost and the organs are emptied by reflex action.

Treatment
The general treatment of tuberculosis of the spine is conservative, and consists of immobilization in extension and measures to

alleviate the distressing symptoms of spastic paralysis. Any sensory stimulus increases spasm and the patient should be kept as still as possible. All nursing care should be done quietly and care must be taken never to jar or bump the bed. The feet are immobilized to prevent deformity and, because immobilization controls spasm, club foot shoes or plaster shells, are used. The involuntary movements of the feet bring about friction between the foot and the splint, thus causing a pressure sore. The pressure sore aggravates the spasm and a vicious circle starts. This is avoided if the plaster shells are well moulded and the plasters or club foot shoes applied with a very thick layer of splint wool and firmly bandaged. Once fixed, they should not be disturbed for washing, nail cutting and heel rubbing. An increase of spasm is an indication of pressure and a readjustment of splints must be made. Should the tragedy of a pressure sore occur it should not be treated four-hourly but covered with tulle gras, and left for a few days. Extremes of temperature also aggravate spasm, the most difficult to combat being cold. The feet must be warm before the splints are applied because even under layers of wool they will not become warm if they are already cold. There is the great danger of bottle burns when there is loss of sensation and this must *never* be forgotten because there may be anaesthesia beyond the costal margins; it is better that bottles are not used. An incontinent patient on a frame or plaster bed is kept clean and dry by leaving the bedpan or urinal in situ. The action of the sphincters can become automatic and regular. A watch must be kept for retention of urine, and retention with overflow. Fluid intake and output is checked.

A paralysed bladder distended with urine is liable to infection and stone formation. With a rigid aseptic technique a urethral catheter of the self-retaining Foley type may be inserted. The urine is tested, prophylactic drugs are ordered and the patient is told to drink at least 4.5 litres a day.

When there is no hope of the paraplegia recovering, the patient is fitted up with an apparatus to enable him to get up — usually a spinal brace and calipers. The calipers are adapted to control the spasm and with crutches, or elbow crutches, the patient gets about with a tripod walk.

Operative treatment

Operations are performed to relieve pressure on the cord by removing pus, tuberculous granulomatous material and sequestra. They are performed under cover of an antibiotic and may consist of costotransversectomy, when the cord is approached through the joints between the ribs and the transverse processes; laminectomy, when the laminae and spinous processes are removed; and lateral decompression when the cord is exposed from the side. The pre- and post-operative nursing care is the same as that described for a spinal graft.

A more radical approach known as the Hong Kong method involves early surgery to eradicate the tuberculous foci; if necessary a bone graft is inserted where the bone has been removed in order to maintain the stability of the spine. Antibiotics are given.

TUBERCULOSIS OF THE HIP JOINT

Tuberculosis of the hip joint used to be largely a disease of childhood and is now getting rarer. From a primary focus elsewhere in the body the synovial membrane of the hip joint is first involved. The infection then spreads and the joint structures are destroyed and replaced by tuberculous granulation tissue. When a child is treated at an early stage of the disease and only the synovial membrane is involved the aim is to induce healing and obtain a joint with full, free movement. When there is destruction of the bone, which is usual in an adult who is rarely seen in the early stages, healing is by fibrous tissue replacing tuberculous tissue. The joint is immobilized in the optimum position and a fibrous ankylosis occurs. This is not regarded as being secure and a sound bony ankylosis is obtained by the operation of arthrodesis.

Signs and symptoms

There are the general signs and symptoms of a tuberculous joint. The onset is insidious. The first symptom may be a limp which is present when the child is tired and disappears after rest. Pain may be present and is often referred to the front of the thigh and inner side of the knee because of the sensory distribution of the obturator nerve. There is restriction of movement in all directions at the early stage. Later, the spasm of the powerful hip muscles is so marked that the joint is quite stiff. Spasm draws the hip first into the position of flexion, abduction and external rotation, and later into flexion, adduction and internal rotation with apparent shortening, and there is lordosis due to the flexion contractions of the hip. The surgeon tests for this with the patient lying on his back. The sound leg is flexed on to the abdomen and the lordosis is then obliterated. In a true flexion deformity the affected leg cannot be kept flat on the couch in line with the body because muscle spasm raises it. This is known as Thomas's test. When there is bone destruction there is real as well as apparent shortening. There is muscle wasting of the whole limb especially of the glutei. On palpation there is tenderness and swelling. Abscesses may be present between the adductor muscles or between the tensor fascia femoris and sartorius. Muscle spasm is protective and is nature's method of keeping the joint still in order to prevent friction between the eroded bone surfaces. During sleep the muscle spasm relaxes and there is friction between the sensitive areas. The child wakes suddenly with a sharp cry and goes back to sleep as the muscles go back into spasm. This is the classic night cry. When the immobilization is adequate night cries do not occur and so are not heard in hospital — at least, we hope not. At first, although clinical signs are present, often there is no abnormality shown up on X-ray examination. Later, there is general rarefaction, diminished joint space and local destruction. When there has been no protection from muscle spasm the head of the femur may press on the softened acetabulum and travel upward or backward (wandering acetabulum) finally causing a pathological dislocation. When the X-ray examination is negative and there are clinical signs of an irritable joint, treatment at first is that given for a proven tuberculous hip.

Local treatment
Immobilization in the optimum position during the active stage with acute spasm of the powerful hip muscles is not obtained without traction. Traction relieves pain and muscle spasm and corrects deformity. The method of applying traction varies with individual hospital practice and the severity of the condition.

Weight-pulley traction is applied to one or both legs as described in balanced traction (see p. 29).

A plaster bed with extension irons and a bar for the groin strap is used when there is a spinal lesion associated with a deformity.

Plaster spica. A plaster spica extending from the nipple line to the foot of the affected side and above the knee of the unaffected side may be ordered. It has to be a double spica in order to prevent an adduction deformity and has the disadvantages of preventing exposure to light and air and of immobilizing unaffected joints. It is used in the acute stage when there is some complicating factor.

Frame fixation gives good immobilization, with the leg abducted at the angle the surgeon desires. Children, as a rule, are more widely abducted than adults and the abduction is wide if there is any possibility of pathological dislocation. In the acute stage the correction of deformity is deferred until spasm subsides. When a Jones's abduction frame is used, the groin strap may at first be on the affected side and later be removed to the opposite side.

Traction by any method must be maintained 24 hours of the day and never released unless by order of the surgeon. It can be maintained while the patient is being X-rayed. The frame is laid on the X-ray table and the bandages undone. One nurse stands at the head and grasps the patient around the shoulders with a hand on each axilla. A nurse holds each leg with a firm steady pull while another holds the pelvis. The groin strap and extension are then undone and the patient gently lifted from the frame and laid on the table. The nurses keep their position holding the pull each way until the radiographer has finished. When the patient is lifted back on to the frame the nurse at the shoulders does not let go until the groin strap is fixed and the nurses keep the pull on the legs until the extensions are tied.

Abscesses are treated (see p. 215).

Later treatment
Later treatment starts when the surgeon is satisfied both by X-ray examination and by clinical signs that the disease is quiescent. When it is hoped to get a freely movable joint mobilization is gradually commenced. This is done without weight-bearing, some-times retaining the extension for part of the day. No forced movements are allowed and full flexion of hips and knees is

obtained before weight-bearing and walking are allowed. Any sign that the disease is not quiescent such as pain, limp and spasm must be reported. Children soon regain mobility and are discharged without splints to resume normal life. The duration of treatment for most adults is longer. They are allowed up, wearing some form of protective splinting, prior to operation. This is good for the general health and morale, which are lowered by prolonged recumbency, and it also ensures that there is no reactivation of the disease before operation.

Plaster spica with weight-bearing will leave the unaffected leg free and extend below or above the knee of the affected side. Preliminary exercises are given. Full knee flexion must be obtained. The patient must be taught to walk distributing the weight on the legs in the normal way.

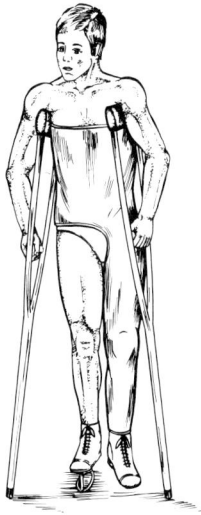

Fig. 112. *A plaster spica with a patten used with crutches.*

A plaster spica with crutches and a patten on the sound side may be used for walking. The patten must be high enough for the affected leg to clear the ground. For a child a height of 5 to 7.5 cm is enough. If it is too high it is difficult for the patient to balance. He is discharged when he is really safe on his crutches. Some surgeons prefer the spica to be made of blocked leather or a plastic material. If there is real shortening of over 1 cm due either to bone destruction or to cessation of epiphyseal growth at the lower end of the femur, this may be compensated by raising the shoe. Unless such compensation is provided the body mechanics are altered and secondary deformities follow. These patients must be reviewed within at least three months. A short spica of plaster or plastic material may be used as an alternative, with the side bars of a caliper incorporated and fitted to the shoe with round spur pieces. The bars are hinged at the knee joint. This controls rotation of the hip and protects the joint from sudden strains.

Operative treatment
Children who do not respond to conservative treatment with full antibiotic therapy are sometimes operated on at an early stage. A partial synovectomy and removal of necrotic bone is done under antibiotic cover in order to give a child a freely movable joint. This is not always possible and does not apply to adults. The operations performed are arthrodesis of the hip, using a bone graft taken from the tibia or ilium to ensure a sound bony ankylosis of the joint if the patient is not under 12 years of age; subtrochanteric osteotomy of the femur for the correction of deformities; and leg shortening or lengthening operations when there has been interference with normal growth.

Pre-operative and post-operative nursing for arthrodesis and osteotomy
The general and skin preparation is carried out as described for spinal graft. After the operation the patient is nursed in a hip spica which has been applied before or at the time of the operation. Some special post-operative nursing points are:

Observation of the toes. Any interference with the circulation, indicated by colour and swelliing or inability to move the toes when the patient is fully conscious, must be reported.

Haemorrhage. Some oozing of blood through the plaster is inevitable and while wet the area should have a sterile covering. If blood is able to ooze out, bacteria can gain an entry. A little blood spreading along a wet plaster can look serious and the nurse must be guided by the colour, pulse, restlessness and thirst of the patient as she watches for haemorrhage. A pencil mark is drawn as a guide around the first area of haemorrhage.

Vomiting may be very troublesome in patients in a double spica and must be reported. Pre-operative preparation helps to prevent it.

When there is sound union the surgeon allows the patient up in a short spica after a preliminary period of immobilization. Later, all splintage is discarded.

TUBERCULOSIS OF THE KNEE JOINT

When the general infection of tuberculosis is localized in the knee joint it first attacks the synovial membrane. Under early treatment it may remain a synovial infection. It may, however, spread to the lower end of the femur or the upper end of the tibia, destroying the articular cartilage and eroding the bone.

Signs and symptoms

These are the general signs and symptoms of a tuberculous joint. The knee joint has a more extensive synovial membrane than any other joint. When this is infected there is an increase of synovial fluid and this effusion causes the normal shape of the joint to be lost. A swollen joint is often the first complaint and a marked symptom. On palpation there is a peculiar 'doughy' feeling. The skin looks white but feels hotter than it does in the opposite knee. The swelling is accentuated by the very marked wasting of the thigh muscles, especially the quadriceps. Pain is not great and usually occurs as the result of some unguarded movement. Muscle spasm limits flexion and extension. Limp is due to the knee being held in the flexed position. In all infected knee joints the patient assumes the flexed position which relaxes the ligaments and enlarges the joint capacity for the excessive fluid. Later, the pull of the hamstrings is so great that flexion increases. Unless protected, outward rotation and subluxation of the tibia follow. There may be genu valgum and destruction of the epiphyseal plates that interfere with growth. The untreated knee is flexed to a right angle with subluxation and external rotation of the tibia. Both knees are X-rayed. The circumference of each thigh is measured the same distance from the patella to assess muscle wasting.

Local treatment
Conservative treatment for adult or child is the immobilization of the joint in the optimum physiological position with correction of deformities if present. This may be carried out by means of:

A plaster of Paris spica including the foot and pelvis. It is bivalved at intervals to inspect the joint.

A Thomas's bed knee splint which controls the joint and allows for exposure to light and air. The joint is easily inspected in order to discover any increase of swelling, heat, deformity and sinus formation. This splint is used with below-knee extensions which are checked daily. Subluxation is prevented by an adequate pad behind the head of the tibia. There is a tendency for the leg to fall into external rotation. This is checked by bandaging inwards or by using guarding splints of plaster or metal. The splints may also be used for restless children to make immobilization more secure. Adults are happier if they are able to sit up against a back rest which should be removed at night unless there is difficulty in breathing. When the acute stage has passed the patient can lie on his face with the foot over the end of the bed for part of each day in order to exercise the back muscles and glutei.

Later treatment
This falls into two parts as given below:
1. When there has been no destruction of bone the patient starts gradual mobilization in bed leading up to weight-bearing.
2. A weight-relieving caliper may be ordered which may be worn night and day or be replaced at night by a moulded splint of leather, plaster or plastic. The caliper may be worn with a guarding plaster. The caliper is discarded and weight-bearing allowed when the bone structure is normal.

Operative treatment
When there is a fibrous ankylosis and limited movement, the operation of arthrodesis is performed to give the patient a safe joint.

Pre-operative care. There is the general preparation already described. Skin preparation includes the whole leg and foot.

Post-operative care. Plaster is applied in the theatre. Nursing involves the care of a wet plaster and the observation of oozing of blood. Circulation and movement of the toes need careful watching. Weight-bearing is started within four to six weeks in order to force the bones into apposition. The patient may walk in a plaster or in a non-weight-bearing (short) caliper with a guarding plaster. When union is sound these may be discarded and any shortening is compensated by raising the footwear.

Amputation. A mid-thigh amputation is performed as a life-saving measure, usually on elderly patients who do not respond to conservative treatment.

TUBERCULOSIS OF THE ANKLE AND TARSUS

The initial focus, when tuberculosis attacks the ankle and tarsus, may be in the bone or the synovial membrane. It often starts in the astragalus and if untreated progresses slowly to all the bones and joints of the ankle and tarsus.

Local signs and symptoms

There is swelling and stiffness which are often the first complaint. Pain is not always present and occurs when there is some unexpected strain on the foot. When the ankle is affected there is swelling on each side of the Achilles tendon and in front of the joint. The foot is held by muscle spasm in equinus. When the tarsal bones are affected there is swelling over the joints and spasm of the muscles that control them. Abscesses are superficial and sinuses easily form.

Local treatment

The foot and ankle are immobilized. The foot is kept in a position that will be suitable for weight-bearing. Ankylosis in an unsuitable weight-bearing position causes a disability that is difficult to overcome. The optimum position is slight equinus with the forefoot in line with the ankle. A girl's foot is placed in slightly more equinus because she wears higher heels. Ankylosis may be obtained by:

Plaster of Paris. A below-knee or sometimes an above-knee plaster is used which gives good immobilization but the ankle cannot be inspected for abscesses or sinuses. A window may be cut in the plaster if there is a sinus and the plaster bivalved at regular intervals. The plaster should be inspected daily and any pain reported.

Later treatment
If the surgeon considers weight-bearing inadvisable, a Thomas's walking splint (patten-ended caliper) may be ordered. Weight-bearing with restricted movement may be allowed and the patient is then fitted with a double iron, having either a square socket or contrary stops. A walking plaster may be ordered and this is later replaced by a moulded leather splint.

Operative treatment
Excision and arthrodesis may be performed followed by plaster fixation. Amputation is performed later if there is no response to treatment.

TUBERCULOSIS OF THE SHOULDER

Tuberculous disease of the glenohumeral joint is comparatively rare. The disease starts in the head of the humerus and there is gradual destruction of the bone that is replaced by tuberculous granulation tissue with little or no pus formation. This 'dry' type, *caries sicca*, is commoner than the type that is accompanied by abscesses. An abscess may point to the front of the deltoid, or track down the sheath of the lattissimus dorsi and point in the region of the sacrum.

Signs and symptoms
There is a dull, aching pain referred to the front of the arm and wasting is apparent in the shoulder muscles, especially the deltoid which gives the shoulder a flat appearance. The patient has difficulty in abducting the shoulder. Limitation of joint movement in this case is somewhat masked because of the movements of the scapula and because the shoulder girdle moves as a whole. There is

swelling and tenderness on palpation.

Local treatment
The glenohumeral joint is immobilized in the best position for ankylosis. The arm is held in abduction of 70° for an adult and about 80° for young children, with 40° flexion and enough external rotation to allow the fingers to meet the mouth when the elbow is flexed. This is obtained by a plaster spica that includes the whole arm and extends to the iliac crest. The elbow is flexed to 90° and the forearm placed in the position midway between pronation and supination. The wrist and hand are usually left free. When the disease is quiescent an arm abduction splint may be ordered to be worn over the clothes. If there is good fibrous ankylosis in a functional position there may be no further treatment as the shoulder is not subjected to the same strain as a weight-bearing joint. There can be a good functional recovery aided by scapula movements.

Operative treatment
Operative treatment consists of an arthrodesis of the glenohumeral joint in 60° abduction, 30° flexion and neutral rotation.

Pre-operative care. The skin is prepared from the fingers to well above the shoulder and the back and front of the body as far as the iliac crests. Sometimes the body part of the plaster is applied previously and completed after the operation.

Post-operative care. There is the care of the wet plaster and observation of haemorrhage. The circulation of the fingers must be observed and any loss of finger movement when the patient is conscious must be reported. When union is sound the plaster is discarded and the physiotherapist teaches the patient to use the scapula muscles.

TUBERCULOSIS OF THE ELBOW

The elbow is the commonest upper limb site to be affected by tuberculosis and is seen more often in adults than in children. The disease usually starts in the elbow and the course is fairly slow.

Signs and symptoms

There is stiffness and swelling at the side of the olecranon process. The swelling is made more obvious because of the evident muscle wasting. Flexion and extension are limited and muscle spasm increases as the disease progresses so that the joint is held in flexion. Tenderness over the olecranon is often an early sign.

Treatment

Early conservative treatment for adults and children usually gives a good functional result, since a fibrous ankylosis is adequate in a non-weight-bearing joint. This, with the general treatment, consists of immobilizing the joint in plaster. An above-elbow plaster extending from the axilla to the metacarpals is used. The elbow is held in a position of flexion a little over 90°, the forearm in the midway position between pronation and supination and the wrist dorsi-flexed. The plaster is supported by a 'collar and cuff' sling. In some cases a plaster shoulder spica may be ordered.

Later treatment

A leather or plastic splint moulded from a plaster cast is used to protect the joint in the quiescent stage, or an elbow cage may be used.

Operative treatment

The operations are arthrodesis and/or excision followed by plaster fixation. The angle at which the elbow is fixed either for splinting or by an arthrodesis is decided by the surgeon who is guided by the occupation of the patient. If only one elbow is affected it is fixed at 60° to 70°; if both are affected the second is fixed at 120° with mid-pronation of forearm.

TUBERCULOSIS OF THE WRIST

Tuberculosis of the wrist is not common at any age, but occurs more frequently in adults than in children. There is swelling at the back of the wrist, pain, spasm and deformity. The wrist is held in flexion with the fingers extended at the metacarpophalangeal joint and flexed at the interphalangeal joints.

Treatment

The wrist is held in 30° dorsiflexion by plaster of Paris. The plaster should not extend beyond the proximal palmar crease because this allows finger movements. If the thumb is included it is held in opposition. If sinuses are present a window may be cut, or a metal splint or a bivalved plaster may be worn. When the disease is quiescent a moulded splint may be used or the operation of arthrodesis performed and the joint fixed in dorsiflexion.

The general treatment of patients with tuberculous lesions of shoulder, elbow and wrist is sometimes overlooked. When they are ambulatory, supervision is needed to see that they do not miss meals or overtire themselves.

TUBERCULOSIS OF THE SACRO-ILIAC JOINT

Tuberculous arthritis of the sacro-iliac joint occurs chiefly in young adults. Frequently there is another lesion present in the spine or lung. The prognosis is not favourable.

Signs and symptoms

The patient complains of pain over the sacro-iliac joint, the lumbar spine and in front of the leg, which may be referred along the course of the sciatic nerve. The pain is aggravated by sudden movement or prolonged stooping. Limp may be due to an abscess in front of or behind the joint. Abscess formation is common and is often the first sign noticed. It may be present over the sacro-iliac joint or may track forward under the iliopsoas muscle and point in the groin. In the later stage there is a well-marked lumbar scoliosis and when the patient walks the feet are shuffled along the ground. In the early stages diagnosis from X-rays is difficult as the outline of the normal sacro-iliac joint is hazy. The earliest sign is erosion of the joint surface and later destruction of the joint which may be limited to part of the joint or involve the whole of it.

Treatment

Since any movement of the spine or legs affects the sacro-iliac joint it is a difficult joint to immobilize. The patient is placed on either a double abduction frame with traction or on a plaster bed.

A careful watch must be kept for abscesses and the patient must be turned at regular intervals for inspection. The action of the bowels puts a strain on the joint and prevention of constipation in this case is particularly important.

Later treatment

When the disease is quiescent the patient gets up in a spica which includes the leg on the affected side to just above the knee or in a sacro-iliac belt. The operative treatment is excision of the diseased bone and arthrodesis.

Although in this country tuberculosis is much less common, it still presents a problem in countries where the social conditions and the level of nutrition is poor. When preparing the plan of care the nurse must remember that this is a chronic condition, and that the patient and his relatives will need support over a long period. The team will need to be involved and the family aware of the part they have to play in achieving the aim of treatment.

10 Tumours of the bone

Neoplasms or tumours are an unwanted increase of tissue. They are classified as being either benign or malignant.

In a benign or simple tumour there is an increase of cells. The tumour is localized and does not spread to other sites. Benign tumours are identified according to the tissue affected, e.g.

Osteoma (bone)

Chondroma (cartilage)

Fibroma (fibrous tissue)

Angioma (blood vessels)

Neurofibroma (nerves)

Lipoma (fat)

A malignant tumour of bone may contain more than one type of cell. It may start primarily in bone and then spread by the blood stream or lymphatic vessels to other parts of the body and secondary growths called metastases are formed. A skeletal metastasis or secondary growth may arise from a primary tumour elsewhere. Carcinoma of the breast in the female or prostate gland in the male may give rise to a secondary deposit in the spine, femur, pelvis or cranial bones. Sarcoma may arise as a primary growth in a bone.

Malignant tumours are treated by surgery, irradiation by X-ray or radium, cytotoxic drugs and hormone therapy. In a long bone a malignant tumour is sometimes first manifested by a pathological fracture.

BENIGN TUMOURS

CHONDROMA

Chondroma is an increase of cartilage cells which may ossify and form an exostosis. The typical exostosis occurs at the end of a long bone often near the knee. There is no need for treatment unless the growth interferes mechanically with the working of adjacent muscles, tendons or joint. It may be excised if a bursa forms under the overlying skin.

OSTEOMA

An osteoma is an increase of bone cells. If it causes symptoms it is excised.

OSTEOCLASTOMA — GIANT CELL TUMOUR

Tumours of this kind form at the end of long bones and involve the epiphyses. The commonest sites are the lower end of the femur, upper end of the tibia and lower end of the radius. Malignant change may take place in cases of large osteoclastomata. The tumour begins in that part of bone that was the metaphysis often extending very near to the joint surface. The bone substance is destroyed, new bone is laid down by the periosteum causing expansion of the bone ends. Pathological fracture is not uncommon.

Signs and symptoms
There is pain, swelling and tenderness on palpation. A pathological fracture may be the first indication that anything is wrong.

Treatment
1. Excision of that part of the affected bone if that is possible, e.g. the clavicle or fibula.
2. Curettage and packing with bone chips. This method has a high recurrence rate; in order to reduce this, some surgeons carry out a more radical excision of bone leaving only a sleeve of periosteum.

3. Excision of the affected part of the bone and replacement with a metal prosthesis to form the joint.
4. Radiotherapy may be used but this is said to increase the risk of malignancy.

MALIGNANT TUMOURS

SARCOMA

A sarcoma is a primary tumour arising in the bone. The growth spreads locally through the bone and can spread by the blood stream to form secondary deposits (metastasis) in the lungs, brain and other organs. In young people sarcoma occurs at the bone ends. Primary sarcomata of bone occur at the upper end of the tibia, the lower end of the femur, the upper end of the humerus and other bones. The tumour may be either osteoplastic in which case bone is formed, or osteolytic, when bone is destroyed. There may be a history of injury. The tumour begins in the metaphysis, destroying the surrounding bone. It bursts through the cortex into the soft tissue seldom crossing the epiphyseal cartilage. Some new bone is laid down in the form of radiating spicules giving a sunray appearance. New bone laid down under the corner of the periosteum is known as Codman's triangle — these typical features are evident on X-ray.

Signs and symptoms
Tenderness and swelling near the end of a bone, commonly the lower end of the femur or tibia, and associated with severe pain, and a sympathetic effusion into the joint.

Treatment
Amputation well above the site of the tumour; some surgeons advocate removal of the whole of the affected bone. This is usually accompanied by the administration of cytotoxic drugs in the belief that there is a strong possibility the tumour has already metastasized although there may be no evidence at the time.

An alternative is a high dose of radiotherapy to 'sterilize' the tumour cells and amputation some six to twelve months later if

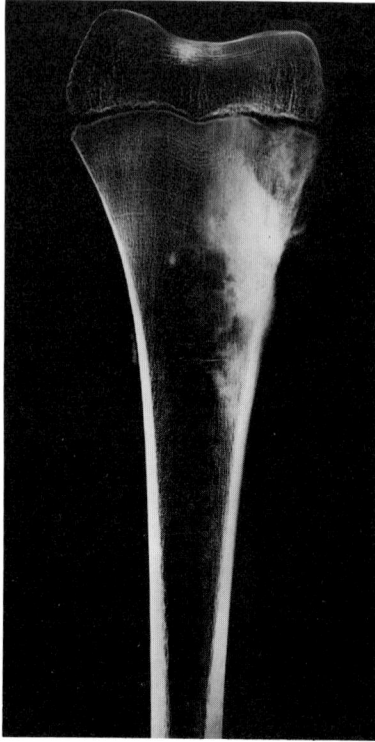

Fig. 113. *An X-ray of tibia showing an osteosarcoma.*

there is no evidence of metastasis. This method is now less
commonly used.

Nursing care
The nursing care of these adolescents or young adults requires
considerable skill. A sympathetic yet cheerful approach is needed
by members of staff knowing that something like 80 per cent have
a life expectancy of less than 5 years. The support will be needed
for the patient and relatives. The growth of the hospice movement
has done much to identify the problems experienced by the family,
and have shown how they can be coped with.

The administration of cytotoxic drugs requires the ability to
learn special techniques designed for the safety of all concerned.

11 Diseases of the nervous system

VOLUNTARY MOVEMENT

There is a continuous stream of conscious and unconscious sensory impulses to the spinal cord and brain. The cerebral cortex contains motor and sensory areas which are linked by connector neurones, so that a sensory impulse will initiate a motor movement. From the cells in the motor cortex arise fibres that pass down the spinal cord. These are called upper motor neurones to distinguish them from the motor neurones of the spinal reflex arc, which are known as lower motor neurones (see Fig. 114).

Upper and lower motor neurones

Fibres pass from the cerebral cortex through the corona radiata, the internal capsule, the midbrain and the pons. In the pyramids of the medulla they cross to the opposite side and run down the white matter in the lateral region of the spinal cord (crossed cerebrospinal or pyramidal tracts). They form synapses with the motor neurones in the anterior horn of grey matter of the spinal cord to form the final common path or lower motor neurone. The fibres of the lower motor neurones emerge from the spinal cord as the motor roots of the spinal (peripheral) nerves to supply the muscles.

Impulses that pass down the pyramidal tract cause voluntary

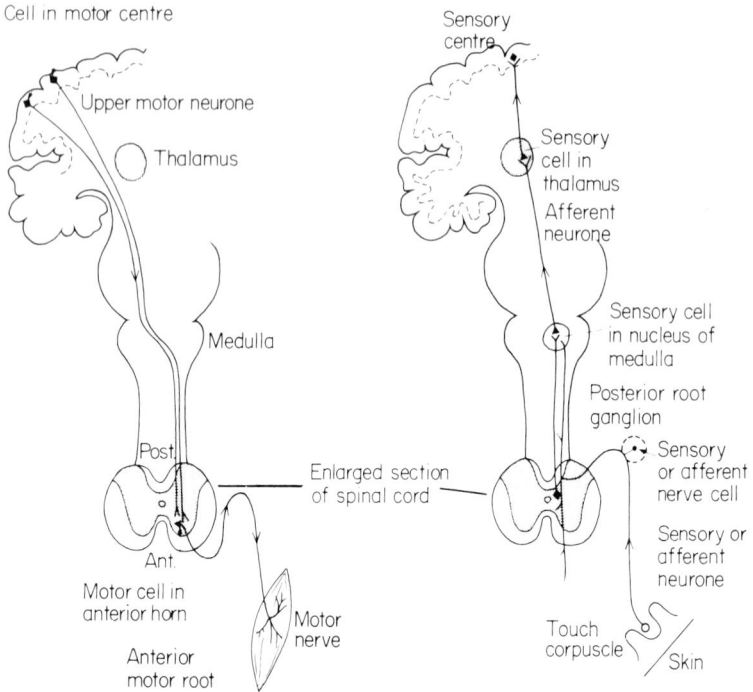

Fig. 114. *The motor nerve pathway* (left); *and the sensory nerve pathway* (right).

movement when the impulse is continued along the lower motor neurone to the muscles.

The upper motor neurone also damps down the activity of the spinal reflexes.

Spastic paralysis is caused by disease or injury of the upper motor neurone. The spinal reflexes are uninhibited and the following symptoms may be observed:

1. An increase of muscle tone.
2. Brisk reflexes.
3. Loss of motor power. This is not complete because some pathways and some fibres are undamaged.
4. Resistance to passive movements.
5. Coldness of the limb unaccompanied by any real trophic changes.

6. Absence of muscle wasting. The condition involves a disturbance of voluntary movement and not a paralysis of muscle groups.

Flaccid paralysis is due to disease and injury of the lower motor neurone and the symptoms seen are:
1. A complete loss of muscle power, voluntary contraction being impossible.
2. Absence of reflexes.
3. Gross trophic changes.
4. Rapid muscle wasting.
5. Absence of resistance to passive movements.

Loss of motor power may be complete or only partial because joints are moved by more than one muscle. The muscles that flex the wrist are supplied by the median nerve; if this is severed a very weak flexion of the wrist is made possible by the action of the flexor carpi ulnaris which is supplied by the posterior interosseous nerve (branch of the musculospiral nerve). The flaccid paralysis of poliomyelitis is often partial and patchy in distribution because only one key muscle or one group of muscles may be paralysed.

ERBS PALSY

Erbs palsy derives from a birth injury which may be caused by a pulling on the arms in a breech delivery; the nerves arising from the lower part of the brachial plexus are affected. The arm lies to the side and is internally rotated with the fingers flexed.

Treatment
The limb may be splinted in a Fairbanks splint or alternatively passive exercises to retain the range of movement in the limb give equally good results.

CEREBRAL PALSY

Cerebral palsy was first described by Dr Little in 1862 and was known for many years by his name. All forms of cerebral palsy are due either to non-development of the cells or to damage to the brain. Injury to the brain may occur during or immediately after birth. It may result from a prolonged or delayed labour followed by a rapid delivery, which predisposes to cerebral haemorrhage, cortical injury and anoxia of the brain cells. After birth the damage may be due to trauma or to measles or to any infection that causes meningitis. Recent figures estimate that there are seven cerebral palsies per 100 000 births. There is no single clear-cut clinical picture of cerebral palsy because the degree and anatomical site of the damage are variable.

The main types of cerebral palsy are:

1. *Spastic palsy* (20 per cent) which follows damage to the motor cortex of the brain. There is disparity of tone in muscles of opposing muscle groups. Often normal muscles are unable to function because the opposing group that would normally reduce their tone offers resistance by increased tone. A common example is when the adductors of the hip have such hypertonicity or spasm that the opposing group cannot abduct the hip. The spasticity varies from a slight awkwardness to complete rigidity which is why children with cerebral palsy are often called 'spastics'. The spastic type is classified according to the region affected: (a) paralysis of one limb — monoplegia; (b) paralysis of one arm and one leg on one side of the body — hemiplegia; (c) paralysis of both arms or both legs — diplegia; and (d) paralysis of both arms and both legs — quadriplegia.

In untreated cases characteristic deformities develop.

In the upper limb the shoulder is adducted and internally rotated, the elbow is flexed, the forearm pronated, the thumb opposed and the fingers flexed over the thumb.

In the lower limb the hips are flexed and adducted, the knee flexed, the foot plantar flexed strongly.

If both legs are involved the adductor spasm causes them to cross and the child walks with a 'scissor gait'. Flexion of the hip and spasm of the erector spinae causes lordosis.

2. *Athetoid palsy* (20 per cent). Athetosis is caused by damage to the basal ganglia and the midbrain and is characterized by distorting involuntary movements, which are worse when the child tries to control them. It is easy to mistake the muscle tension for spasticity.

3. *Ataxia* (10 per cent). There is incoordination of muscles and no appreciation of the position of the limbs.

4. *Rigid*, with tremors (5 per cent)). These are infrequent and

the lesion, which is believed to be in the midbrain, is obscure.

The remaining 45 per cent display signs of two or more of the types described. Children with cerebral palsy may have other handicaps. They may be wholly or partially deaf or blind, or may suffer from fits of a convulsive type. Speech may not be normal and the child may have no control over salivation. Loss of muscle sense makes it hard for the child to learn the ordinary skills of life such as dressing. He may be incontinent.

Mental and psychological difficulties

Intelligence tests have shown that half the children with cerebral palsy have an intelligence quotient within the normal range. Intellectual ability may be handicapped if the child has been restricted, for instance if he has been kept in a cot and not given the opportunity to see and feel everyday objects like other children.

The other half range from being slightly sub-normal and emotionally unstable to complete idiocy. Psychological difficulties may arise from damage to the brain or may be due to the behaviour of over-protective and fussy parents. There may be overt or masked rejection on the part of the parents. The child may seem to be normal at birth, but it is later noticed that he does not follow the normal pattern of development in grasping, head control, sitting, and attempting to walk and talk.

Treatment and management

Under specialist advice the treatment and management are essentially the work of a team consisting of a physiotherapist, nurse, speech therapist, teacher, social worker, occupational therapist, parents and family doctor. The child may be in a special residential school or have home treatment under supervision.

No treatment will replace nerve cells that have been destroyed, but the child can be trained to help himself. Some of them may be trained to be economically self-supporting; others may attain only a limited degree of self care.

Physiotherapy plays a major role. The physiotherapist aims at teaching the child voluntary control of movements by forming a new pattern of movement for the spine and limbs. Muscle relaxation and training of individual groups of muscles towards their correct function and strength are taught in short, frequent treatment sessions. Progress is unhurried and the child should not be fatigued. As control improves training in balance and posture starts.

Special equipment. For home and hospital use special chairs and tables are used as aids to acquiring the ability to stand and balance. The chair is similar to a high baby chair and is altered as the child progresses and grows. A special standing table has been designed so that the child can use his arms and legs without fear of falling.

Educational plastic toys, such as pegs and boards, are used for teaching coordination.

Splints. Calipers may be used for some children to help them in the control of their legs. They are of the cuff-topped type and may be fixed to a pelvic band in order to keep the legs abducted. Plaster or plastic night splints may be worn for the prevention of foot deformities. A light, short, cock-up splint for the wrist may be worn to help the child to acquire grasping power.

Nursing

A sense of security is needed by every child and is needed even more by a child with cerebral palsy, who performs every movement with difficulty and is handicapped by a lack of balance. As soon as the child is admitted to hospital every effort must be made to allay his fears and gain his confidence. Everything that is done for him should be done calmly. He should never be hustled or frightened. He should enter into ward life but must not be teased by other children or be allowed to get over-excited.

When such a child is bathed he should be lowered gently into water at 38°C and washed with even movements. There must be no running water or undue splashing while he is in the bath. These children are sensitive to cold and very easily develop splint sores and bed sores.

The child must learn to dress, feed and wash himself. The nurse and physiotherapist cooperate in helping him to achieve those skills. The physiotherapist will teach the movements that are needed by giving him practice in lacing boards and button frames. Washing is taught by first letting the child put his hands in water to play with floating toys. Then the movements of washing are shown and he is encouraged to imitate them. Feeding is best done with the aid of light-weight, large-handled cutlery and the child must be allowed to feed himself however long it takes or however much mess is made. Once he has learnt to feed himself the nurse must see that he does not bolt his food. Nothing is learnt quickly by a child with cerebral palsy. Patience, kindness and a smoothly running ward routine can help a lot.

Parents
The value of an ordered routine is explained to the parents who are told that these children need extra daytime rest. The physiotherapist selects exercises for the child to perform at home. Clothes that he can manipulate himself must be provided. It is very tempting to help a struggling child but the best help that parents can give is to encourage their child to do things for himself.

Surgery
Operations are performed only on selected cases and they include:

1. Tenotomy — a division of the tendon of an over-active muscle in an attempt to restore the balance between groups.
2. Elongation of tendon — the tendo calcaneus to allow the foot to be placed in the plantar grade position is the best example.
3. Neurectomy — to divide the nerve to an over-active spastic muscle. An example is the obturator nerve supplying the adductors of the hip.
4. Tendon transfer — carried out to change the pull of a muscle so that it is no longer a deforming force but a correcting one. The transfer of the insertion of the hamstrings into the back of the femoral condyles is an example.
5. Arthrodesis — after growth has ceased a joint may be arthrodized in a position of function to correct a persistent deformity; the ankle is an example.

POLIOMYELITIS

Poliomyelitis is an acute infectious disease of the central nervous system caused by a filterable virus which has an affinity for the motor cells in the anterior horn of the spinal cord (see Fig. 114). It is endemic in most countries, and in the past epidemics were not uncommon. However, since the advent of the Salk vaccine in 1954 the incidence has dramatically receded, nevertheless, sporadic cases do occur and therefore could continue to present an orthopaedic problem where residual paralysis persists.

The poliomyelitis virus gains entrance to the body either through the nasopharynx or alimentary tract; the exact route taken by the virus is uncertain but thought to be via the blood stream. There are two stages: (1) the invasive or *preparalytic stage* with signs of a generalized illness often accompanied by meningeal symptoms; and (2) the *acute paralytic stage* with selective involvement of the motor cells in the brain stem or cord.

The motor cells in the anterior horn of the cord bear the brunt of the attack. The cells may undergo neurosis (death) and be completely and permanently destroyed, or they may sustain only temporary damage which accounts for the early and dramatic recovery often encountered in the early weeks of the disease. The extent of the residual paralysis depends on the number of nerve cells which undergo complete destruction.

SIGNS, SYMPTOMS AND TREATMENT

The incubation period is variable but is commonly seven to ten days. Many patients give a history of general malaise, with slight headache and fever, lasting a day or so and preceding the acute onset of poliomyelitis by several days. Many cases will never proceed beyond this stage to recognizable polio and this probably explains the apparent irregular spread of the disease.

It is difficult to divide the clinical course and treatment of poliomyelitis into clear-cut stages, but for simplicity it is justifiable to describe the following stages provided it is remembered that there is a certain amount of overlap. The treatment employed at different stages is outlined but it must be emphasized that the clinical progress of the patient is the only deciding factor and each patient must be considered individually because of the great variability in the degree of paralysis, rate of recovery and response to treatment:

1. Preparalytic stage — patient's home or isolation hospital
2. Acute paralytic stage — isolation hospital
3. Convalescent stage — orthopaedic hospital
4. Residual stage — home.

PREPARALYTIC STAGE

The preparalytic stage varies in severity of symptoms. It is the acute and critical stage of the disease with the virus multiplying in the central nervous system. Muscle fatigue in this stage definitely invites a heavy attack on the anterior horn cells supplying those muscles.

The patient develops fever, headache, nausea pains in the back and limbs. The most constant sign is spinal rigidity on attempting neck or spinal flexion. This illness lasts a few days and may continue into the paralytic stage or the temperature may drop and the patient may feel better only to be followed by the paralytic stage a day or so later. Some cases are fortunate however in not progressing to the paralytic stage.

Treatment

Treatment consists of ensuring that strict bed rest and quiet are enforced — if symptoms are marked the patient should be admitted to an isolation hospital. If the diagnosis is in doubt, lumbar puncture should be performed.

ACUTE PARALYTIC STAGE

Development of lower motor neurone paralysis is the hall-mark of the disease. The muscles become flaccid and the deep reflexes are abolished. In most cases the paralysis is of rapid onset and at its maximum in a few days. The temperature is usually normal by the end of the first week. Spinal stiffness or meningism (stiff neck) is common during the first week, pain and muscle tenderness may be marked in some cases.

Passive movement of the limbs may be limited by an exaggerated muscle contraction which is usually called muscle spasm. This term is not really accurate as observation shows that these muscles are relaxed until an attempt is made to move the joint beyond a certain range, whereupon muscle contraction resists further movement and pain is produced if force is used. If the muscles are severely paralysed and incapable of contraction, full passive movement may still be limited by pain alone.

Early recognition and treatment of respiratory complications are of major importance at this stage. Bulbar poliomyelitis affects principally the muscles of deglutition leading to pooling of saliva, inability to swallow and flooding of the lungs. Respiratory distress due to the spinal polio is manifest by diaphragmatic or intercostal weakness shown by rapid shallow breathing and the like.

Treatment

Respiratory complications. Bulbar poliomyelitis in which there is slurring or nasal speech or inability to swallow fluids should immediately be treated in the head-down prone position, thereby ensuring that secretions will escape; in addition to this postural drainage, suction may be necessary. Diaphragmatic or intercostal weakness is treated in a respirator (see p. 254).

General nursing care. When preparing a plan of care for this child (although it is likely to be a child, adults are also affected) it must be appreciated that it is very distressing suddenly to find one cannot move a limb. Both child and parents will need support from the nursing staff. Although it is difficult to know what the final outcome will be the nurse must maintain a positive, cheerful outlook when giving the care that is necessary. The patient should be kept quiet and all essential nursing carried out with the minimum of disturbance to the patient before the acute first week. Sedation and analgesics may be ordered providing there are no respiratory complications. Paralysis of the bladder may necessitate catheterization.

Care of the limbs. Lower limbs should be supported by a small pillow behind the knees and the feet resting on a sandbag or footboard in the neutral position. The arms if affected should be maintained in comfortable abduction with slings or pillows, the wrist and hand in the position of function (Fig. 115). Passive movements should be carried out once or twice daily after the patient has settled down, usually about the end of the first week. The movement must be within the painless range; moist heat is useful in the acute stage for alleviating pain. The patient is visited by an orthopaedic surgeon who estimates and charts the affected muscles and supervises the treatment of the limbs.

By the end of the third week the patient usually is free from pain and stiffness and has a satisfactory range of painless passive movement.

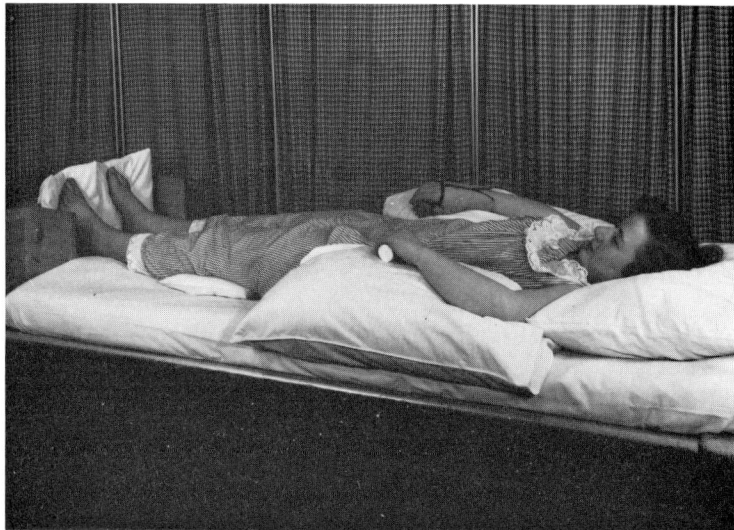

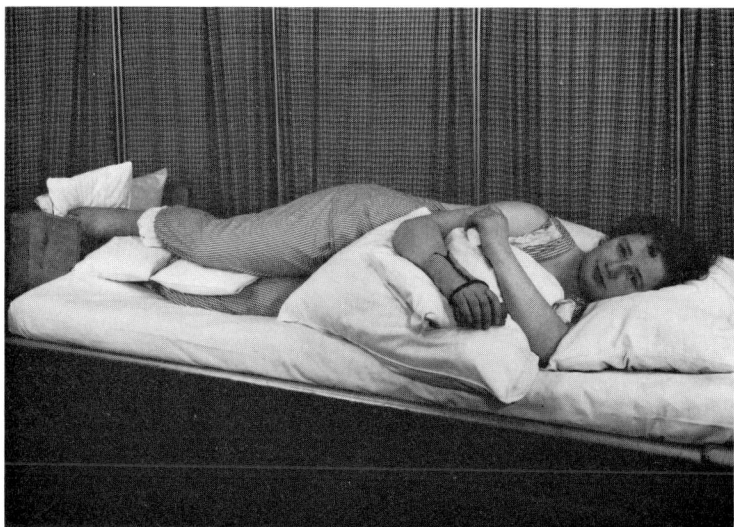

Fig. 115. *Correct postural positions.*

Principles of treatment: (1) prevention of stretching of paralysed muscle; (2) prevention of over-use of paralysed muscle in early stages which may cause a set-back; (3) preservation of mobility of joints; and (4) re-education of affected muscles.

CONVALESCENT STAGE

The convalescent stage can be divided into a natural recovery stage and a stage of muscle development and rehabilitation.

Natural recovery

Motor cells which have sustained only temporary damage may come to life even during the isolation stage, but most recovery usually takes place in the early months of the convalescent stage. In the orthopaedic hospital passive movements are continued and active movement commenced, at first assisted, and then against gravity, depending on the degree of paralysis. After six weeks from the onset the patient commences pool therapy, which is of great benefit because of the heat and the elimination of gravity by the water. Good coordination of movement is the aim and trick movements are not encouraged at this stage.

Muscle development and rehabilitation

When it is estimated that most of the natural recovery has taken place and the patient's general condition is satisfactory, efforts are directed to developing the muscle strength of partially paralysed muscles and healthy muscles by more strenuous forms of exercise. The patient progresses gradually from movements against gravity to progressive resistance exercises with the help of slings and increasing weights. Rehabilitation in walking or the use of the upper limbs in the occupational therapy department is assisted by splints and supportive apparatus as required. The aim by the end of this stage is to equip the patient for life in the outside world — the assistance of the medical social worker may be necessary to arrange training in a different occupation.

RESIDUAL STAGE

When the patient is discharged from hospital he is kept under supervision as an outpatient and may attend for further physiotherapy where necessary. Residual weakness and instability are controlled by apparatus which may be worn permanently or until function can be improved by surgical procedures.

Apparatus

Severely paralysed — motor chair

Unstable spine — spinal brace or corset

Unstable hip — caliper

Unstable foot — leg irons, Fritt toe-raising spring, if drop-foot

Upper limb — abduction splint for shoulder. Opponens splint for thumb.

Surgical procedures

Surgery is usually postponed till two years after the onset as late improvement does occasionally occur. Bone operations are not carried out in children until approximately the end of the growth period.

Stabilizing operations — fusion of the shoulder for paralysed deltoid with good scapular muscles. Sub-taloid mid-tarsal arthrodesis (triple fusion) is a very useful procedure and can be varied to improve drop-foot or TEV deformities, etc.

Tendon transplants. Very useful in the hand to improve finger function, or thumb opposition. In the foot tendon transplant may increase power in calf and so improve foot stability.

After-care

A long-term outlook is essential involving suitable education and employment as well as training in the care of splints and warnings against excessive heat and cold, over-fatigue and respiratory infection. Patience and work are called for from both patient and hospital team.

Respirators. When there is respiratory failure and the spinal cord only is involved, the mechanical respirator is of life-saving value. Bulbo-encephalitis and bulbo-spinal cases may have paralysis of swallowing combined with paralysis of breathing. The student is referred to one of the textbooks, dealing solely with acute poliomyelitis for detailed care of such patients.

PARALYTIC SPINAL POLIOMYELITIS WITH RESPIRATORY FAILURE

Any patient with paralysis of trunk and shoulder girdle muscles should be constantly watched for early signs of respiratory failure. The relief of a respirator should be provided before the patient has cyanosis, dyspnoea or difficulty in speech. The early signs are a rise in pulse rate, difficulty in breathing, anxiety, inability to sleep and use of accessory muscles for respiration. The nurse can observe these signs as well as keeping a correct record of pulse and respiration.

Breathing is affected when the phrenic nerve is involved, since the action of the diaphragm is impaired. The patient then breathes only with the intercostal muscles and uses accessory muscles of respiration, such as the sternomastoid, scaleni and platysma. If the diaphragm is normal and the intercostal muscles are paralysed, the outlook is better because diaphragmatic breathing can be adequate for a patient in bed. Usually both diaphragm and intercostals are in some degree paralysed as well as there being some limb paralysis. Respiratory power is measured by a spirometer. After breathing in the patient blows into a tube attached to the instrument and the expired air is recorded on a dial. This is called the vital capacity. When the vital capacity is lowered assistance in respiration is required.

Nursing care

The positive-pressure type respirator, e.g. the Radcliffe respirator. An electric motor drives in air, or a mixture of oxygen and air, through a cuffed intratracheal tube, at rhythmic intervals 12 to 20 times per minute according to the needs of the patient. In bulbo-spinal cases, when the patient can neither swallow nor breathe, the intratracheal tube is passed through the tracheotomy tube. This allows the respiratory tract to be blocked with a cuffed tube so that saliva and other secretions cannot trickle into the air passages and be sucked into the lung where they would cause aspiration pneumonia. These cases are severe but the patient may recover some ability to breathe and swallow again.

A daily blanket bath is necessary, and the position should be changed two hourly to relieve pressure. Nursing appliances such as sheep skins are used where appropriate to prevent pressure sores.

Feeding. Small sips of water or fruit juice must be given at first and a fluid intake chart kept to ensure that the amount provided is adequate. An angular glass tube makes this easier for the patient and allows him to sip without turning his head. Appetite is often poor and all efforts must be made to encourage feeding. A well-balanced diet must be given even if the quantity of food taken is small.

Constipation. Glycerin enemas or glycerin suppositories given on alternate days are usually satisfactory for preventing constipation. The treatment of constipation can be difficult with a patient with poor abdominal musculature.

CONCLUSION

Since the advent of vaccination the incidence of the disease has been spectacularly reduced. Nevertheless when it does occur the principles of treatment still apply and the care given by the nurse would still be of prime importance.

LOW BACK PAIN AND SCIATICA

Low back pain is the term used to describe acute and often crippling pain in the lumbar region, but pain in the back varies from a continuous or intermittent nagging ache to pain of great severity. Chronic back pain is very common and has many causes. It may be due to a disorder of the abdominal or pelvic organs and will then be treated by the general surgeon or gynaecologist.

Other causes may be:
1. Disease of the vertebrae, such as tuberculosis, tumours, ankylosing spondylitis, osteo-arthritis and Paget's disease.
2. Strain of muscles, ligaments and joints, such as sacro-iliac strain or lumbosacral strain.
3. Protrusion of an intervertebral disc.
4. Postural defects and muscle weakness.
5. Trauma.
6. Congenital or acquired deformities.
7. Spondylolisthesis.
8. Tumours of the spinal cord or nerve roots.

A psychological factor may complicate any of the above but to put a 'psychological' label on a patient could mask an undiagnosed pathological condition.

Sciatica is the term used to describe pain along the course of the sciatic nerve. It is not a disease but a symptom arising from pressure on ligaments or the trunk or roots of the sciatic nerve. A prolapsed intervertebral disc is the commonest cause of sciatica. More rarely there is another cause, such as a tumour affecting the spine itself or invading the sacral plexus, e.g. from the rectum or uterus.

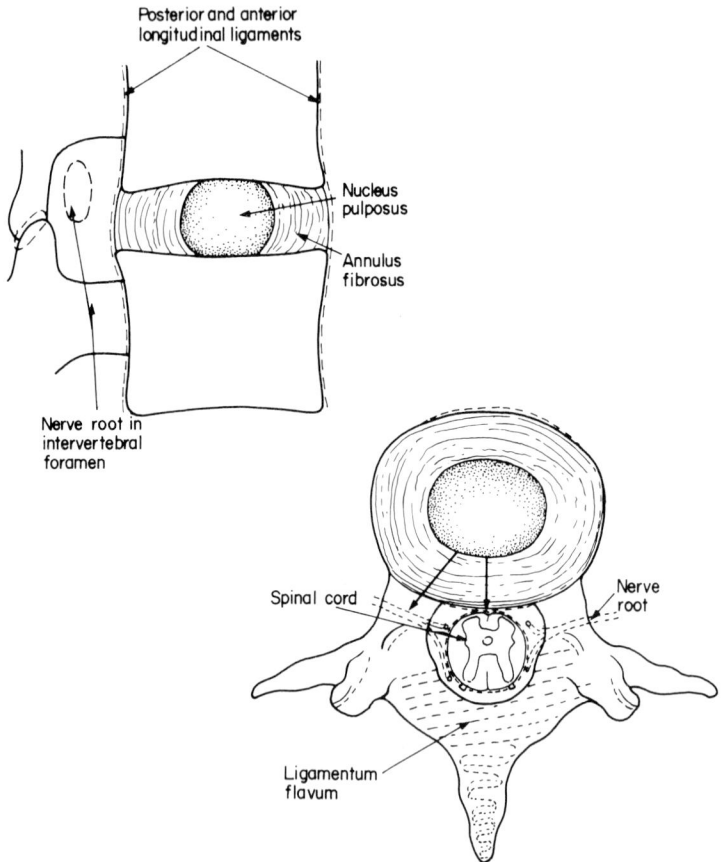

Fig. 116. *Invertebral disc as seen in longitudinal section of the spine* (top); *top view of intervertebral disc and its relations* (bottom). *The arrows indicate the usual sites of nuclear protrusion. Dotted lines and closely dotted areas represent sensitive structures which can cause lumbago or sciatica if pressed upon.*

Lesions of the intervertebral discs

Lesions of the intervertebral discs are now recognized as one of the most common causes of sudden, painful interference with the function of a joint. The discs separate the vertebral bodies and have a tough ring of fibrocartilage (annulus fibrosus) around a soft centre of nucleus pulposus (Fig. 116). This structure plays an important part in spinal movements but once it has begun to degenerate (early in adult life) slight but definite abnormalities of spinal movement can occur and may cause anything from mild 'rheumatics' or 'twinges' to acute torticollis or a crippling attack of lumbar pain. There is often a previous twist or strain but attacks may start quite unexpectedly. As the annnulus fibrosus degenerates it is liable to crack and the nucleus pulposus becomes forced (or prolapsed) through the crack to bulge into the spinal canal. It may cause sciatica, numbness, tingling or weakness in the legs, depending on whether it presses on a nerve root or some sensitive structure such as the dura mater or spinal ligaments. Cervical disc lesions also occur, but prolapse is more common in the lumbar region.

Signs and symptoms of a prolapsed intervertebral disc

The most important symptom is pain in the back or neck and it may or may not radiate down the leg or the arm. The onset may be sudden, with pain rapidly becoming severe, or there may be a dull ache gradually getting worse, with pain in the limb. Attacks of pain may occur with long periods freee of symptoms. Pain is aggravated by stooping, and weight lifting and often by sitting for long periods. Apart from pain the patient looks and feels well.

Clinical examination

The normal lumbar curve is absent in many cases. The patient stands with the spine inclined to one side. This list of the spine, although not a true curvature, is known as sciatic scoliosis. The mobility of the spine is impaired. Flexion is limited, but the lateral movements are free. There is muscle wasting, or flabbiness, especially of the gluteal, thigh and calf muscles. Sensation is altered and the ankle jerk (tendon reflex) diminished or absent. Raising the leg with the knee straight is a diagnostic test in sciatica. The patient can raise the limb to only about 45° or less because of the pain caused by stretching the nerve roots. Radiographs may show up no abnormality. Myelogram — the injection of an opaque fluid into the subarachnoid space followed by X-ray examination may show the prolapse.

Treatment

There are many cases of spontaneous recovery. Conservative measures are usually adopted in the majority of cases — rest in bed on a firm mattress for a period of three weeks, possibly with analgesics to relieve pain. If ambulant some form of support, corset or plaster jacket may be beneficial. If no relief is obtained from these measures the patient will be admitted to hospital for treatment by traction, usually continuous pelvic traction, or traction applied to both legs using adhesive strapping bandaged to the limb. The strapping is carried some 5 cm beyond the plantar surface of the foot and incorporates a spreader from which a cord passes over a pulley, and the amount of weight ordered by the surgeon, is attached. The foot of the bed is elevated.

Operative treatment

Preparation for operation. It is important that the patient fully understands what is to be done to him, and what is expected of him when he returns to the ward, such as how he will be moved and why. This will help to allay his fears.

Post-operative care. The patient will be received into a bed with fracture boards and a firm mattress, and sufficient pillows to achieve the required position. This may be on his side with two pillows down his back and one between the legs, and either one or two under the head, whichever is more comfortable. If the patient is lying on his back a small pillow is placed under the lumbar spine and pillows to flex the knees. The position should be changed 3-hourly by log rolling the patient, keeping the spine in one piece to avoid twisting.

The temperature, pulse and blood pressure should be observed and recorded, also whether the patient has passed urine or not, and whether he can move his limbs. After about 3–4 days the patient should be able to move himself, after which he will soon be allowed up. It is important when preparing the patient for discharge that he is given clear instructions regarding what he can do and what should be avoided. He must be aware of the need for a good posture and how to lift properly when he is allowed to do so.

12 Deformities

Before considering children's orthopaedic conditions, it is essential for the nurse to take into account the modern approach to children in hospital. There are still some people who are not sure what is needed for their care.

Orthopaediccs started as a speciality with the treatment and care of crippled children. Dame Agnes Hunt, the first and probably the greatest orthopaedic nurse, said of the hospital which she founded — 'Baschurch with its splendid voluntary service, its joyous carefree atmosphere, its absolute certainty that the good of the patient was the paramount aim of the hospital, taught the world what could be done for cripples despite lack of money, inadequate water supply and very poor drainage.' Later, when Robert Jones and G. R. Girdlestone were planning regional services for the whole country, the establishment of a properly recognized and funded education service was incorporated at that early stage.

That this splendid beginning was not recognized and appreciated by all who were caring for children in hospital, prompted the setting up of the Platt Committee who reported on the welfare of children in hospital in 1959. The report stressed that children should not be admitted to hospital if they could be treated elsewhere, and if skilled medical and nursing care was needed then it was essential that the atmosphere and facilities provided should meet the child's need for love, affection and security. Other organizations such as The National Association for the Welfare of Children in Hospital have worked tirelessly for this cause; their promptings have done much to improve conditions for children in hospital. The Court Report and many DHSS circulars have reinforced this policy that the service should be directed at satisfying the whole needs of the child and not just his need for treatment.

In recent years this philosophy has been further reinforced by research. Dr Pamela Hawthorn's book *I want my Mummy* highlighted many discrepancies in the care of children in hospital. Isabel E. P. Menzies Lyeth from the Tavistock Institute of Human Relationships in her research study carried out at the Royal National Orthopaedic Hospital showed how important it is to consider the environment from the child's angle, that it needs to be confined to a manageable size. Staff should be trained in child development. The skills required for adequate psycho-social care of such patients and their relatives are beyond those which one should reasonably expect of a student nurse. They should be there only in a learning situation.

The child needs a person to relate to, so we should consider not patient assignment or mother and child, but family assignment. The father, seldom mentioned in research projects or reports, is very important in the eyes of the child. He is the person who picks the child up, throws her in the air and catches her. If the plaster gets a little chipped in the process it can be repaired — children are not made of cotton wool and do not wish to be so treated.

If orthopaedic nurses are aware of this wealth of knowledge which is now available, and of the changes which are taking place, then the pioneering work of our predecessors should bear fruit. Children with orthopaedic conditions are often having treatment for quite a long time, but for most of that time they will be at home. It is, therefore, vital that proper communications are established with the family. Many children admitted to orthopaedic wards have on discharge been more advanced with their school work due to the individual attention the child gets from the teacher and, as Isabel Menzies Lyeth pointed out, the potential of the experience was 'to help some mothers become in some sense better mothers.'

The introduction of the 'Play Lady' has made a significant contribution to the happy yet controlled atmosphere of the children's ward. To surround the child with toys is not enough — they need help to enjoy them. Adolescents are best cared for in their own section of a children's ward; their needs are different from those of children and adults — their world is that of the pop star with more noise than that which is expected in a hospital ward. Given the opportunity, junior nurses will cope very well with them.

Parents want the very best treatment and nursing care for their child — they believe they can get this by sending them to one of the Regional Orthopaedic Centres, which have a reputation of being centres of excellence. It could mean that some parents have to travel some distance to visit their child. Flexibility of visiting times is essential, and financial help may be needed. Home Helps can assist the mother by relieving her of some of her domestic work, giving her more time to care for her child. They can also look after the other children when she is visiting hospital.

The two main categories of deformities are the congenital and the acquired.

CONGENITAL DEFORMITIES

Congenital deformities are due to a failure of development in the skeleton and soft tissue structures. Suggested causes are malposition or pressure on the embryo in the uterus, maternal malnutrition and certain toxic substances taken during pregnancy. They are found to occur in members of a certain family stock, which means that the genetic factor responsible for the deformity is transmitted from one generation to another, and in certain geographical areas. Three principles are followed in the treatment of congenital deformities:

1. To commence treatment as soon as possible.
2. To overcorrect the deformity, avoiding the use of force and to hold it in the position of overcorrection which gradually stretches the contracted soft tissues.
3. To continue treatment by other means such as physiotherapy, splints and surgery until the optimum position can be maintained by muscular action.
4. To surgically divide tight structures which are preventing correction.

ACQUIRED DEFORMITIES

Acquired deformities are due to changes which first take place in the soft structures. Muscles adapt themselves to the changed position of a joint or joints. They soon shorten, and in long-standing cases, there is shortening of ligaments, fasciae and joint capsule. Changes later occur in the bone structure of the joint. These contracture deformities start early in the course of disease and injury and are insidious. The emphasis is on prevention by careful splinting in the optimum position, daily active exercises of the unaffected joints and putting the joints through a full range of passive movements daily when the muscles are paralysed. The nurse must ensure that the correct posture and attitude in bed or chair are maintained. Much can be done to gain the cooperation of the patient by a simple explanation. The patient will gladly lie flat part of the time when the danger of stiff hips and knees caused by being in a bent position is explained. The seated position in armchairs or wheelchairs, overstrains both the glutei and quadriceps muscles, the important anti-gravity groups, and there is always a tendency to sit with the spine sagging. Posture is important while the patient is unconscious. Adequate support is necessary during sleep and the bed should be firm and not sag in the middle. When the patient is supine pillows must be carefully arranged to fill up the hollow between the neck and shoulders and maintain the head in its natural relation to the neck. A supporting pillow in the lumbar hollow may save much strain and discomfort.

Under modern anaesthesia, which frequently involves the use of muscle relaxants, joints and ligaments can be badly strained from lack of support on the operating table or on return to the ward. If the arm is abducted for intravenous therapy it must be supported at such an angle that the brachial plexus is not tightly stretched over the head of the humerus.

DEFORMITIES OF THE SPINAL COLUMN

KYPHOSIS

Kyphosis is an exaggeration of the normal dorsal curve (Fig. 117) and may result from:

    1. *Congenital conditions.* This type is due to an abnormality in

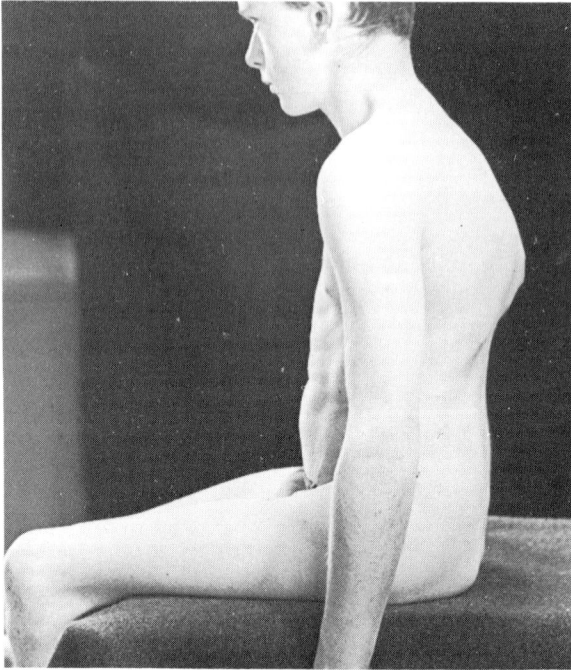

Fig. 117. *Kyphosis showing prominent dorsal curve.*

the formation of the vertebral bodies, two or three of which may be partially fused. There are no symptoms and no treatment is possible except exercises.

2. *Inflammatory disease of the spine*, e.g. tuberculosis or osteomyelitis.

3. *Anterior poliomyelitis*, when the abdominal and gluteal muscles are affected.

4. *Adolescent kyphosis* (Scheuermann's Disease) (see p. 201).

5. *Ankylosing spondylitis* (see p. 191).

6. *Kümmell's disease* which is the crumbling and collapse of one vertebra following injury and is seen in adults.

7. *Rickets* which is now rare (see p. 323).

8. *Senile kyphosis* which is caused by degenerative changes in the intervertebral discs and bodies of the vertebrae. It occurs in the elderly and is associated with osteo-arthritis. It is a fairly

common condition in women in the post menopausal period.

9. *Postural kyphosis.* There is the typical appearance of bad posture as the child stands with sagging shoulders and an increased lumbar curve. Often the condition is associated with flat feet and knock-knees. Predisposing causes such as defective sight and hearing are treated. The postural defect is corrected by exercises but the child must enjoy them and develop a desire to stand correctly.

General treatment of kyphosis
The treatment consists of treating the cause, building up the general health and giving remedial exercises. Plaster beds or straight frames may be used for correction and spinal braces to maintain posture.

LORDOSIS

Lordosis is an exaggeration of the normal curve in the lumbar region (Fig. 118).

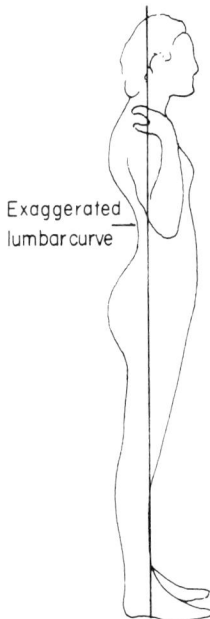

Exaggerated lumbar curve

Fig. 118. *Lordosis.*

Causes

Lordosis may be due to the following causes:

1. It may be compensatory to a kyphosis.
2. It may be due to bad posture.
3. It may be secondary to other deformities such as congenital dislocation of the hip, hip deformity, or spondylolisthesis.
4. It may result from muscle imbalance, e.g. contracture of the hip flexors and stretched hamstrings, causing the pelvis to tilt forward.
5. It may follow frequent pregnancies with little or no rest.

Treatment

The cause of the condition is treated by correcting the primary deformity. Other treatments are remedial exercises, plaster beds, corrective supports.

SPONDYLOLISTHESIS

Normally each vertebra articulates with the vertebra above and the vertebra below by the articular processes. If there is defective ossification of the pedicles and laminae the neural arch between the articular processes is incomplete, and the vertebra has no bony attachment to the vertebra below and is joined only by fibrous tissue. This is known as *spondylosis*. In spondylolisthesis (Fig. 119) the affected vertebra slides forward, together with the whole vertebral column above it, leaving the inferior articular process in situ. In 9 per cent of the cases the fifth lumbar vertebra is defective and slips forward on the sacrum. More rarely the fourth lumbar vertebra slips forward on the fifth. The degree of displacement may be slight or so great that there is a complete dislocation. The onset of the symptoms may be gradual. There may be a history of injury but it is believed that the accident excites the symptoms in a pre-existing painless displacement. The patients are usually seen in early adult life.

Signs and symptoms

The trunk is shortened and there is marked lordosis. The patient complains of backache. The pain may be referred over the distribution of the sciatic nerve.

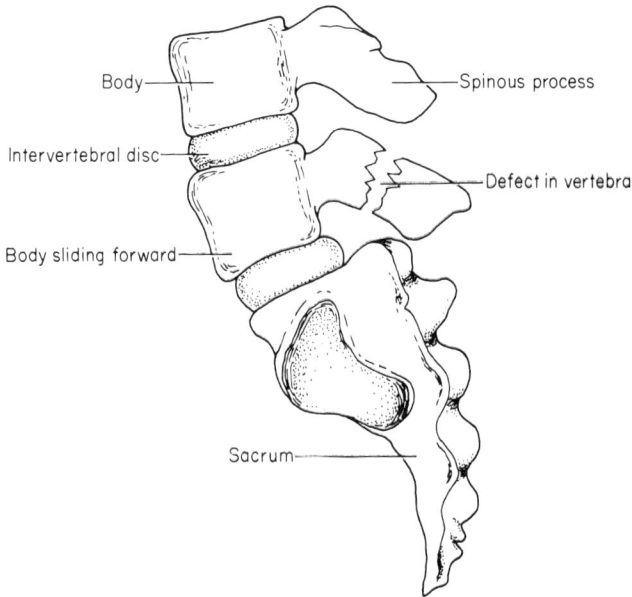

Fig. 119. *Sagittal section of the spine showing spondylolisthesis.*

Treatment

Treatment may be conservative. If the displacement is slight the symptoms may be relieved by rest and lumbo-sacral support. If severe, operative treatment will be necessary.

Operative treatment. Spinal fusion is performed to stabilize the spine. Post-operatively the patient may be nursed on a plaster bed as described for tuberculosis of the spine or alternatively may be free in bed and rolled gently from side to side. The latter method is more commonly used — this is made possible because of better grafting techniques; it avoids the risk of decalcification and other complications which occur with a more rigid form of immobilization.

SCOLIOSIS

Scoliosis is a lateral deviation of the spine to one side of the midline (Fig. 120). Deviation of the spine to one side is known as a

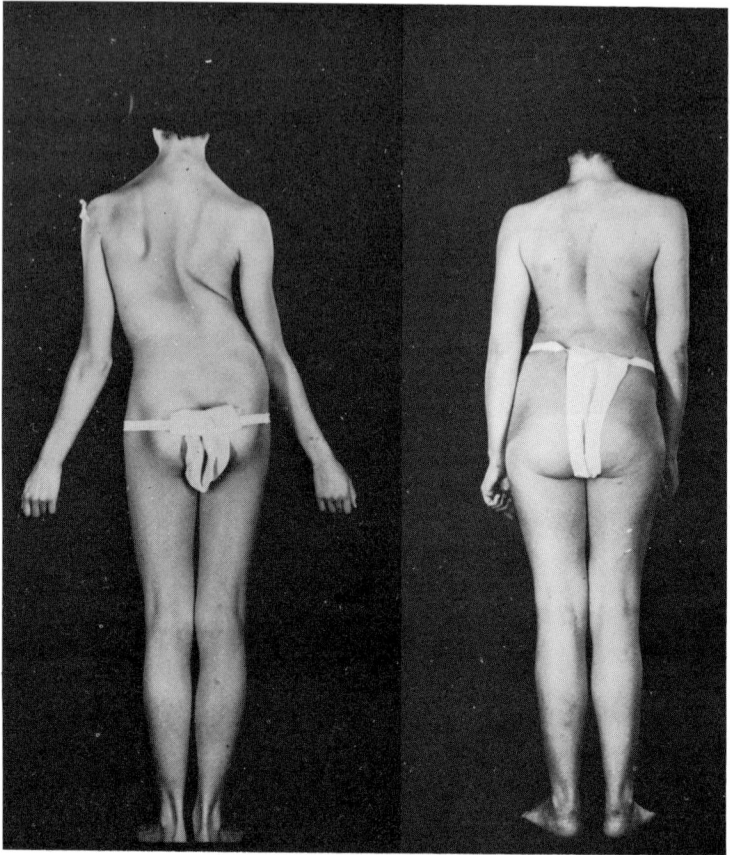

Fig. 120. *Scoliosis showing curve to the left.* (a) *Before;* (b) *after surgery.*

C curve. The deformity is described according to the region affected and the direction of the curve. When the convexity is to the right of the midline in the dorsal region it is known as a right dorsal scoliosis. The curvature is seldom single. When there is a primary dorsal curve, there will be a compensatory curve in the lumbar region possibly and in the cervical region. This is an S-shaped curve. In a structural scoliosis the lateral curvature of the spine is combined with rotation of the vertebrae and the vertebral bodies become compressed and altered in shape.

In a dorsal scoliosis the ribs rotate with the vertebrae and there is a projection of the chest wall on the side of the convexity. Sometimes the angles of the ribs are bent so sharply that the deformity is described as 'razor back'.

Classification
1. Non-structural   Postural
                                 Compensatory
2. Structural   Congenital
                                 Paralytic
                                 Idiopathic

Postural scoliosis
Postural scoliosis can be corrected by voluntary muscular effort. There are no bony changes and the curve disappears when the spine is flexed. A radiograph will distinguish it from an early structural scoliosis. The prognosis is good and it corrects itself when the general health and emotional adjustment are satisfactory.

General exercises for the whole body to improve balance and poise are given.

Compensatory scoliosis
Compensatory scoliosis is said to occur when the curve develops as compensation to a short leg or hip adduction or abduction. The deformity disappears on equalizing the leg lengths by blocks or operation (Figs 121 and 122).

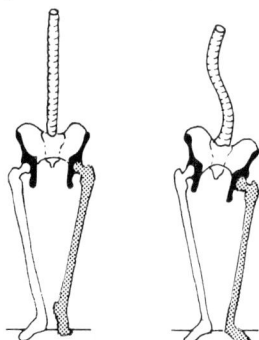

Fig. 121. *Scoliosis secondary to a short leg.*

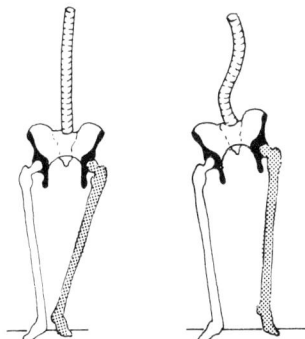

Fig. 122. *Scoliosis secondary to an adducted hip.*

As the name implies structural scoliosis is said to occur when structural changes in the vertebrae produce wedging and consequent rotation of both vertebrae and ribs.

Congenital scoliosis
Congenital scoliosis is very seldom noticed at birth but becomes evident due to late development in sitting and obvious when the child is held in the sitting position. The treatment given is to let the infant sleep at night on a Murk Jensen bed (Fig. 123) and later wear a Milwaukee brace until old enough for a stabilizing operation.

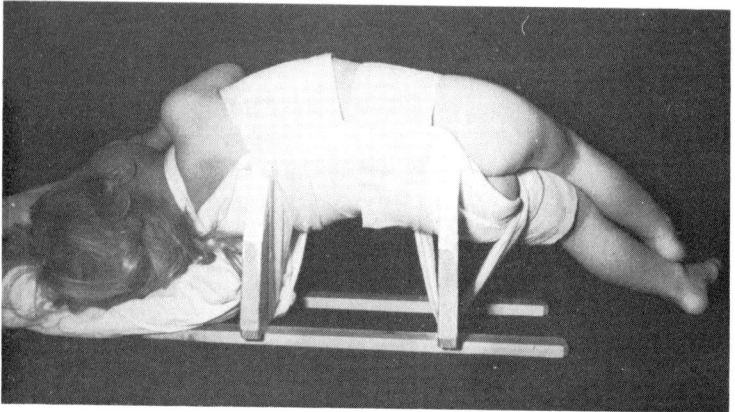

Fig. 123. *Murk Jensen plaster bed showing the patient lying on his side with convexity of the bed approximating with the concavity of the curve.*

Paralytic scoliosis
Paralytic scoliosis is due to muscle imbalance as a result of poliomyelitis. Treatment is to prevent increase of deformity by splinting, usually with a Milwaukee brace (Fig. 124) and possible grafting at a later stage.

Idiopathic scoliosis
Idiopathic scoliosis is the commonest type about which least is known. It is commoner in girls and commences in childhood or during the pre-adolescent period. There is a fixed curve which is not corrected by flexion of the spine. Radiographs show distortion of the vertebrae. If untreated it may progress to gross deformity.

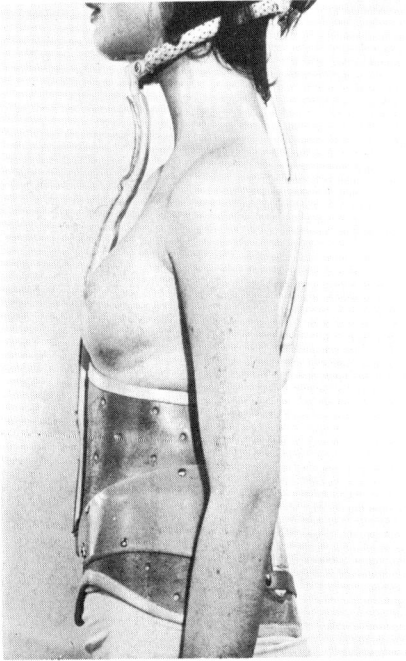

Fig. 124. *The Milwaukee brace modified by Moe showing distraction obtained between the pelvis and the head.*

Early treatment especially during growth is essentially to control the progress as far as possible and prevent respiratory complications.

Methods of treating scoliosis

Exercises aim at increasing mobility, improving muscle strength and teaching the patient the best compensatory posture and correct breathing. If the deformity is slight exercises will prevent it from increasing. When the spine is mobile and compensatory curves develop together with a good sense of posture, improvement can be gained even with a severe scoliosis. During the recovery stage there should be a definite period of rest. Exercises are also given during plaster treatment, when a support is worn, and after a spinal fusion.

Supports are of various kinds. A moulded block leather corset, spinal brace or skeleton splint may be worn with the object of: (1) preventing an increase of deformity while the child is too young for a spinal fusion; (2) following a corrective plaster and spinal fusion; or (3) as a permanent support, e.g. Milwaukee brace worn during the growth period (Fig. 124). The Coltrell and Boston braces fit more closely to the trunk, and are largely hidden by clothing. They are, therefore, cosmetically more acceptable to the patient, and some surgeons think they are as effective as the Milwaukee brace.

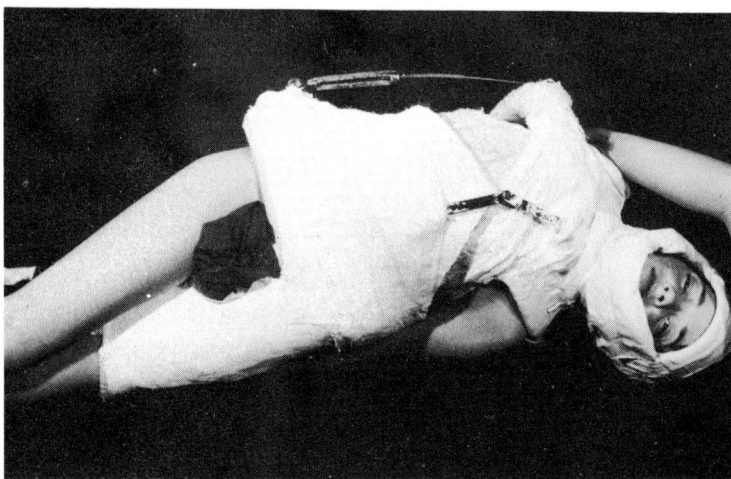

Fig. 125. *A patient in a Risser jacket showing some correction, the turn-buckle having been considerably unscrewed on the convex side.*

Methods of correcting the curve

1. *Risser's jacket and spinal graft* (Fig. 125). Treatment by this method is carried out only when the compensatory curves are mobile. The patient is prepared by being given a light diet the previous day and, if necessary, an enema. A sedative is usually ordered. It is advisable to keep the patient in bed for 48 hours prior to application.

The jacket is applied on the Hawley table or similar apparatus. Felt padding is applied to the areas that are subjected to direct pressure. Felt is applied in layers on the convex side so that it can be pulled out as the angulation is altered. The plaster extends to the head, includes the shoulders and terminates above the knee on the concave side. The other leg is left free. When the plaster is dry it is split all round at the level of the apex of the curve. Hinges are then incorporated front and back and a turn-buckle fixed on the concave side of the primary curve. The turn-buckle is adjusted each day and gradually bends the spine in the opposite direction. Daily care must be given to the skin under the turn-buckle. In this type of plaster jacket regular change of position to prevent plaster sores and give comfort to the patient is essential.

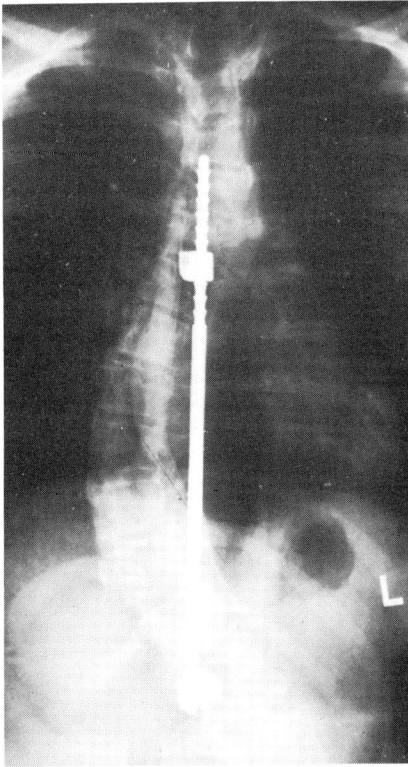

Fig. 126. *The Harrington rod in situ.*

When the surgeon is satisfied that maximum correction has been reached plaster bandages are applied to convert the plaster into a complete jacket. A window is cut out at the back so that the operation of spinal fusion may be performed. The graft may be taken from the patient or from the bone bank. A plaster jacket or support is worn until fusion is satisfactory. When the patient is ambulatory he wears a support until growth is completed.

2. *Correction by the use of an elongation derotation and lateral flexion cast (EDF).* Pads are placed over the point of maximal convexity of the curve 48 hours after the cast is applied. When the child's condition is satisfactory she may be allowed home for 3 months. The child is then re-admitted, the plaster cast is bivalved, and a cast taken for the splint maker to produce a Coltrell brace. A new EDF cast is applied for 6–8 weeks when the brace is being made; the child is then re-admitted for fitting the brace or for surgery.

Alternatively Coltrell's method of auto elongation may be used (Fig. 127) in which case the child will go on traction at night and morning — this helps to correct the curve, strengthen the muscles, and keep the spine mobile.

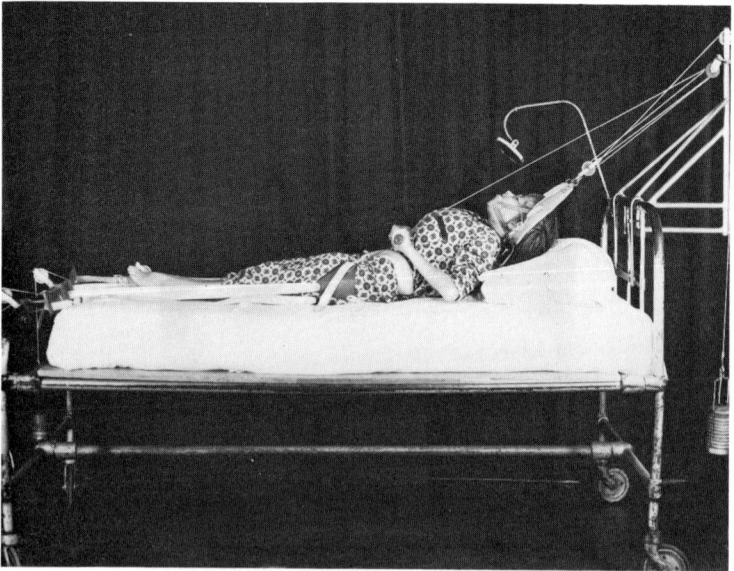

Fig. 127. *Child in Coltrell traction.*

Surgery. This may be carried out in two stages — a thorocotomy and auto-lateral fusion — followed 3 weeks later by a posterior fusion using Harrington rods and a bone graft.

Preparation for spinal fusion
Tests carried out prior to fusion:

1. Lung function
2. Electrocardiogram
3. X-ray and myelogram
4. Blood taken for count, electrolyte estimation, grouping and cross-matching

The pre-operative nursing care will include an explanation of what is to happen, given to the child and to the parents. The operation is not without risk and this should have been fully explained by the surgeon when planning the management.

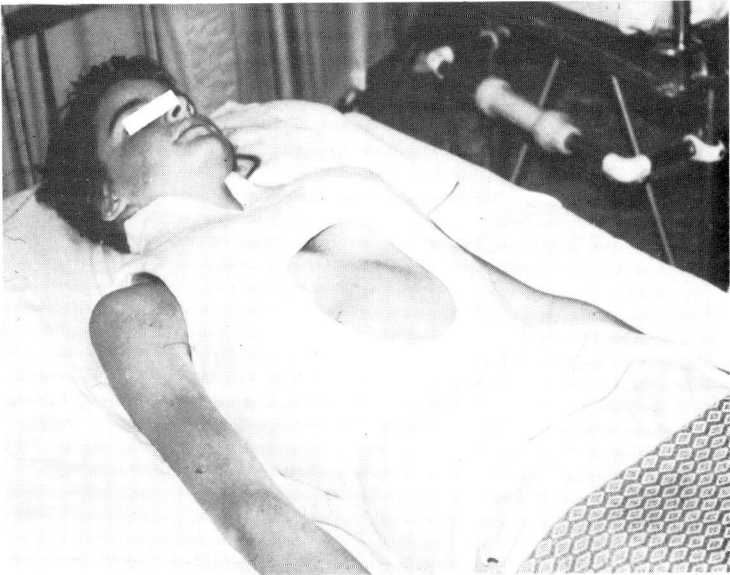

Fig. 128. *Localizing jacket showing abdominal window.*

Post-operative care. The child will need careful observation during the early post-operative period. Blood pressure, temperature, pulse and respiration will be recorded. A catheter will remain in situ for 4 days. Blood transfusion to replace the loss may be administered into both ankles, followed by Hartman's solution. The Zimmer drains are removed after 48 hours. Antibiotics are given intravenously, then orally until the sutures are removed. The child is 'log rolled' by two nurses – a third nurse is needed to control the head if the lesion is a high one or the legs if the level is low. Stitches are removed after 12 days, and an EDF cast is then applied. Allowing 2 days for the cast to dry, and a further 2 days resting in bed, the child may then get up and go home, providing she is walking satisfactorily to return after 6 months for the removal of the cast and the application of a plastic or Coltrell brace.

Before embarking on the plan of management it is important to see that it fits into the child's schooling and does not clash with examinations. The cooperation of all members of the team, together with that of the child and her parents, is essential for success.

WRY NECK — TORTICOLLIS

Torticollis may be congenital or acquired (Fig. 129).

Congenital torticollis

In congenital torticollis there is a contraction of one sternomastoid muscle. It may be noticed that the baby holds his head to one side. The mother tries passively to straighten the head, and fails to do so. Sometimes there is a swelling; a so-called tumour, possibly a haematoma, can be felt in the sternomastoid. It is now considered that the swelling is due to some interference with the blood supply resulting from a kinking of the neck before birth. Deformity is not apparent until the child is one year old and then it slowly increases as the child grows.

The contracted muscle stands out like a cord. The head is pulled to one side and tilted so that the face looks upward and to the opposite direction. If untreated a compensatory scoliosis develops and the face becomes asymmetrical. The half of the face on the same side as the affected muscle becomes smaller and shorter and the eye is lower than the other. The shoulders are elevated which makes the appearance ungainly. Treatment may be conservative or operative:

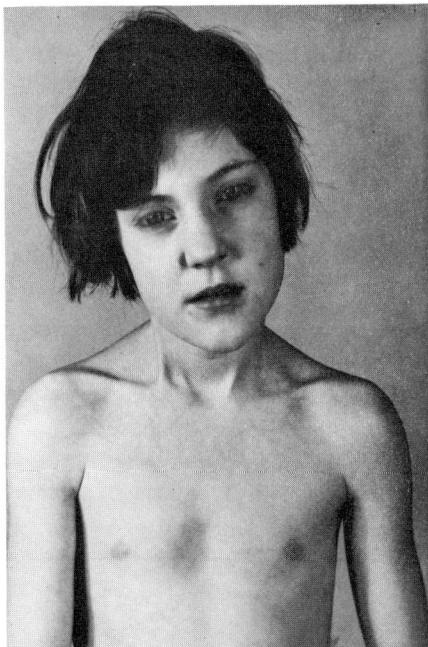

Fig. 129. *A patient with torticollis showing contracture of the light sternomastoid muscle.*

Conservative treatment. A mild case may be treated by the physiotherapist giving gentle passive stretchings. The baby is put in the lying position while an assistant fixes the shoulders. Holding the head gently but firmly, the physiotherapist flexes and rotates the head in the opposite direction. Even if good correction is obtained by this method the baby must be kept under observation for at least a year.

Operative treatment. If surgical treatment is intended a radiograph of the cervical spine is first taken in order to exclude any bony abnormality.

If the deformity is corrected before the child is eight or ten years old the asymmetry of the face corrects itself. In older neglected cases it will not do so, and is so disfiguring that most surgeons consider operation inadvisable at this stage.

The operation may be a subcutaneous tenotomy or open

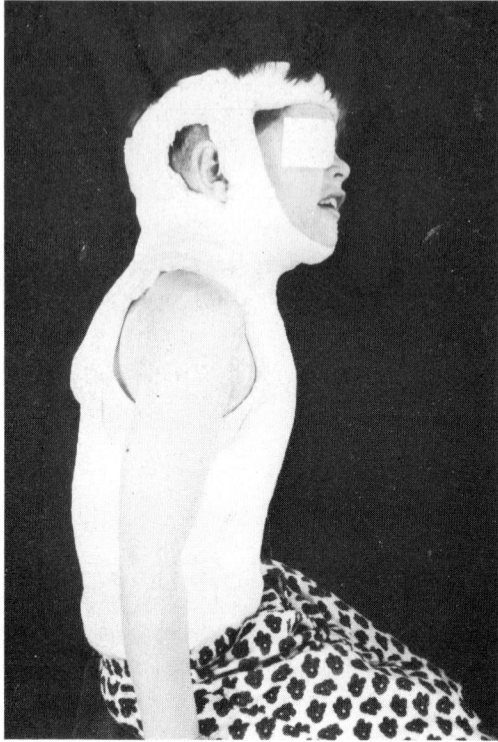

Fig. 130. *Minerva plaster showing side flexion from, and rotation towards the released sterno-cleido-mastoid muscle.*

division of the upper or lower end of the sternomastoid, followed by fixation of the head in the overcorrected position. The head is flexed away from the affected side and rotated towards it. This may be obtained by:

1. Plaster fixation applied in the theatre which is worn for about six weeks (for preparation and care of plaster, see Chapter 6) (Fig. 130).

2. Placing the child flat on the bed with the head in the over-corrected position. A folded hand-towel is placed over the forehead and the head held by sandbags of a suitable size placed on the ends of the towel. The child must not be allowed to sit up and is washed and fed by a nurse. Passive stretchings and active

exercises are started as soon as the child is fully conscious and fit enough. After about ten days the stitches are removed and the child is allowed up. Short periods of head traction with a head halter may be ordered. A collar padded higher on the affected side may be worn to remind the child to keep the head straight.

3. An alternative method is to fix the child in head traction, which is released only for meals and treatment. Re-education in front of a mirror is given until the child has the postural sense to keep the head straight by a reflex. Supervision is continued after discharge.

Acquired torticollis

Acquired torticollis is secondary to a pathological condition which must be treated. Some of types are:

1. *Postural.* This may be due to a habit of holding the head to one side for no obvious reason and is treated by re-education. The head may be held on one side because of defective hearing or vision, or incoordination of ocular muscles.

2. *Paralytic.* Paralysis of one sternomastoid muscle due to poliomyelitis or injury to the spinal accessory nerve causes unopposed action of the other sternomastoid.

3. *Bony abnormality* of the cervical vertebrae, such as hemivertebrae or destruction following an inflammatory condition.

4. *Spasmodic*, which is psychogenic in origin.

5. *Referred irritation*, due to inflammation of the cervical glands, otitis media or parotitis.

Treatment consists of treating the cause.

SPRENGEL'S SHOULDER

Sprengel's shoulder is due to the raising of one scapula. It results from a developmental abnormality of the shoulder girdle. Sometimes a fibrous or bony ridge joins the scapula to the spinous processes. Occasionally the treatment is operative. If the physiotherapist can teach the child good muscle control he can have a useful arm even if the scapula is not in its normal position.

COXA VARA

Normally the angle between the neck and shaft of the femur is between 120° and 140°. A decrease of this angle is the deformity of coxa vara (Fig. 131).

The causes of coxa vara are:

1. Malunited fracture of the neck of the femur.
2. Metabolic diseases, such as rickets and osteomalacia, that cause softening of the bone.
3. Slipped femoral epiphysis in adolescence (see p. 196).
4. Congenital. This is a rare condition in which there is a congenital defect in the development of the neck of the femur. It is often bilateral. The treatment is operative.

An osteotomy is performed to restore the angle of the neck. This is followed by a period of fixation in a double hip spica.

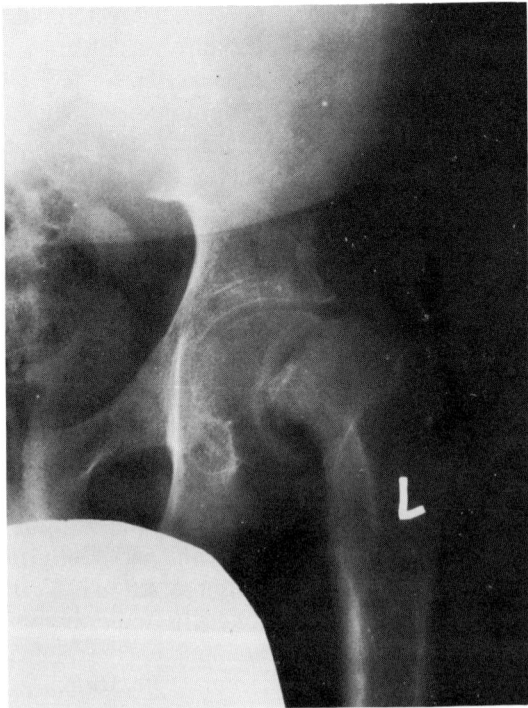

Fig. 131. *Adolescent coxa vara: X-ray showing left slipped femoral epiphysis.*

COXA VALGA

If the angle is increased the deformity is coxa valga which is an uncommon condition. It is usually secondary to congenital dislocation of the hip or infantile paralysis.

Treatment is that of the cause if possible. If the condition causes a severe limp, osteotomy may be resumed, with fixation till union occurs.

OTHER CONGENITAL DEFECTS

Congenital defects are seen in a variety of forms. Often they are multiple.

Some varieties of congenital defects include:

1. Congenital absence of the ulna. There is an ulnar deviation of the hand. The deformity can be partly checked by splintage and later corrected by surgery, sometimes fusing the lower end of the radius to the carpus.
2. Congenital absence of tibia. Amputation is usually necessary in order to fit a prosthesis.
3. Radio-ulnar synosteosis. Pronation and supination of the fore-arm is impossible, due to fusion of the radius and ulna. There is surprisingly little disability because of compensatory shoulder movements.
4. Syndactylism or webbing of the fingers which is corrected by plastic surgery.
5. Polydactylism. An extra finger or part of a finger is present and may be removed surgically.

SPINA BIFIDA

Spina bifida occulta

Spina bifida occulta is a developmental failure of the spine, usually seen at the lumbosacral level. It is the least serious of the neural arch defects. It may be symptomless but it could account for deformities of feet (Fig. 132b).

Meningocele

Meningocele is more serious where the gap is wide and the dura

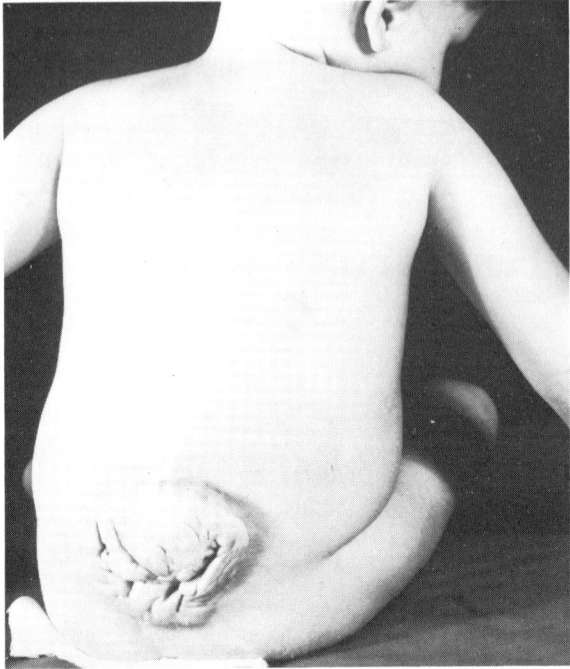

Fig. 132a. *A child with meningocele.*

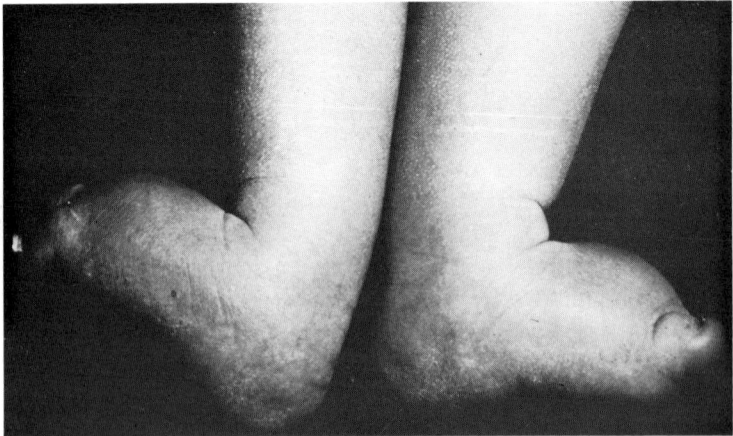

Fig. 132b. *Feet of the child with spina bifida showing calcaneovalgus.*

mater protrudes forming a sac containing cerebrospinal fluid (Figs 132a and 133).

Treatment is by surgical removal of the sac and closure of the defect.

Myelomeningocele

Myelomeningocele is the commonest and most severe anomaly of the spinal defect and involves the spinal cord, membranes and nerve roots; it is seen as a large bulge, usually in the lumbar region. This delicate mass can easily be damaged, and become infected causing meningitis. Hydrocephalus is very often present (see Fig. 133).

Assessment. Careful assessment is needed by experienced doctors, including a paediatrician, neurosurgeon and an orthopaedic surgeon. This team of specialists will ascertain the degree of damage to the spine, the extent of the neurological involvement, and whether other systems are defective; abnormality of the urinary system is not uncommon. Whether or not treatment is possible will be based on the assessment. One member of the team will then discuss the outcome with the parents, keeping in mind that it is the quality of life that is important.

Associated problems
1. Paralysis of lower limbs affecting mobility.
2. Loss of sensation accompanied by poor blood supply, leading to pressure sores.
3. Urinary involvement with loss of bladder control and the risk of kidney infection.
4. The loss of bowel function leading to constipation.
5. Accompanying deformities such as congenital dislocation of the hip with flexion deformity and deformities of the feet.
6. Hydrocephalus needing early drainage and possible review later.

Treatment and nursing care
The aim will be to ensure that the child is able to lead as full a life as possible and that the family is supported to help to achieve it.

NORMAL VERTEBRAE
Showing intact neural arch

SPINA BIFIDA
Least serious
defect

MENINGOCELE
Failure of fusion
allows protrusion
of the membranes

MYELOMINGOCELE
Sac containing spinal
cord

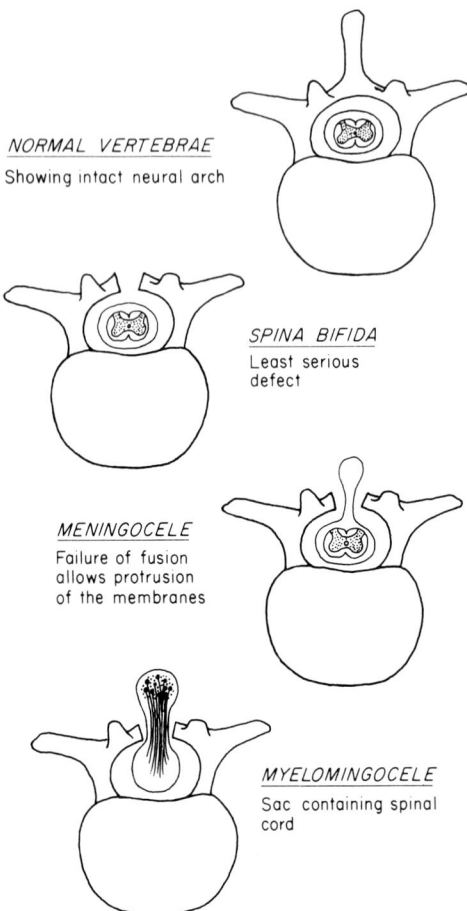

Fig. 133. *Congenital abnormality in which the vertebral arch fails to fuse thus allowing protrusion of the underlying membranes or even the spinal cord.*

The plan of management will be drawn up in the light of the clinical assessment, and the situation in the family. It will be modified if necessary as the child develops, or if any new problems arise. Closure of the defect in the back will be undertaken within a few hours of life. The child needs to be nursed prone to avoid pressure on the wound. To support the child on a sling is a convenient method.

Surgery is often necessary to drain the developing hydrocephalus with the insertion of either a Spitz Holter or a Pudenz valve. Paralysis of certain muscle groups and the over-pull of the opposing group leads to deformities, usually flexion of the hip, extension of the knee, and either talipes equinovarus or talipes calcaneovalgus (Fig. 132b). Surgery is usually necessary to correct the deformity, tenoromy or muscle transfer, such as the transfer of psoas to the back of the trochanter. Splints may be used to prevent, but not correct, the deformity — the insensitive skin will not tolerate the degree of pressure needed. Movement every two hours is essential to prevent pressure sores in these children; with loss of sensation they must be kept clean and their limbs protected from damage.

Management of the paralysed bladder. A high fluid intake is necessary, and gentle and regular pressure over the suprapubic region to produce emptying. Transplantation of the ureters from the bladder into a loop of the ileum which is brought to the surface of the abdomen at the right iliac fossa is a tremendous help in dealing with all the consequences of incontinence. The urine drains into a specially adapted bag and the surrounding skin is suitably protected. This method is particularly suitable for females; the alternative is a urinal attached to the penis in the male.

Management of the bowel. In management of the bowel, training can be helpful, but in practice an enema given every second day is often found to be satisfactory; alternatively suppositories may be preferred. Manual evacuation may be necessary — the older child can be taught this procedure.

Dislocated hips are treated as described later in this chapter. Ilio-psoas transplant may be performed to counteract the hip flexion and restore the muscle balance; soft tissue release to correct talipes equinovarus. Calcaneovalgus may also require surgical treatment.

Because of the complexity of this condition the child will need to be monitored by the team. The nurse has a very important role in observing changes in the condition and caring for the child, and at the same time teaching the mother how to observe whether the valve is functioning or not.

Genetic counselling is needed and tests may be carried out in future pregnancies. The medical social worker will play an important part in coordinating community care. The families of these children need a great deal of support, especially as the child grows up and goes through the adolescent years.

GENU VALGUM OR KNOCK-KNEE

Knock-knee is a common disorder of childhood. It was one of the common deformities of rickets but since this is now rare the usual type seen is idiopathic. The growth of the internal femoral condyle is more rapid than that of the external condyle and this alters the line of the knee joint. Normally when a child stands erect the internal femoral condyles and internal malleoli touch each other. When knock-knee is present the malleoli cannot be brought together without overlapping the knees. The degree of knock-knee is estimated by measuring the distances between the internal malleoli. When the child is lying flat with knees straight and the patellae facing forwards the legs are brought together and any intermalleolar separation becomes apparent.

The child is often of the heavy type with valgoid flat feet and poor posture. The internal lateral ligament of the knee is slack as the strain falls on the inner side of the joint. In a great many cases genu valgum is spontaneously corrected as the growth of the condyles becomes equalized and no treatment is needed.

Conservative treatment
The inner side of the soles and heels of the shoes may be wedged to relieve strain on the inner side of the knee joint. If this is to be effective the shoes must be worn continuously and the child not even allowed to get out of bed to go to the lavatory without wedged shoes.

If there is no spontaneous decrease and the separation reaches 7.5 cm or more and continues to increase, other measures are taken.

GENU VARUM OR BOW LEGS

In bow legs neither the knees nor internal malleoli can be brought together. Real bow leg with an incurving of the tibiae is rare since the abolition of rickets.

Mild cases are sometimes seen and are due to a slight epiphyseal defect combined with poor posture. The deformity corrects itself with growth and postural education.

GENU RECURVATUM (OR HYPEREXTENSION OF THE KNEE)

Hyperextension of the knee may be due to paralysis of the hamstrings when the quadriceps have recovered and the splintage has been inefficient. It may follow any long period of recumbency when the knee is kept fully extended so that the posterior part of the capsule of the knee joint is overstretched. This is prevented by immobilizing the knee joint in slight flexion and supporting the head of the tibia.

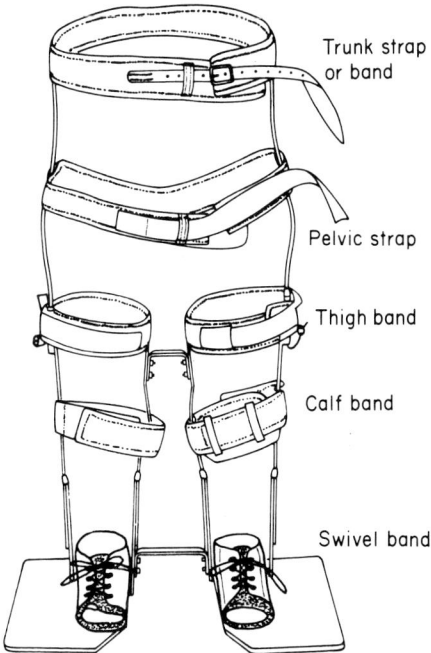

Fig. 134. *The Shrewsbury splint designed to give stability to the lower back, hips and feet, at the same time allowing a swivel gait.*

DEFORMITIES OF THE FEET

The foot has three functions — to support the weight of the body, act as a lever to raise the body and move it forward in locomotion, and to be concerned with balance. For these purposes it must be both mobile and stable.

Conditions for mobility and balance are provided by the arrangement of the small bones in a series of arches. There is no real arch on the lateral side of the foot but the supporting bones, the calcaneum (or os calcis), the cuboid and the fourth and fifth metatarsals, are slightly bowed to give them spring.

The medial longitudinal arch is definite and consists of the calcaneum (os calcis), the talus (astragalus), the navicular (scaphoid) and three cuneiform bones. The highest and weakest point of the arch is the gap between the sustentaculum tali of the calcaneum and navicular. This is bridged by the spring ligament upon which the astragalus rests.

A series of arches, formed by the metatarsal and midtarsal bones, run transversely across the foot. The slight curve that forms the transverse arch is flattened during weight-bearing.

The factors that maintain the arches are:
1. The structure and shape of bones. The articulating surfaces are curved.
2. The interosseous ligaments.
3. The structures that span the sole of the foot, which are the short foot muscles, long and short plantar ligaments, and plantar fascia.
4. The long tendons of the tibialis posterior and peroneus longus muscles are attached to the bones of the foot so that they act as supporting slings.

The height of the arches varies with individuals and with the constant change of posture. Good function of the foot depends on mobility and muscular control so that the arches can easily be formed. Balance of the foot is maintained by the tension between evertor and invertor muscles.

MOVEMENTS OF THE FOOT

The foot works as a unit.

At the ankle joint the movements are:

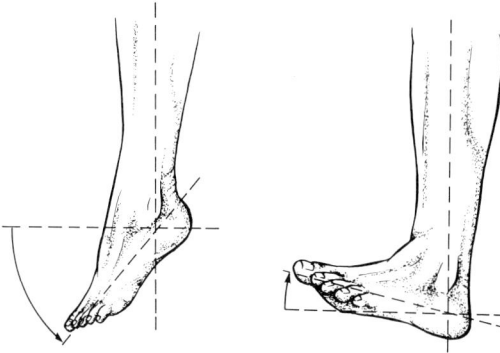

Fig. 135. (a) *Plantar flexion;* (b) *dorsiflexion.*

1. *Plantar flexion* (toes pointing downward, Fig. 135a) by the action of the gastrocnemius, soleus, plantaris, tibialis posticus, peroneus longus and brevis.

2. *Dorsiflexion* (toes pointing upwards, Fig. 135b), is performed by the action of tibialis anticus, peroneus tertius, extensor digitorum longus and extensor hallucis longus.

The joints between the calcaneum and talus — the sub-talar joint and the talonavicular joint function as one for the movements of:

3. *Inversion* (plantar surface of foot turned inwards), accompanied by adduction and plantar flexion by the action of the tibialis anterior, and posterior.

4. *Eversion* (plantar surface turned outward) accompanied by abduction and dorsiflexion is performed by the peroneus longus, brevis and tertius.

(For the foot in walking, See Chapter 14)

PES PLANUS

The term 'flat' foot is used for many conditions when there is a weak or painful foot held in the valgus position.

VALGUS FEET IN CHILDREN

Valgus feet are common in children with the slender type of feet.

The condition is associated with knock-knees or some postural defect. There may be no symptoms but the mother consults a doctor because the child's gait is clumsy.

Treatment
Exercises are given when the child is old enough to cooperate. Since they mist be repeated for a few minutes several times a day, the mother must be interested and supervise them. They should be simple exercises that the child will enjoy, such as picking up marbles with the toes. If inside wedging to the heels of shoes is ordered the shoes must be worn constantly. For example a 5 mm wedge of the heel on the inner side of the shoe may be fitted and in severe cases combined with a Thomas heel which is an elongation of the inner border of the heel. An alternative is a wedge heel and sole on the inner side.

CONGENITAL FLAT FOOT

In congenital flat foot there is a congenital abnormality in the structure of the tarsal bones. The symptom of acute pain appears in adolescence when the strain on the feet is increased. Conservative treatment is of little use. Operative treatment is usually the triple arthrodesis. In Dunne's triple arthrodesis the talocalcanean and calcaneocuboid joints are fused and the entire navicular removed, the talus being joined to the cuneiforms. Many surgeons prefer not to remove the navicular but fuse the talonavicular joint using a cancellous graft.

FOOT STRAIN

Types of foot strain vary in degree rather than in kind. They are due to the inability of the feet to meet strain. When the muscles of the foot and leg are fatigued they relax and the foot rotates into a valgus position. This causes an aching pain in the foot. If the foot is rigid, strain is thrown on the ligaments which causes severe pain. A mobile foot is seldom painful but there is pain when the muscles are weak and ligaments which are not designed to take strain are stretched.

At first the patient complains of pain over the inner side of the foot which is relieved by rest. Later it becomes a constant nag and radiates over the whole foot and up the calf. On examination tender spots may be found over the affected ligaments and passive movement is painful. At the end of the day the feet become swollen.

A radiograph is taken to reveal any arthritic changes.

Causes
Causes may be:
1. Muscle weakness and habitual poor posture.
2. Prolonged or unaccustomed standing.
3. Increase of body weight.
4. Long or short period of bed rest.
5. Unsuitable and ill-fitting shoes.

Treatment
Treatment varies with severity of the condition and may consist of:
1. Rest and plaster fixation, if the condition is acute.
2. Manipulation under anaesthesia.
3. Physiotherapy in the form of active exercises.
4. Reduction of body weight.
5. Supports. If possible, supports are used only as a temporary measure until the muscles have improved. A resilient type made of sorbo rubber is suitable. It can be discarded if the patient performs the exercises assiduously and wears the shoes prescribed. It will be necessary to retain supports and adjust them from time to time if there is chronic arthritis, chronic ligamentous strain or if the patient is very obese. This type of patient needs a more rigid support.

Exercises are given to increase the mobility of the foot, to strengthen the muscles, especially the intrinsic foot muscles, and to improve general posture. Faradic foot baths may be given for muscle stimulation and contrast baths to relieve swelling.

PARALYTIC FLAT FOOT

Paralytic flat foot is an uncommon condition. Treatment consists of supporting the affected muscles.

SPASMODIC FLAT FOOT

In spasmodic flat foot the foot is held in the position of eversion and slight dorsiflexion due to spasm of the peronei. The cause is unknown. Usually it is unilateral. Sometimes there is an abnormal bar of bone between the calcaneum and navicular which is seen only on an oblique radiograph. The onset of symptoms occurs between the years of fourteen and seventeen, often after starting an occupation that involves standing. At first there is pain only at the end of the day. Later, spasm increases so that walking or standing even for a short period is painful. In an untreated case the spasm may disappear but there will be secondary bone charges in later life and a painful foot.

Treatment
Treatment is by manipulation under general anaesthetic with the foot in as much inversion as possible and immobilized in plaster of Paris, usually retained for six weeks, non-weight-bearing. On removal the patient is given invertor exercises, wedge heels on inner sole and possibly an inside T-strap and outside iron (see Fig. 23).

Operative treatment
Operative treatment may be by:
1. Tenotomy of the peronei followed by plaster fixation.
2. Excision of abnormal bone.
3. Triple arthrodesis when other treatments are unsuccessful.

PES EQUINUS (DROP-FOOT)

Inability to dorsiflex the foot (Fig. 136) may be due to:
1. Muscle weakness and contracture of the tendon, pressure from bedclothes, or lack of suitable splints following a faulty position of the foot due to exercises. This type is prevented if the patient receives adequate care.
2. Paralytic drop-foot as a rsult of anterior poliomyelitis or injury to or pressure on the external popliteal nerve.
3. Spastic paralysis due to spasm of the calf muscles and the unopposed action of gravity.

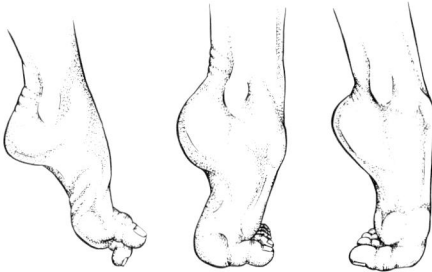

Fig. 136. *Various forms of talipes equinus (pes equinus).*

Treatment depends upon the cause. Postural and paralytic drop-foot require support in plaster of Paris with the foot in neutral. Later if the dorsiflexors remain weak, below knee irons and a toe raising device may be worn (Fig. 23).

PES CAVUS (CLAW FOOT)

Claw foot is characterized by a raised longitudinal arch caused by a dropping of the forefoot (Fig. 137). The interphalangeal joints are flexed, the metatarsophalangeal joints extended and the metatarsal heads dropped.

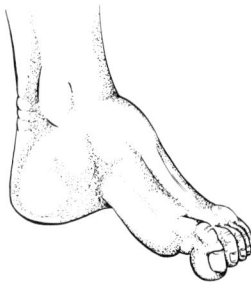

Fig. 137. *Pes cavus (claw foot).*

Causes
The condition may be due to:
  1. Paralysis (see Poliomyelitis).

2. Disease of the central nervous system, e.g. spina bifida or Friedreich's disease.

3. Prolonged exposure to wet and cold causing contracture of the ligaments and intrinsic muscles.

4. Idiopathic causes. The idiopathic types may be symptomless and require no treatment. There is seldom complaint of pain from a child with claw feet; there is a complaint from the parents about the rapid rate at which the uppers of the shoes and the soles under the metatarsal heads wear out. Later pain is caused by abnormal pressure on the ball of the foot. There is pain in the metatarsal region over the dorsum of the foot and the metatarsal heads are tender. Callosities form over the dorsum of the toes and under the metatarsal heads.

Conservative treatment
If the condition is mild, foot exercises are given to strengthen the intrinsic foot muscles. A metatarsal bar or pad may be worn to relieve pressure. The patient is advised to wear shoes with a very low or no heel and stout soles. Footwear made specially with a moulded cork insole do not correct the deformity but give considerable comfort to the patient.

Operative treatment
Operative treatment may be:

1. Tenotomy of the plantar fascia, possibly combined with an elongation of the tendon Achilles and plaster fixation for six weeks. Weight-bearing in plaster is allowed after a few days. When the plasters are removed, foot exercises are taught and footwear prescribed.

2. Steindler's operation. The short muscles of the foot are divided at their origin and brought forward. Sometimes this is combined with Lambrinudi's operation.

3. Triple arthhrodesis or similar stabilizing operation.

METARTARSUS VARUS

Metartarsus varus is a congenital adduction of the forefoot in the metatarsal region. The disability is slight.

Treatment

Treatment consists of:

1. Wearing the shoe on the opposite foot — right shoe on left foot and left shoe on right foot.
2. Outside wedging to shoes.
3. Applying a series of moulded plaster.
4. Applying a plaster with Kite's wedging similar to the wedging used in talipes.

CORNS AND CALLOSITIES

A callosity is a horny layer of skin formed where there is intermittent pressure and friction. Where there is pressure over a bony prominence a hard corn is formed. The horny layer becomes deeper and there is often a central core. Soft corns occur when there is friction between skin between the toes. Corns and callosities are caused by pressure resulting from foot deformities or the wearing of ill-fitting shoes. They may be cured with local treatment by the chiropodist but will return unless the cause of the pressure is removed.

Temporary relief can be obtained by using felt pads or rings to relieve pressure.

HALLUX VALGUS

In hallux valgus the big toe is abducted from the midline of the body (Fig. 138). Predisposing causes may be a short first metatarsal or footwear that interferes with the function of the intrinsic foot muscles. Neither of these causes is proven but it is a commoner deformity of women than men and does not occur in races that go habitually unshod. The first metatarsal is adducted and is in the varus position (towards the midline). The phalanges are abducted towards the second toe into the valgus position (away from the midline). The big toe lies over or under the second toe. This combined deformity makes the metatarsal head prominent on the medial side of the foot and friction occurs between this and the shoe. An exostosis forms over the inner side of the prominent metartarsal head. Often an enlarged bursa, known as a bunion forms over the exostosis and a painful corn develops in the overlying skin. Pressure on the enlarged bursa causes pain and the

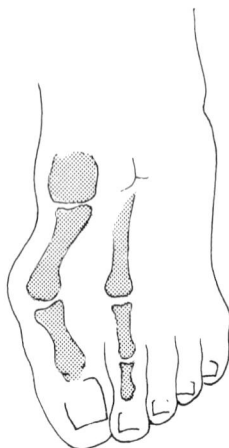

Fig. 138. *Hallux valgus showing marked lateral deviation of the great toe.*

bunion may become inflamed and suppurate. The deformity interferes with the function of the intrinsic foot muscles; there is a dropped arch, metatarsalgia and a displacement of the second toe. Later osteo-arthritic changes occur in the metatarsal head. The symptoms may be slight with quite a marked deformity but pain from the bunion and the secondary deformities can be so severe that walking is almost impossible.

Conservative treatment
Conservative treatment is advised in mild cases which consists of felt padding to relieve pressure on the bunion, the wearing of wide shoes with a straight inner border, foot mobilizing exercises and supports.

Operative treatment
Operative treatment may be a simple trimming of the metatarsal head or an arthroplasty. The type of arthroplasty may vary; a common one is that described by Keller when the proximal half of the proximal phalanx is removed. The importance of the after-care is always stressed. The operation may be followed by plaster fixation. Pulp traction with a pin or nylon suture may be used. The plaster is removed after three or six weeks.

Some surgeons prefer to bandage the foot so that the toe is held in the varus position. In this case gentle exercises are started on the third or fifth day. Stitches are removed and weight-bearing started after about a fortnight.

When walking starts foot exercises are given for mobility and to re-educate the intrinsic foot muscles especially the interossei. Wide-fitting shoes must be worn and correct walking must start straight away, often a metatarsal bar is ordered. This requires effort on the patient's part as weight must be taken on the ball of the big toe. There must be no shuffling about in bedroom slippers. Correct footwear must be continued after discharge.

HALLUX RIGIDUS

In hallux rigidus the normal range of movement of the great toe is limited. At first dorsiflexion is limited and then the whole toe stiffens. The patient complains of severe pain on using the foot; walking becomes difficult and even pressure from the bedclothes is painful. The adolescent type occurs in children with long narrow feet. In the older patient it may be due to osteo-arthritis or repeated minor injuries.

Treatment
Shoes of the correct length are advised with a metatarsal bar outside or metatarsal dome inside. If the symptoms are not relieved operative treatment is needed and it is the same as that carried out for hallux valgus.

METATARSALGIA

Metatarsalgia is a painful condition affecting the metatarsopha-langeal joints. The metatarsal heads are painful and tender. The pain varies in intensity at different times. Callosities develop on the ball of the foot. The condition occurs when the feet are not correctly taking the body weight.

It may be due to:
1. Deformity that disturbs the mechanism of the foot, such as hallux valgus, hammer toe or flat foot.
2. Weakness of the intrinsic foot muscles.
3. Shoes that are too short, or the type of shoe that slides the foot forward crushing the metatarsals.

Treatment

The patient is told to wear low-heeled, laced shoes and instructed in the re-education of the intrinsic foot muscles. A metatarsal bar or dome placed immediately behind the metatarsal heads may be ordered in order to relieve pressure.

MORTON'S METATARSALGIA

In Morton's metatarsalgia there is acute pain between the third and fourth toes due to a neuroma of the digital nerves. The affected part of the nerve is excised.

HAMMER TOE

A hammer toe has the metatarsophalangeal joint extended and the proximal interphalangeal joint flexed to right angle (Fig. 139). The distal interphalangeal joint may be extended, flexed or straight. It may occur in several toes, but usually only in the second toe. Pain is due to a corn forming on the dorsum of the toe and the associated metatarsalgia. The patient will say that it is impossible to find comfortable shoes.

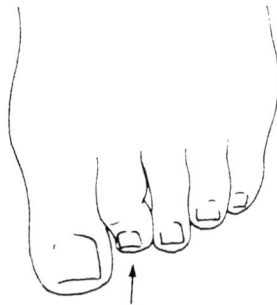

Fig. 139. *Hammer toe.*

Treatment

Conservative treatment is advised when the condition is very mild, or the patient very young, and consists of strapping, gentle stretching and wearing a night splint.

Operative treatment

Operative treatment involves arthrodesis of the affected joint or filleting of the toe.

DUPUYTREN'S CONTRACTURE

The palmar fascia lies immediately beneath the skin of the hand. The proximal border into which the palmaris longus muscle inserts is attached to the transverse palmar ligament. The distal border is divided into four bands which are inserted into the skin at the level of the web of the fingers. It is joined to the deep fascia. In Dupuytren's contracture the palmar fascia is thickened and contracted so that one or more fingers are drawn into a position of flexion. The cause is unknown.

Clinical features

The condition occurs in middle-aged and elderly people. Men are affected more commonly than women. The ring finger is always involved, then later the little finger, the middle finger and forefinger become flexed. In severe cases the fingers may touch the palms. The rate at which the deformity progresses varies and it may take months or years to become severe.

Treatment

Treatment is operative. A mild case can be corrected by a tenotomy of the palmar fascia. In a more severe case the fascia is excised.

TALIPES EQUINOVARUS (CLUB FOOT)

The term talipes is applied to congenital deformities of the foot and ankle. The commonest type of talipes is talipes equinovarus (taken from *equus*, a horse, *varus*, inverted), in which there is plantar flexion of the ankle and forefoot, the forefoot being adducted and inverted (Fig. 140).

Causes

The hereditary factor is now regarded as negligible. Two well-known theories are:

1. Abnormal intrauterine pressure.

2. Failure of the tarsal bones, especially the talus and the navicular, to develop, followed by contractures of muscles and ligaments.

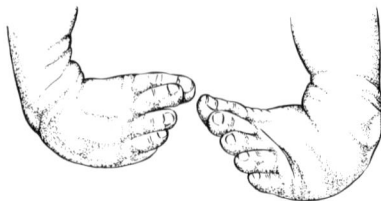

Fig. 140. *Double congenital talipes equinovarus.*

Clinical features

Both sexes are equally affected. When the condition is bilateral the deformity is more severe on one side. In a severe case the bones may be smaller than normal and distorted in shape. When the bones are normal in shape and size the deformity of plantar lexion, inversion and adduction at the mid-tarsal joint is maintained solely by contracture of the soft tissue. The muscles and tendons on the inner side are contracted; those on the outer side are stretched. The deltoid ligament, the spring ligament, the capsule of the ankle joint and the plantar fascia are all contracted. Secondary bone changes take place if the deformity is not corrected. These make correction more difficult. The talus is displaced forward out of its normal socket between the malleoli. It becomes thickened in front which makes the correction of equinus difficult. The calcaneum is tilted inwards. The navicular may be projected upwards in front of the external malleolus; the cuboid may also be displaced. The tibia may be medially rotated. The calf muscles are contracted and the Achilles tendon acts as an invertor of the foot. If walking has started, callosities and bursae develop over the outer side of the foot.

Prognosis

If treatment is started as soon as possible and persisted with, there is the prospect of getting a normal or nearly normal foot. Much of the success will depend on the intelligence and perseverance of the mother, since these children are treated as outpatients. Correction is more difficult when there is a tiny heel and marked adduction.

Treatment

Treatment begins as soon as the condition is diagnosed; it consists of a series of manual manipulations to stretch the contracted tissues and steps to retain the foot in the over-corrected position until there is no likelihood of relapse. Manipulation is performed without an anaesthetic. It is done gently and rhythmically in two stages. There should be no break between the two stages in practice. An assistant protects the epiphyses of the tibia and fibula by holding the ankle. The ligaments on the inner side of the knee joint must also be protected or a knock-knee may result from the continuous stretching of the internal lateral ligament. This protection is achieved by keeping the knee flexed and the hip externally rotated. The operator first corrects the adduction deformity by abducting and plantar flexing the forefoot while the heel is fixed. The foot is then dorsiflexed taking care that there is dorsiflexion of the whole foot and not only in the talar-navicular phase. The foot is then held in position by adhesive strapping. The strapping is designed to correct the deformity and maintain the correction by gentle stretching of the tight structures towards the opposite over-corrected position.

The strapping programme continues until the child is 6 weeks old — it is changed twice a week for the first week to ensure no allergies to the strapping have developed; then at weekly intervals until the child is 6 weeks old. A prepared template is used to cut out the three felt sections. The felt is split lengthways to halve its thickness. The backing is peeled off the adhesive felt. Two 16 in. lengths of 1 in. zinc oxate tape are cut ready. Tincture of Benzoin compound is applied to the child's lower limb.

The surgeon places his index finger and thumb on one hand on top of the thigh, holding the knee at 90°, the other hand correcting the foot (Fig. 141a). The prepared adhesive felt is applied above the knee. The foot section is attached to the sole, and the lateral section is stretched along the side of the leg, and this adducts and everts the heel. The medial section is smoothed into place. A strip of tape is attached to the skin above the medial felt section and taken downwards across the point of the heel and then up and over the knee. Care must be taken to ensure that the tape is not positioned too far forwards at the knee as this can cut into the skin as the child attempts to extend the knee.

A second strip of tape is applied in a similar manner but passes

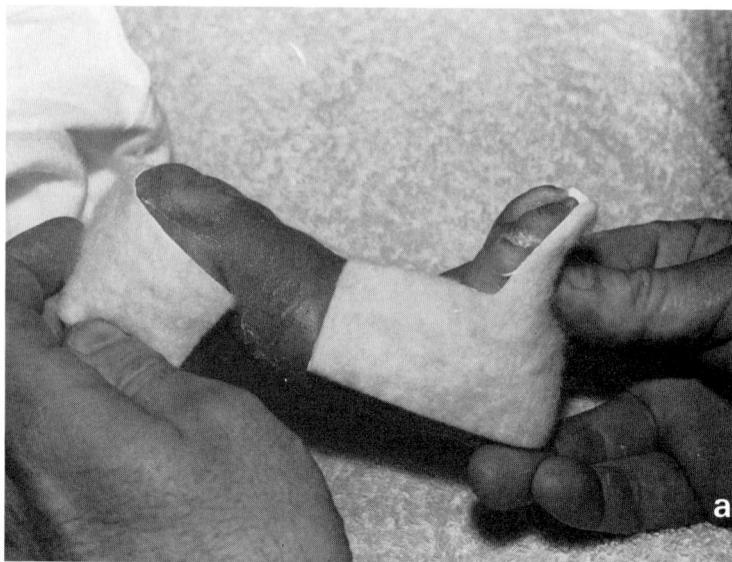

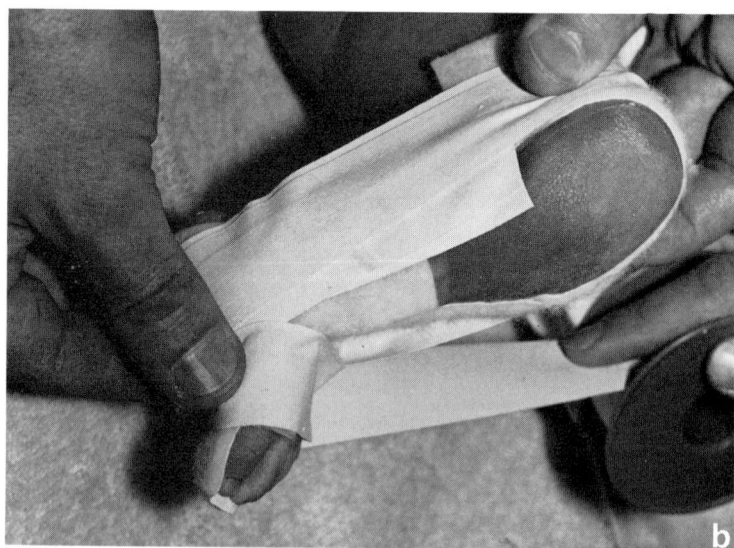

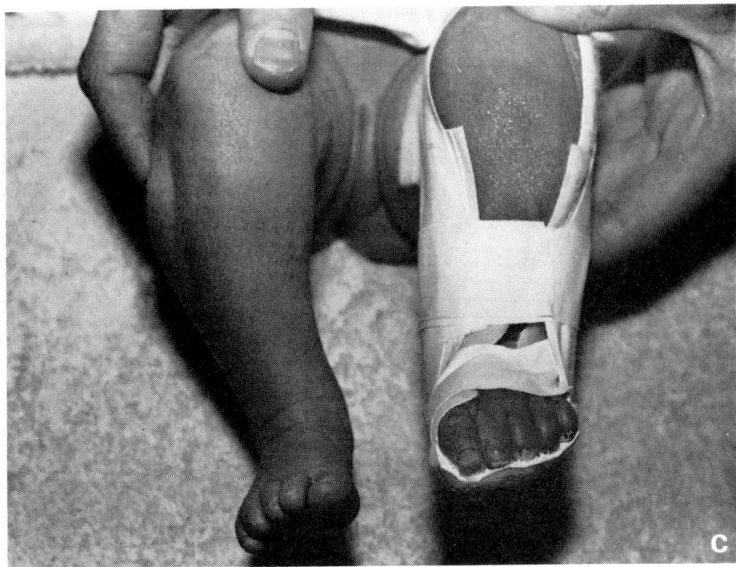

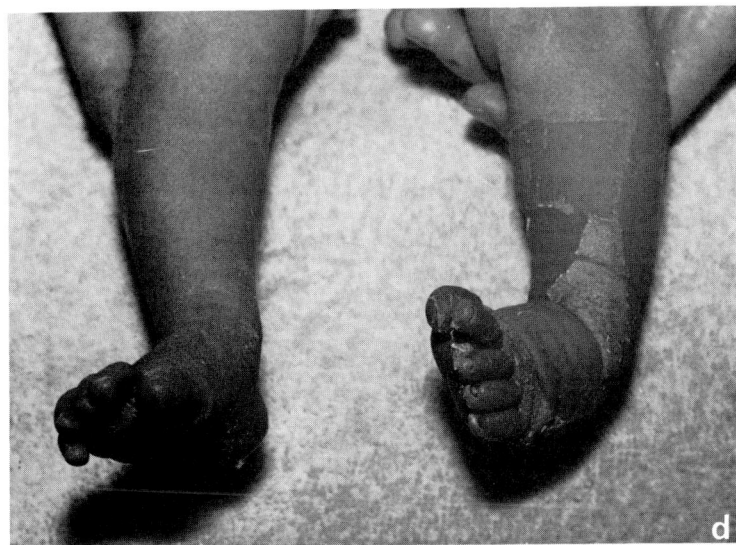

Fig. 141. *Strapping a club foot.* (a) *Positioning the limb and application of the adhesive felt,* (b) *application of the plaster strapping,* (c) *final position of the foot, and* (d) *compared with the free foot.*

slightly anteriorly so that there is a dorsiflexing and everting force on the hindfoot.

The first metatarsal head is protected by the small piece of adhesive felt which is applied medially and superiorly. A third piece of strapping is applied directly from the heel to the sole of the forefoot and this tape is passed over the front of the foot from lateral to medial, then under the foot and finally over the knee. This procedure is illustrated in Fig. 141b.

All strapping is secured using a circumferential band of tape around the calf. The first postion is demonstrated in Fig. 141c and this should be compared with the free foot in Fig. 141d.

The circulation of the toes is checked. Initially the fifth toe may blanch and if this occurs the tape must be cut back until blood flow is restored. This tendency for toe circulatory embarrassment is not usually a feature of subsequent strappings. Corrective strapping applied in this way hardly ever causes pressure areas but if any do arise extra felt patches should be used.

If the child has a strong kicking thrust, if surgery has to be delayed, or if the child is allergic to the strapping, below knee serial plasters are used as an alternative. The advantage of this early treatment programme is simplicity. The strapping is changed in a few minutes and the corrective force is readily controlled.

Correction by Denis Browne splint

If the deformity is mild a Denis Browne splint can be applied straight away. If severe it will have to be corrected by serial plasters of Paris until overcorrection is obtained and then the Denis Browne splint can be applied. It should be remembered that the Denis Browne splint maintains the correction and does not correct the deformity. This splint holds the foot in the overcorrected position and at the same time allows the child to kick and use the leg muscles (Fig. 142). The splint (Fig. 143) consists of two Duralumin sole plates which can be screwed securely to a cross bar of the same material. The sole plates have a side plate that fits up the lateral side of the leg. Before application the sole plates are detached from the cross bar. They are padded with triangular pieces of adhesive felt, so fixed that the base of the triangle will be under the lateral border of the foot and increase eversion. After manipulation the foot is secured to the sole plate with 2.5 cm adhesive strapping. When the foot and heel are secured the side

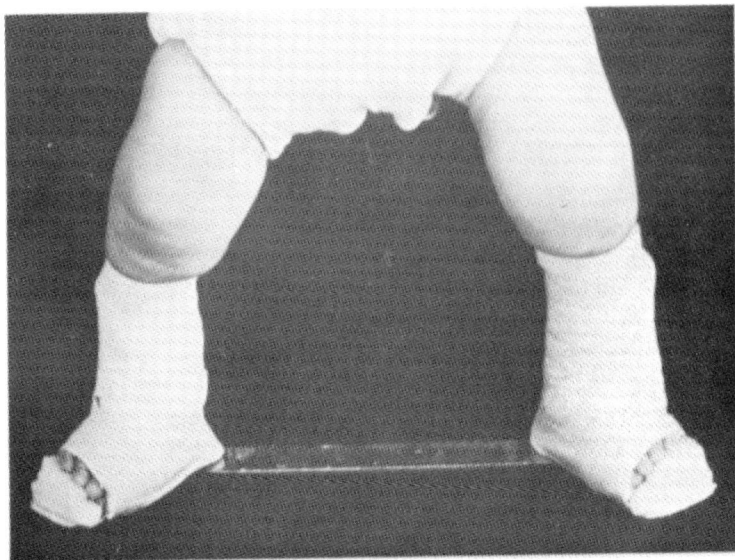

Fig. 142. *Denis Browne splint applied showing felt and strapping. Note that the felt pad is too far forward.*

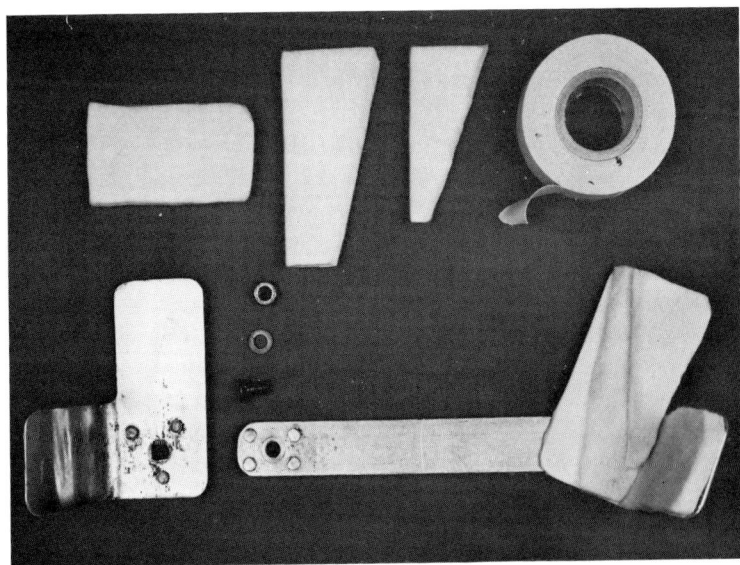

Fig. 143. *Denis Browne splint. Requisites for applying the splint.*

plate is strapped to the leg. The cross bar is then attached and the feet turned into as much eversion as possible. If one foot is normal the sole plate is covered entirely with felt and the foot held in a neutral position. Remanipulation and reapplication are done once or twice every week. The adhesive felt under the outer side of the foot and forefoot is readjusted to maintain the valgoid position. An extra pad may be placed under the calcaneocuboid joint. The child is encouraged to kick and crawl about, and when he is old enough to be standing and the foot goes readily into the overcorrected position (calcaneovalgus), Denis Browne boots or 'hobble' splints are worn. These are open-toed boots made of soft leather and reinforced with a metal sole plate. They are laced to well above the ankle and the leg is encircled by a leather band and buckle. On the sole plate is fixed a metal bar with screw adjustments. This is connected to the leg band by a leather strap. The screws are adjusted to alter the valgoid position. Two metal bars at the back join the boot to the leg band. These splints may be worn continuously and removed only for toilet of the feet. Later they may be retained as night splints while the child is walking in ordinary boots with an outside raising or an inside iron and outside T-strap.

Plaster fixation

The surgeon manipulates the foot and the over-correction is held by plaster. The plaster extends from the toes to the mid-thigh with the knee flexed. This prevents the child from kicking off the plaster, which is not left on for more than four to six weeks.

When it is finally removed, plaster night splints or the above-knee 'hobble' splint may be worn (Fig. 144).

Kite's plasters

Kite's plasters are well-padded plasters which, twice weekly, are wedged to the pain limit in order to obtain a gradual and unforced manipulation.

The first wedge is removed from the inner side of the foot to correct the varus forefoot, and a dorsal wedge is made to correct equinus.

Operative treatment

Following the 6 weeks treatment by the strapping technique, if the

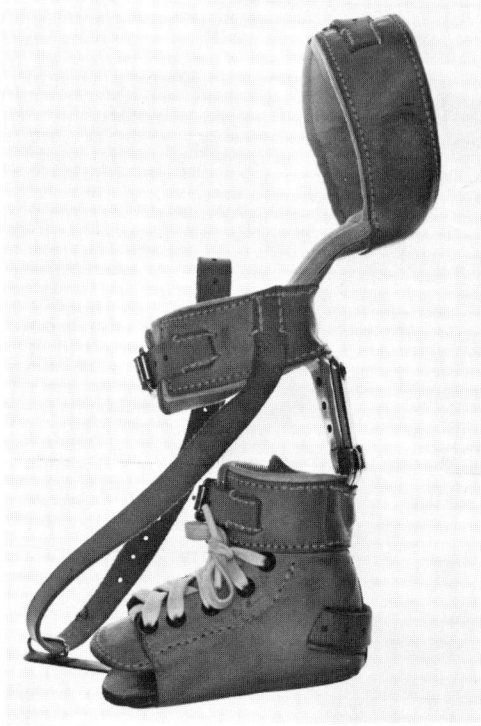

Fig. 144. *The above-knee hobble splint. Adjustment of the strap produces and maintains the corrections.*

result is not satisfactory surgery may be necessary to:
1. Correct the equinus.
2. Restore the correct relationship between the talipes and calcaneum.

Lengthening of the Achilles tendon is followed by the application of a plaster cast for 6 weeks.

Release of the ligaments which bind the bones together will be necessary in order to place the foot in the correct position. They are then transfixed by passing wires upwards through the heel and subtalar joint. A well padded plaster is applied for 3 weeks when the wires are removed and a new plaster is applied.

Operations on the bones are usually deferred until the 'teens in order to avoid interference with growth. Operations carried out include:

1. Wedge tarsectomy.
2. Triple arthrodesis which is the fusion of three joints: talo, calcaneo-navicular and calcaneo-cuboid (Fig. 145).

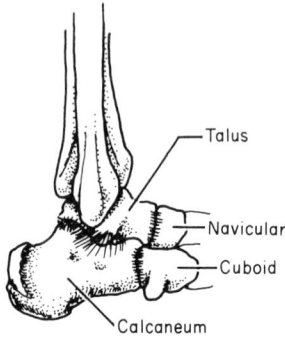

Fig. 145. *Lateral view showing the three joints fused in triple arthrodesis.*

Tendon transplantation
When overaction of the tibialus anticus produces a deformity the tendon may be transplanted to the cuboid as a corrective.

After-care
Splints are retained until the foot can be pulled into eversion and dorsiflexion by muscular action. Strong evertors and dorsiflexors are essential. Muscle re-education and walking is started as soon as the child is old enough. There is a tendency for talipes to relapse. Supervision is continued until growth is completed.

TALIPES CALCANEUS

Usually this deformity is milder than talipes equinovarus. The bones are normal at birth and the deformity is due to the soft tissues being contracted. There is a dorsiflexion at the ankle joint and eversion at the subtaloid and mid-tarsal joints (talipes calcaneovalgus); occasionally there may be inversion at these joints (talipes calcaneovarus). The foot is manipulated and held in the over-corrected position of equinus by a straight splint of plaster of

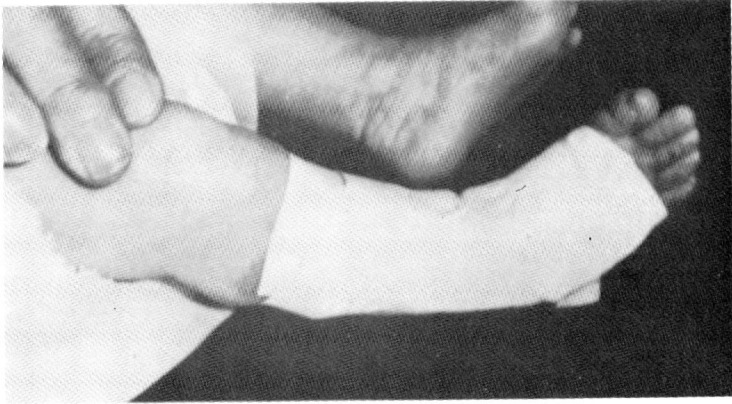

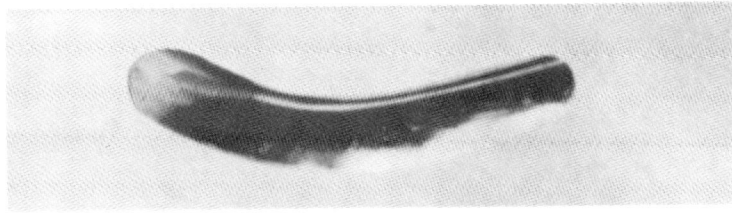

Fig. 146. *Baby with a banana splint strapped to the outer side of the foot and ankle.*

Paris or a malleable metal splint, or banana splint fixed with adhesive strapping (Fig. 146). If the condition is treated early the prognosis is good.

CONGENITAL DISLOCATION OF THE HIP

In congenital dislocation of the hip the femoral head is dislocated with a varying degree of displacement (Fig. 147). It is more often unilateral than bilateral and is commoner in girls than boys. The cause is unknown. The incidence is greater in parts of France and Italy, which suggests an hereditary factor.

Pathology
The acetabulum is shallow and tends to be oblique. The head of the femur ossifies late and is small. After weight-bearing it becomes displaced upwards and backwards so that it lies on the

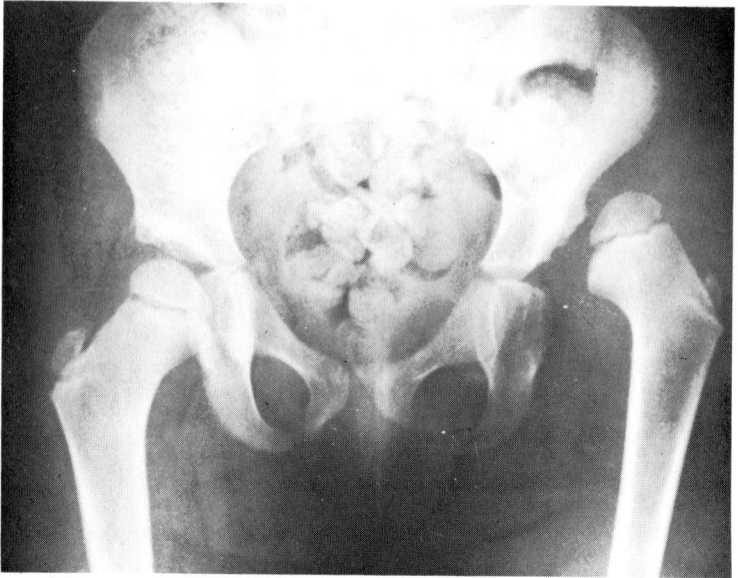

Fig. 147. *Congenital dislocation of the hip.*

dorsum of the ilium, eventually forming a false acetabulum. The attachment of the joint capsule is normal but as the dislocation takes place the capsule becomes elongated and with weight-bearing is further stretched. It becomes thickened and forms an 'hour glass' constriction which is an obstacle to reduction. The normal acetabulum is filled with fatty-fibrous tissue. The neck of the femur is anteverted (tilted forward) 60° to 90°.

The altered position of the trochanter and ilium also alters the line of pull between the origin and insertion of the hip muscles which have to work at a mechanical disadvantage. The adductor muscles are shortened and the action of the abductors is weak.

Clinical features

Prognosis depends on the age at which the diagnosis is made. If treatment is started before the child is two years of age the prognosis is fairly good. There is always a possibility of osteo-arthritis early in adult life, especially in untreated cases.

Early diagnosis is considered very important and any suspicion of a similar condition in the family history would necessitate careful examination. Soon after birth it is the practice to perform the 'click test' (Ortolani's sign). This test is carried out with the child lying on a table, knees flexed towards the abdomen, then gentle abduction and rotation of the affected hip joint. A 'clunk' rather than a 'click' is experienced as the head slips back into the acetabulum. Barlow's test is the reverse movement. The surgeon applies gentle pressure with his thumbs over the lesser trochanter with the child's hips and knees flexed. A clunk is felt as the head slips out over the acetabular ring — the unstable joint is now dislocated.

Clinical features are:
1. Asymmetry of the legs, which cannot be fully abducted.
2. The level of the gluteal folds is uneven with the creases more marked on one side.
3. There may be swelling in the gluteal region due to the displacement of the femoral head.
4. Broadening of the perineum.

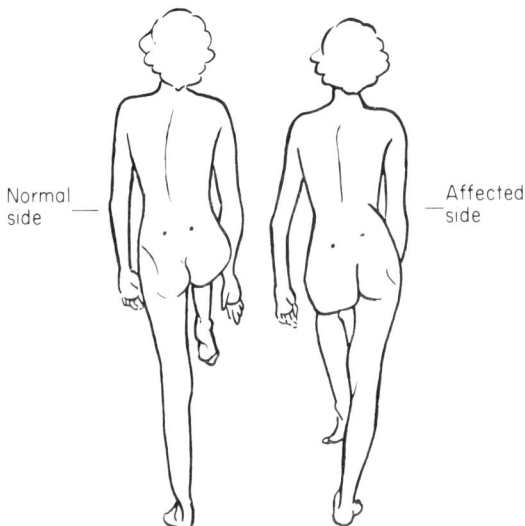

Fig. 148. *Trendelenburg's sign. Positive for right hip, negative for left.*

After weight-bearing advice is sought because the child is late in walking, or walks with a limp. The characteristic single or double limp increases as the child grows older. In a unilateral case the child dips to the affected side when walking and there is real shortening of the leg. In a bilateral case the legs appear short in comparison with the trunk. A waddling gait is caused by the child dipping alternately to each side as he walks. It may be single or double. Trendelenburg's sign is present (Fig. 148). Normally when a person is asked to stand on one leg and raise the other knee as if marking time the buttock of the raised leg is at a higher level than that of the standing leg. Trendelenburg's sign is positive when the buttock of the raised leg is lower than that of the standing leg. When standing on one leg the centre of gravity is shifted to a position above that foot because the gluteus medius and minimus contract and fix the hip in abduction. When the hip is not stabilized in slight abduction the centre of gravity is moved to the supporting leg by bending the lumbar spine laterally so the pelvis is tilted towards the side of the supporting leg. Inabilty to abduct and so stabilize the leg while weight-bearing may be due to:

1. Paralysis or weakness of the abductor muscles, gluteus medius and minimus.
2. The absence of fulcrum as in congenital dislocation of the hip.

The sign is elicited in an infant by watching him climb up on to the mother's knee. The abnormal position of the head of the femur tilts the pelvis forward and so lordosis is marked. On examination the surgeon may palpate the femoral head in the abnormal position and demonstrate a telescopic movement by moving the leg upwards and downwards in the longitudinal axis of the thigh. Movements are pain-free with limitation of abduction and of external rotation. A radiograph is taken and usually also an arthrogram using 5 ml of 37 per cent solution of diodone to show the cartilaginous outline of the femoral head and acetabulum and the position of the capsule.

Treatment
The aim of treatment is reduction of the head and keeping it in the acetabulum until normal growth has taken place. The presence of the femoral head in the acetabulum stimulates growth both of the acetabulum and the head and helps the fatty fibrous tissue to be absorbed.

Divarication. If the displacement of the head of the femur is slight and the infant is treated soon after birth simple abduction of the hips may be successful. This can be achieved by:

1. Double nappies — this is a simple method but not very reliable after the first few weeks.
2. Pavlik harness (Fig. 149). This maintains the position and allows movement of the hips which is necessary for normal development. The harness can be adjusted as the child grows. Most children diagnosed early can be treated as out-patients by this method.

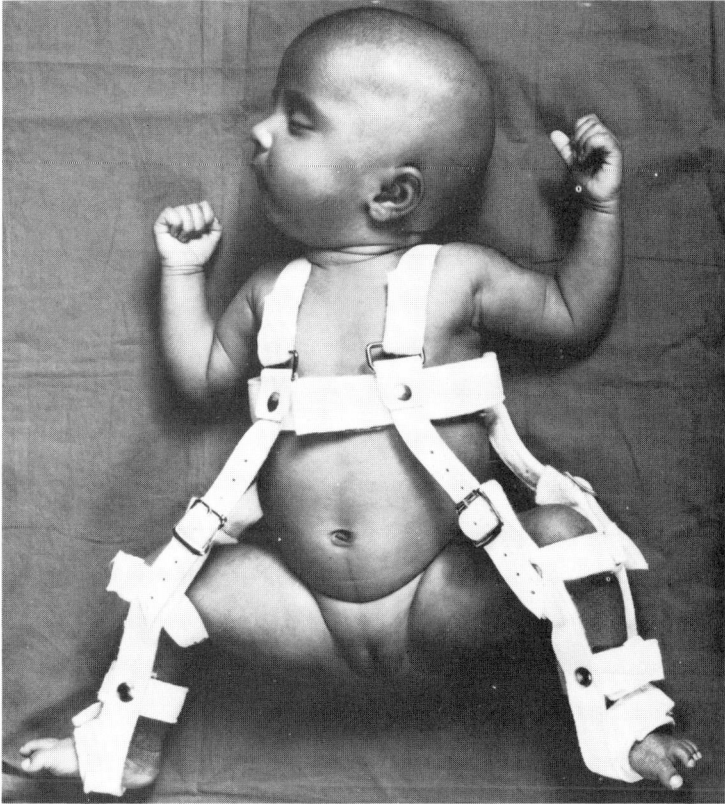

Fig. 149. *Pavlik harness used for the treatment of congenital dislocation of the hip.*

3. Von Rosen splint (Fig. 150). The splint maintains the hip in abduction and external rotation by the padded metal extend-

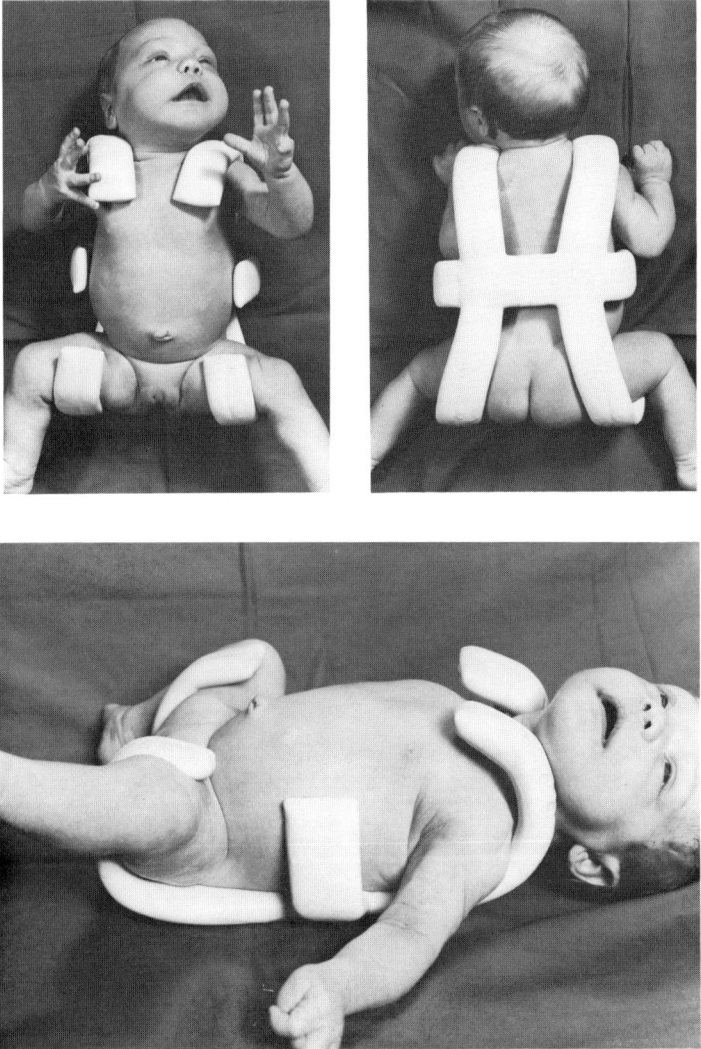

Fig. 150. *A child in a Von Rosen splint.*

ing over the shoulder and round the thigh. Care must be taken to see that the splint is well moulded and not cutting in, and that the skin under the splint is clean and healthy.

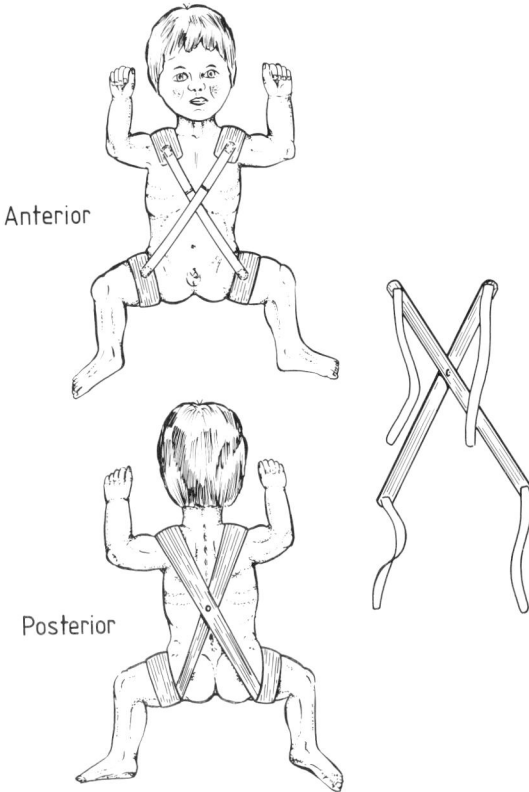

Fig. 151. *The Barlow splint applied to child.*

4. Barlow's splint (Fig. 151) is similar in principle and the child needs the same care.
5. Putti's mattress which is a triangular wedge placed between the child's legs secured by straps and worn continuously. It is removed daily for washing and reapplied so that the legs are in abduction and external rotation. A Frejka pillow is a similar device.
6. Forrester-Brown abduction (basket) splint which is a modification of Putti's divaricator (Fig. 152). In this the legs are abducted gradually until they are nearly in a straight line with each other. The splint is now less commonly used. The

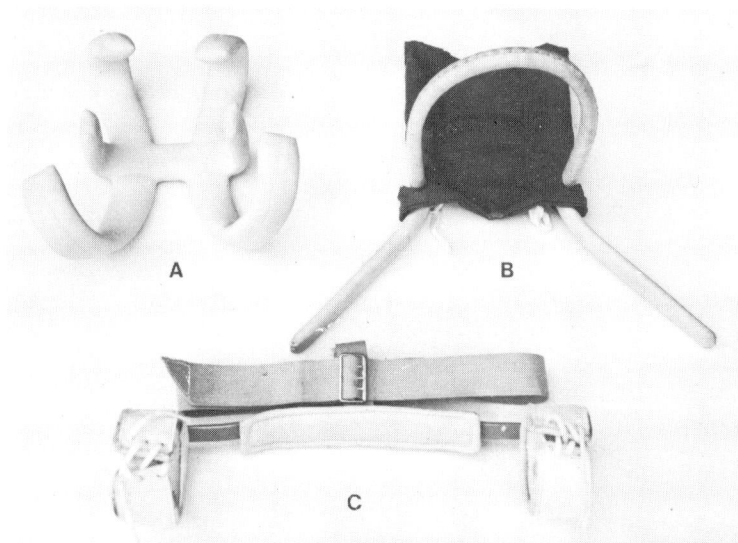

Fig. 152. (a) *Von Rosen C.D.H. splint;* (b) *Forrester Brown C.D.H. splint; and* (c) *Denis Browne C.D.H. splint.*

position of the hips is checked frequently by X-ray examination and later treatment may be by means of plaster of Paris or a Denis Browne splint.

Reduction by manipulation. This method is seldom used after the first few months because of the risk of damage to the blood supply to the developing femoral head. If reduction can be obtained by simple Ortilani's manoeuvre then one of the splints previously mentioned can be used. Following the reduction of the hip of a slightly older child a 'frog' plaster may be applied. This is a double hip spica with the hips fixed in 90° flexion and 90° abduction. The hip is externally rotated. The knees are flexed to a right angle and the feet left free. Until the plaster has dried out it should be supported on a waterproof-covered pillow, and the child should be turned over at intervals (see Care of wet plaster, p. 91).

Every effort must be made to prevent the plaster from being soiled. When the plaster is dry the buttocks are supported on a wooden box in which a hole has been cut for nursing purposes.

Sandbags are placed under the thighs and the rest of the body is supported on pillows.

A bedpan or dish is easily placed in position. This box goes with the child on discharge and the uses explained to the mother, who is told to use it and not to use napkins. The child should be trained in regular habits and attention given to the bowels. The buttocks should be kept scrupulously clean and well 'greased'. The child must spend part of each day prone. The feet must be kept warm. The child will be allowed as much activity as possible — a platform with castors (Fig. 153) is a good method of achieving this.

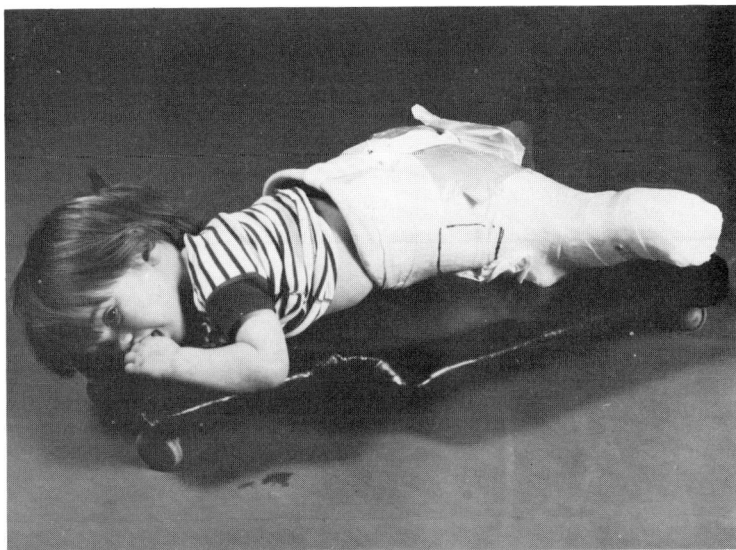

Fig. 153. *Child on platform with castors to allow mobility.*

Batchelor plaster. Application of a Batchelor plaster is an alternative method. After reduction plaster of Paris is applied extending from groin to ankle on both legs which are held in full abduction and internal rotation. The plasters are attached to a cross bar of wood. This type of plaster allows greater activity. It holds the hips in abduction while allowing flexion and use of the abdominal muscles (see Fig. 154). It is important that the child should spend a short time, about two hours, lying prone to prevent hip flexion contractures.

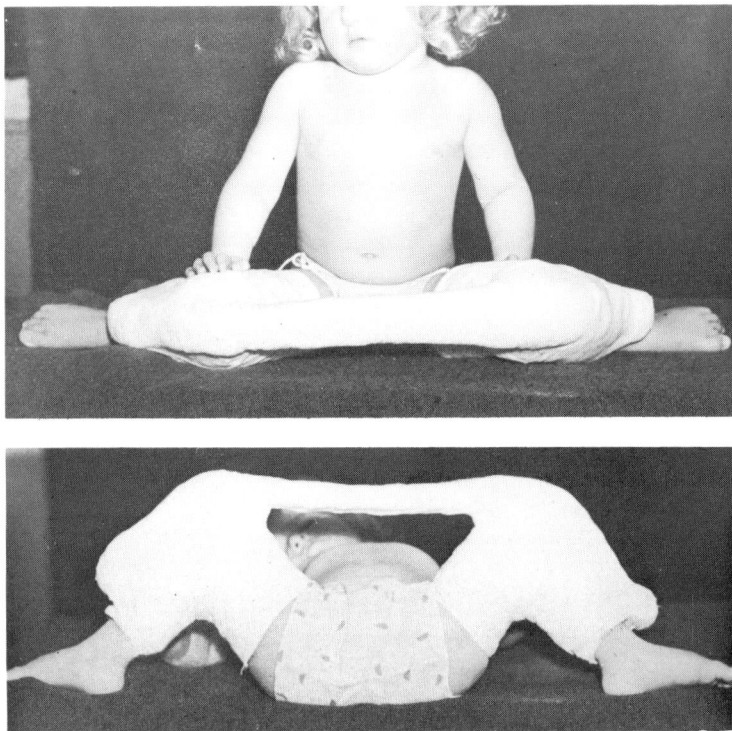

Fig. 154. *Batchelor plaster showing wide abduction maintained by the broomstick incorporated in the plaster.*

Gradual Reduction. If the hip is not reduced and the position maintained after six months, gradual reduction is undertaken in order to prevent damage to the blood supply of the head already mentioned. This method also allows gentle stretching of the tight structures which may be preventing reduction.

Methods used:

1. Gallow's traction.
2. Pugh's traction.
3. Abduction frame.

Gallow's traction (Fig. 65). This form of traction is modified in order to allow the hip to be abducted, and at the same time maintaining the pull on the legs with the child's weight providing the counter pull. The buttocks must be kept just clear of the bed to allow this to happen.

On admission about 36 hours will be needed for the child and the mother to adapt to the hospital routine. If the child is being breast fed the mother must be encouraged to continue. This can be done in spite of the child being on Gallow's traction, especially if weights and pulleys are used instead of the legs being tied in a cross beam. The legs are examined daily to see that there is no skin reaction to the strapping, and the circulation to feet should be checked. Abducting the legs will commence after one week and should be fully abducted by three weeks. Half-way, the hips will be X-rayed to check the position. Arthrogram is usually carried out after full abduction is achieved.

Surgery. Following arthrogram an open reduction and limbusectomy will be performed if necessary. A 1½ hip spica is applied, with the hip on the affected side internally rotated, abducted and the knee flexed to maintain the position. The plaster is retained for one month when the child is re-admitted for rotation osteotomy. The rotation osteotomy allows the head to stay internally rotated and in the stable position while the shaft is realigned so that the patella is facing forwards. Following this operation another hip spica is applied with the leg in a neutral position and the knee slightly flexed. This stays on for 6 weeks.

The child is re-admitted 6 weeks after surgery. The spica is bivalved, X-rays are taken, the child is blanket bathed and the skin is examined. She may stay in either the anterior or posterior shell for a few days while a decision is taken regarding the need for further treatment. Usually the child is then allowed up in a 'lobster pot' for about one week, then discharged home to normal activity.

Care of the child in plaster. The plaster can be dried in the normal way in a warm room with air circulating (see Chapter 6). Heat cradles should not be necessary. Care must be taken to avoid strains that would produce cracking or pressure from fingers that could cause sores. The child can be placed on protected pillows with a towel or similar substance under the plaster to absorb the moisture. The child should be turned every 2 to 3 hours. It is essential to check the circulation to the toes every time the child is turned. When the plaster is dry in approximately 3 days, waterproof strapping is applied to the edge of the plaster in the toilet area to prevent soiling. A runner is applied to the back of the spica next to the skin — this ensures that the skin is clean.

The child is usually allowed home in the plaster, in which case the parents must be given clear instructions and shown how to care for her. This will include the observations to be made and how to get in touch with the hospital if necessary. A trolley may be loaned to the parent so that the child can be pushed out in order to have contact with other children; that the child is allowed to live as normal a life as possible is essential for everyone.

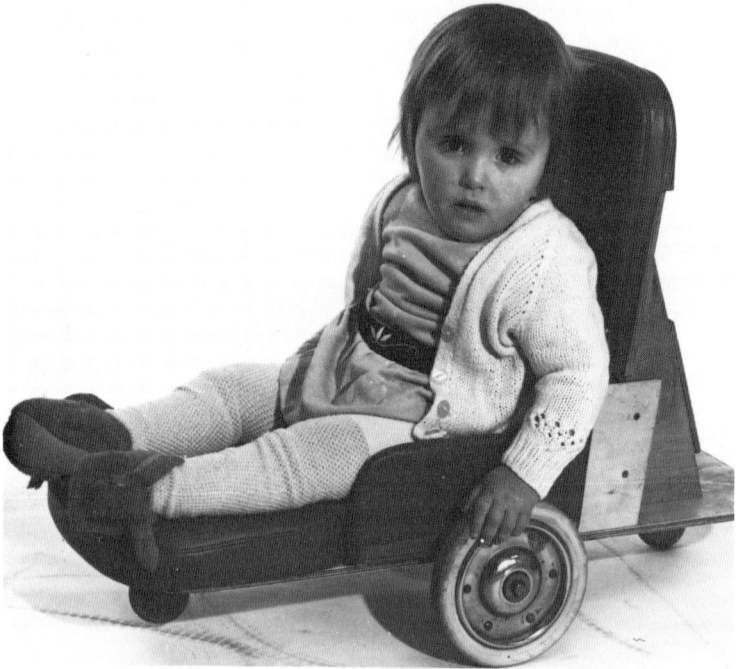

Fig. 155. *Childs Trolley.*

If the child is over one year when treatment is commenced, Pugh's traction may be used instead of Gallow's, but the principles of management are similar. The child on Pugh's traction is allowed off traction for cuddles each day, the skin is checked and the legs rebandaged.

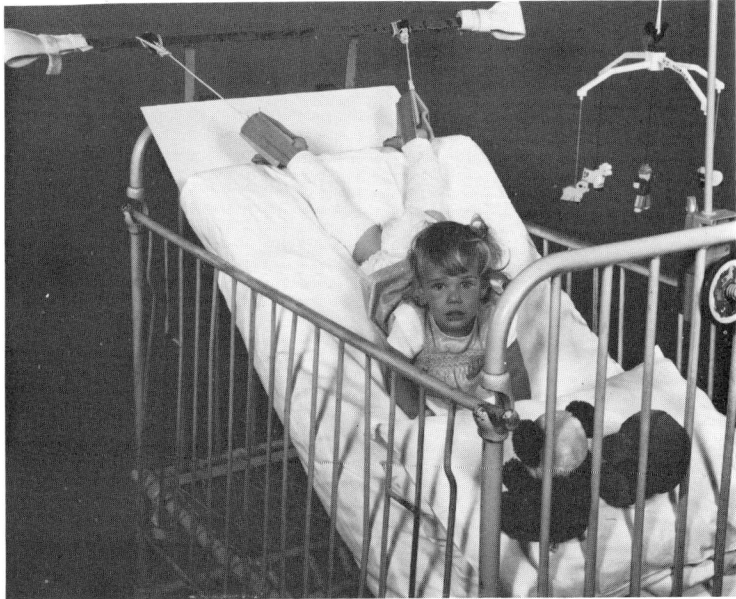

Fig. 156. *Pugh's traction used to reduce a congenitally dislocated hip.*

Gradual reduction on a double abduction frame in which the dislocated hips are gradually reduced with the minimum of trauma to soft tissues. The frame has a C-shaped cross bar and the leg portions of the saddle are made as separate pieces so that the saddle can be adjusted with the frame. Skin extensions are applied and the child is placed on the frame as previously described. At first the legs are abducted about 20°. Three or four days are allowed for the child to settle on the frame and when he has done so each leg is abducted one hole at a time on alternate days. After two to three weeks both legs will be widely abducted. If the radiograph shows that the femoral head is not coming down satisfactorily or is still outside the acetabulum cross traction is applied. The thigh of the affected leg is padded with sorbo or felt below the great trochanter and the padding held by a strap or extension strapping to which is attached a length of cord. The cord passes over on the opposite side of the bed with a weight of ½ to 1 kg. Reduction may be obtained in three to four weeks.

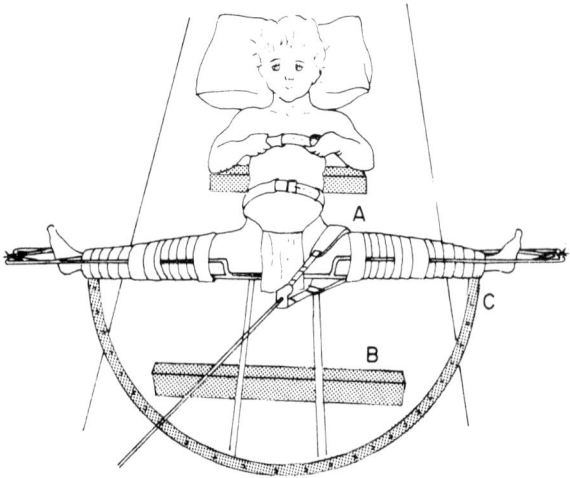

Fig. 157. *Cross-pull with a Jones abduction frame:* (a) *cross-pull applied over felt;* (b) *bar-raising frame for nursing purposes:* (c) *abduction bar allowing 180° of abduction.*

In addition to the *nursing care* of a patient on an abduction frame previously described, the special points to remember are:

1. Strong traction is needed so the extension tapes must be taut. Equally strong counter-traction is needed to relieve the pressure under the groin straps; for this it is advisable to elevate the foot of the bed after first securely tying the frame.
2. It must be ensured that the line of cross pull is just below the trochanter and not on the knee.
3. Watch must be kept to see that neither straight pull nor cross pull is causing sores.
4. Pressure on blood vessels and nerves must be avoided. Supervision is continued until adolescence.

13 Metabolic bone disease

RICKETS

Rickets is a disease affecting the development of bone, in young children, due to lack of vitamin D in the body. It usually occurs in children of six months to two years of age and is due to poor or inadequate diet. It is rarely seen in this country nowadays but cases have been reported among poorly nourished coloured immigrant children.

Vitamin D helps in the deposition of calcium salts in the bones. Where it is lacking the bone-forming tissue (osteoid) near the ends of the bone still keeps on growing but does not become calcified. The osteoid tissue grows quickly and irregularly and the epiphyses becomes wider than normal. The lack of calcium also causes a general softening of the bones.

During recovery from the disease the osteoid tissue becomes calcified and the rest of the bones return to their normal hardness. If the bones have become bent by reason of body weight they can be corrected in the early stages of recovery, but if they are left until the bones have recalcified the deformities are permanent.

Besides being taken in food, particularly in animal fats, vitamin D can be formed in the body by the action of sunlight. consequently children in sunny climates rarely get the disease, even though their diet may be deficient.

Signs and symptoms

Acute stage. The child is off colour, pale, not wasted, and may have a large abdomen. His teeth are late in appearing, and the epiphysis of the wrists, elbows, ribs and legs are thickened and widened. There may be softening of the bones of the skull just behind the ear.

Late stage. Deformities are present and are mainly knock-knee, bow leg (genu valgum and varum), bowing of the tibia and femur, chest deformities and spine deformities. X-rays show up general lack of calcium — the bone does not look as dense as normal, and at the ends of the long bones there is a lot of uncalcified osteoid tissue and the end of the bone is very wide. During the healing stage a dense line appears in the cartilage — this is the new calcified bone being formed. Minor degrees of all deformities will correct spontaneously if the diet is sufficient, with adequate vitamin D.

Deformities

Bow legs. In mild cases wedges may be added on the outer side of the shoes to prevent the child turning the toes in. Mermaid splints may be applied at night.

Knock-knee (or genu valgum). Both femur and tibia may enter into this deformity, or the lower end of the femur only. Wedges on the inner side of the shoes and exercises are usually sufficient with the general treatment.

Treatment

Early. (1) rest in bed, good food including those rich in vitamins; (2) sunshine and cod liver oil; and (3) prevent deformities by avoiding body weight on legs, and splinting if necessary.

Late. It may be necessary to correct deformities by: (1) manipulation and plaster application; and (2) bone operation, e.g. osteotomy followed by plaster fixation.

RENAL RICKETS

Renal rickets is a defect in calcification of bones due to impaired renal function, which results in upsetting the calcium balance producing changes in bone metabolism. The disease becomes apparent about the age of puberty, and the child is dwarfed. Treatment includes administration of vitamin D and prevention of deformities.

OSTEOMALACIA

Osteomalacia is adult rickets — softening of the bones due to calcium deficiency and lack of vitamin D. The latter is derived from fish oils but it can also be manufactured in the body by ultraviolet radiation of the skin — deficiency therefore may be due to inadequate diet or lack of sunlight. Both factors can tend to be somewhat neglected in the elderly and although osteomalacia is considered rather rare in this country instances in patients are seen in special clinics. If due to faulty diet treatment on dietetic lines and administration of vitamin D will be required.

ADULT COELIAC DISEASE

Adult coeliac disease is due to inability of the intestine to absorb vitamin D, resulting in osteomalacia. The bowel is also unable to absorb fat (steatorrhoea). A special gluten-free diet is given.

PARTIAL GASTRECTOMY

A possible consequence of partial gastrectomy operation could be an impaired absorption of vitamin D resulting in osteomalacia. Administration of vitamin D and calcium is given in treatment.

OSTEOPOROSIS

Osteoporosis is a condition in which there is softening of the bone due to a reduction in the calcium and phosphate content. Deficiency of calcium and protein in the diet is probably the main cause of senile osteoporosis — it is more common in women than in men. The presence of this condition is often quite symptomless, although some patients have bouts of backache which occur at intervals and are probably associated with some sort of occupational strain. In the general treatments calcium and steroids may be prescribed. Local treatment may take the form of some type of back support, e.g. brace or surgical corset. Immobilization of a limb or prolonged bed rest can produce osteoporosis, hence the importance of mobilization.

HYPERPARATHYROIDISM

Hyperparathyroidism is usually due to an adenoma (benign tumour) of one or more parathyroid glands. The resulting upset in the calcium balance causes decalcification of the skeleton. Treatment is by surgical removal of the tumour. Administration of vitamin D during the post-operative period is beneficial in skeletal repair.

PAGET'S DISEASE

Paget's disease usually occurs about the age of 40 and over. The bones most commonly affected are the lumbar spine, sacrum, skull, pelvis, femora and tibias. Perhaps two of the most striking features are the progressive enlargement of the skull and bowing of the long bones. The disease may be quite symptomless and not be diagnosed until the patient seeks advice on account of bone pain, osteo-arthritis or increasing spinal deformity, e.g. kyphos. There is no specific treatment for Paget's disease. Osteo-arthritis or fractures receive the appropriate treatment.

OSTEOGENESIS IMPERFECTA OR FRAGILITAS OSSEUM

This is an hereditary defect in the normal ossification of the skeleton. The disease may be severe or mild, and there are three recognized varieties:

The *fetal* variety is the most severe. The child is stillborn.

In the *infantile* variety multiple fractures occur in infancy resulting in deformity and stunted growth.

The *adolescent* variety is the mildest form associated with multiple fractures during growing period which rights itself at puberty.

It is quite usual to see blue sclera in these patients. There is no specific treatment, the fractures are treated along the usual lines. The children may have to attend special schools for physically handicapped children.

14 Rehabilitation: an introduction

Rehabilitation is the whole process of restoring a person to normal life after illness or injury. For those who have to accept permanent disability rehabilitation aims at achieving normal functional recovery. Many orthopaedic patients make a full recovery without special arrangements for rehabilitation, but their recovery can often be speeded up and enhanced with the help of rehabilitation procedures. Much of rehabilitation depends upon planning the stages of recovery as soon as definite treatments (e.g. operative procedure or drug therapy) are decided upon. Good rehabilitation means ensuring that physical recovery is kept up to the optimum timetable for each individual patient in each individual set of circumstances. Some patients recover quickly, others are less resilient. The rate of recovery and the ultimate functional capability of a disabled person depends upon personality, the physical disability and the incentive to recovery. Rehabilitation has to exploit these factors, assessing the patient and the disability, and providing the incentive and the means of achieving physical and functional recovery.

Rehabilitation is a team effort. The team comprises the orthopaedic surgeon, nursing staff physiotherapist, occupational therapist, social worker, clinical psychologist and the patient, together with his relatives — the patient being the most important member. In some circumstances the rehabilitative practice is a special unit, with a consultant in physical medicine leading the team, and then providing a service to the other specialized teams. In some disabilities, such as spinal injuries, multiple injuries, the severely physically disabled, head injuries and rheumatological disorders there may be a call for specialized rehabilitation units. Rehabilitation signifies all those measures which help to restore optimum function, and is a continuous process from the onset of disability until the achievement of the greatest potential, whether the activities are undertaken in the wards, in special units or at home.

One of the important factors in the patient's recovery is his own motivation. If this is present a good functional result is likely although the injury may be severe. The nurse who is caring for the patient over the whole 24-hour period has a key role to play in rehabilitation; by her cheerful manner she is able to encourage him and help him to achieve his long-term goal and his more immediate objectives. The nurse also has a very important coordinating role: she is able to observe the effects of the various procedures on the patient, which she must report to the surgeon or the consultant in physical medicine, or whoever is in charge of the patient, and to other members of the team.

When considering rehabilitation one must consider the whole patient in his environment. The major areas of concern may be listed as:

The diagnosis
Medical and surgical treatment
Psychological adjustment and motivation
Self-care activities
Income
Housing
Transport
Occupation
Recreation
Sexual activity

Each of these areas requires special consideration. Their diversity indicates the need for a team approach and emphasizes the need to coordinate the various activities of the team. Plans have to be drawn up and decisions made. All must be directed to achieving the common aim, which is to restore the patient to as full a life as possible, and to help him to adjust to his disability.

The nurse's role

The role of the nurse is a very complex one; she needs a knowledge of basic anatomy and physiology, and of the condition affecting the patient; she will need to remember that people react differently from the same condition; she will have to be flexible, able to adapt quickly as her role changes, which may be nurse, counsellor, teacher, pupil or coordinator. In carrying out her duties there will inevitably be some overlap with other team members — in some cases this may be desirable. What is not acceptable is that some of the patient's needs are not met, or that there is confusion or wasteful duplication. Good communications should avoid this.

The caring aspect. The basis reason why most people join the nursing profession is because they want to care for people, and in the acute phase of the disease when the patient is dependent, that kind of care is needed. The nurse must appreciate, however, when it is time to move towards self care — it will vary in different conditions and with different individual patients. It is for this reason that the care plan must be adjusted as the patient progresses.

Counselling. The role of the nurse as counsellor is becoming more appreciated. She is often the first person to meet the patient and his family who may be in a very distressed state. The nurse will be able to pass on valuable information to other members of the team, especially the social worker, who has special training for this role. A newer and extended role of the nurse is that of counsellor in sexual matters — this aspect of the patient's needs has for too long been neglected by nurses.

Teacher. The nurse has an important role to play in teaching the patient and his relatives, and especially junior nurses. Teaching is not confined to passing on new knowledge or skill but includes helping to change attitudes and helping the patient to adjust to a new way of life. He may never work again, in which case recreation is of prime importance. It is also as well to remember that a good teacher is also a good learner, and that we all have much to learn.

Communication. The nurse, because she is in contact with the patient the whole day, must be a good communicator. She will need to think carefully what is to be communicated, and what is the best method to do it. She will need to use both formal and informal methods. The Kardex is the usual method of formal communication; the treatment and up-to-date knowledge of his case will be recorded and available to other members of the team. In the case of a patient with major injury undergoing a process of rehabilitation, the overall plan of management may be drawn up by several members of the team and presented at a case conference, each having carried out his or her own assessment of the patient. The case conference is usually repeated at intervals throughout the stay in hospital and progress recorded. This information can then be passed on to the general practitioner and to the community team. If the communications have been good and the treatment and care carried out as planned, then the patient will have benefited from his period of rehabilitation, and the nurse will have made a significant contribution to that care.

Physiotherapy is nearly always an essential part of orthopaedic treatment. The term itself, healing by physical means, covers a number of therapies. It is no more descriptive to say that a patient is 'having physiotherapy', than to say he is having medicine or hospital treatment. If the nurse can appreciate the aims of the physiotherapist they can both work more effectively to help the patient in his own efforts to regain as much health and function as possible. The nurse has a more continual contact with the patient and has many opportunities of helping the patient to follow intelligently the physiotherapist's instructions. The following is of necessity little more than brief and by no means comprehensive. It takes three years of intensive training at one of the schools approved by the Chartered Society of Physiotherapy — some physiotherapists working in orthopaedic centres have undertaken training and passed the Orthopaedic Nursing Certificate, the examination set by The Joint Examination Board of The British Orthopaedic Association and the Central Council for the Disabled.

Physiotherapy techniques can be broadly divided into those which are active, involving the patient in a moderately active part in the treatment, and those in which the patient plays a passive role. Passive treatment includes the use of heat, electrical current, manipulative procedures and massage. Most of these are used as preludes to active therapy; the basis of all active therapy is exercise.

EXERCISE THERAPY

The two main groups of movements are passive and active.

Passive movements
Passive movements are performed on the patient by the physiotherapist. They are used only when the joint is no longer under control because the muscles are paralysed. In poliomyelitis and peripheral nerve lesions the joint is normal, but unless it is moved from the start stiffness and contractures develop. The physiotherapist carries the joint through the full range of normal movement without force or overstretching.

Passive movements are not to be confused with the manipulations performed by the surgeon with the patient under general anaesthetic and followed later by active movements. Stiff joints are never treated by passive movements as there would be much resistance. As a result of the force used a reaction would occur in the joint that would increase the stiffness.

Active movements
Active movements are the basis of modern remedial exercises. It should be explained to the patient that exercises are a definite and important form of treatment. The prolonged inactivity (see Chapter 5) resulting from injury or a disease running a long, chronic course can have a devastating effect on physical and mental health. Self-activity, with a definite aim and planned to a schedule, not only restores physiological function but prevents mental lethargy, despair and self-pity. Even patients for whom there is no complete cure find they are able to do more than they ever thought possible. The aims of active exercises are:

1. To conserve function of joints and muscles controlling them during periods of immobilization or bed rest.

2. To strengthen weak muscles and restore mobility in stiff joints.

3. To re-educate neuromuscular control. After a period in bed the sense of balance is lost and the 'link up' between brain and

muscles must be regained in order to walk. Patients with flaccid and spastic paralysis are taught in such a way that they can regain the maximum control possible. The physiotherapist selects the exercises and arranges them so that they can be adapted to the different phases of recovery. Muscle power will not increase unless the muscle is given progressively harder work to do.

A series of exercises is a number of exercises for one part of the body, i.e. hand exercises after a Colles' fracture. A table of exercises is a set for the whole body, following a balanced order, breathing, leg, arm, head, etc. A scheme of exercises is the whole course of exercise treatment working through weak, medium, and strong series of exercises.

Types of exercises

Local or specific exercises are used to develop a particular muscle group or to mobilize a particular joint. These apply for instance in the case of the weak muscles of a limb when there has been a fracture. General exercises are given to move the body as a whole. For a good functional result both are essential, since the body works as a whole and not in parts.

Static muscle work. A muscle group is said to work statically when it contracts without producing joint movement. For example the quadriceps extensors can contract voluntarily while the knee is fully extended. Static contractions are used as an early form of treatment because they can be carried out while a limb is immobilized in plaster or a splint. The quadriceps can be contracted during the healing stage of a fractured femur or within 48 hours after a meniscectomy of knee. Each contraction should be followed by a period of relaxation. A sustained contraction is when the muscle is 'held' in the contracted state for a short period. The period of 'holding' is brief because it is very fatiguing. This form of exercise is used in the treatment of deformities and to correct posture. The patient is taught the position and instructed to 'hold' it and gradually learns to sense when he is standing well or badly.

Free movements are performed by the patient without assistance or resistance. They range from bending and stretching the fingers or foot exercises on a frame to difficult gymnastic exercises.

Range of movement. A muscle is said to work in full or whole range when it contracts from the greatest possible lengthening to the greatest possible shortening such as when the fully extended elbow is flexed as far as possible. A muscle works in the inner range when it works from a point mid-way between full extension to full contraction, for example when the elbow is brought to full flexion from the right angled position. When the fully extended elbow is brought to right angle it is said to work in the outer range (Fig. 158). When possible, exercises are given to work the muscles

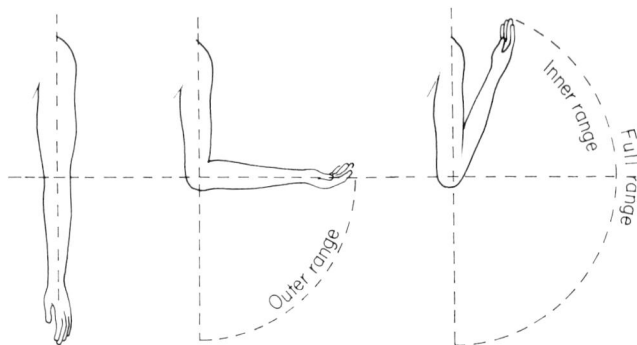

Fig. 158. *Range of muscle movements.*

in their full range and each movement taken to its limit. In the early stages of recovery, when muscles are weak and tire easily, exercises are confined to the inner and middle range. If the quadriceps are weak and a heel-raising, knee-bending exercise is given to strengthen them, knee flexion is not carried as far as a right angle. Later as the quadriceps improve the knee is allowed to flex as far as possible. This is muscle re-education. Exercises of normal feet and fingers should be as full as possible and not just a feeble waggling.

Active assisted exercises are performed by the patient assisted either by the physiotherapist or by apparatus.

The apparatus may be a polished board, water, suspended slings of the Guthrie Smith type, a spring cord and pulley circuit or weight and pulley. When the limb is supported and suspended, muscles that are too weak to overcome the force of gravity can be used.

Resisted movements. In these the muscles work against resistance supplied by the physiotherapist, gravity or apparatus such as springs, weight and pulleys.

Re-education in walking. The patient is prepared for walking while he is still in bed. Exercises are given to strengthen the anti-gravity muscles, such as the anterior tibialis, quadriceps, glutei, spinal and abdominal muscles. Training in balance whilst sitting with correct posture is an essential preliminary to walking.

Walking is the most continuous form of remedial exercise. To walk if only a few steps is the greatest possible stimulation for a patient after a period of inactivity. It is most important that he should walk correctly from the start. A limp and trick movements such as pelvic swinging are not only ugly but throw strain on normal joints. Walking periods should at first be short and followed by a period of rest with the legs elevated to check reactionary oedema. Before actually walking the patient is taught to stand, taking the body weight equally on each foot. The toes must point forward and be kept pointing forward when short steps are taken. The steps must be of equal length and each leg moved at the same pace.

Heel and toe walking is done as follows:
1. The patient stands correctly.
2. The right foot is moved forward and lowered to touch the ground.
3. The weight is then taken on the right foot and the knee pressed back by the quadriceps.
4. At the same time the left heel is raised from the ground and the left knee relaxed.
5. The left leg is brought forward and the same process repeated.

Walking in calipers, crutches and sticks has already been described (see Chapter 5).

Class exercises. Patients may not only be treated individually but also in small groups or exercise classes. Working with other people is stimulating and patients enjoy a sense of friendly competition. Organized games and competitions also encourage effort.

Home exercises. Since it is only by repeated voluntary movement that muscles can be strengthened, patients must continue their own treatment at home. The physiotherapist selects a few, not too many, free exercises for homework. She sees that the patient knows exactly how they should be performed, and if possible gets a member of the family to cooperate.

Breathing exercises and rest. Apart from the special technique used for respiratory disorders, breathing exercises are always included in an exercise scheme, as well as periods of relaxation to prevent fatigue.

TREATMENT BY HEAT

Infra-red irradiation, radiant heat from an electric lamp, an electrically-heated pad or a hot water-bottle, heat the surface of the body. This surface heating produces a dilatation of the superficial blood vessels, and if properly applied can be very soothing. An overdosage is definitely harmful. The heat waves themselves have no healing powers but, because they relieve pain and muscle spasm, are a useful adjunct to other treatments.

Diathermy
Short-wave diathermy involves the use of an electric current with a high rate of oscillation. This form of heat, in certain circumstances, can heal tissues somewhat deeper than can be achieved with heat lamps or pads.

Paraffin wax
Paraffin wax of a low melting-point is used as it can be heated to a liquid state that is tolerable to the skin. The hand or foot is dipped in the melted wax several times in order to obtain a thick coating which is covered and allowed to remain on the part for 20 to 30 minutes. The melted wax may be painted over a joint, several layers being applied in rapid succession. The wax coating prevents normal heat loss from the skin and the retention of heat raises the internal temperature. After the wax is removed the part is bathed with copious perspiration and is much more supple. Wax treatment is used for the stiff and painful joints of rheumatoid arthritis or after injury.

Ice

Some patients find that heat tends to make painful joints more painful and there is a current tendency to use ice in the management of painful stiff joints. Ice is usually applied in the form of a cold compress using towels packed with ice chippings. This form of treatment seems to be particularly useful for stiff painful shoulders, for painful spastic conditions (e.g. hemiplegia and paraplegia) and for knees which are painful and stiff after operation (e.g. patellectomy). As with heat, ice treatment is usually used as a prelude to active mobilization of the joint.

HYDROTHERAPY

Hydrotherapy is treatment by water.

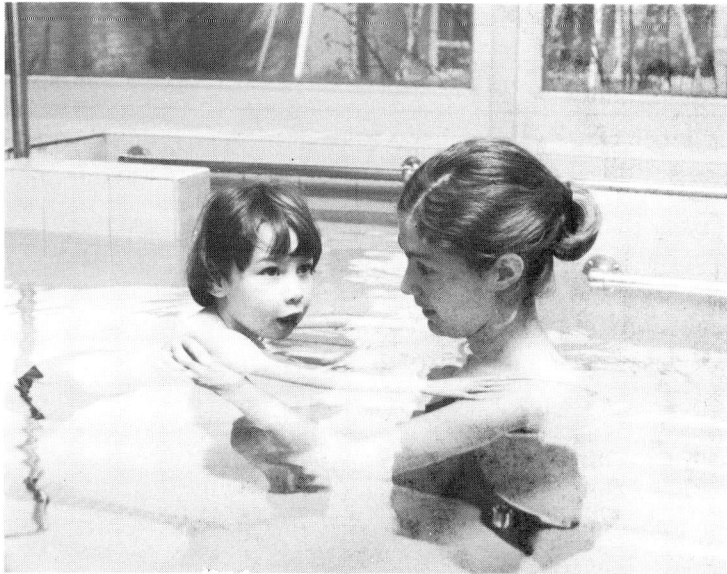

Fig. 159. *Hydrotherapy treatment (by courtesy of The Spastics Society).*

The warm water pool

The keynote of treatment in the pool is movement, active or passive, aided by the buoyancy and warmth of the water. The partially paralysed patient with poliomyelitis may be able to float and exercise not only the weak muscles, but the unaffected ones as well. Passive movements can also be carried out under water. The mineral content of the waters used in spas helps only in that it increases the buoyancy, thus making it easier to move stiff and painful joints.

There are several local forms of specialized hydrotherapy. A useful one that can be employed as a home treatment is that of contrast baths. They are used to stimulate the peripheral circulation which can be built up to resist cold. The feet or hands are placed in hot water 40 to 43°C for five to ten minutes. They are then placed in cold water 15.5 to 21°C for one minute and then returned to the hot water for four minutes. This is repeated several times.

ULTRAVIOLET RAYS

Ultraviolet rays, similar to those of the sun, can be produced by lamps such as the carbon arc, mercury arc, and by more powerful ones, such as the electronic arc tube mercury vapour lamp. Ultra-violet radiation is only of value when it is given with accuracy and is used more for its localized counter-irritant action than as a general treatment.

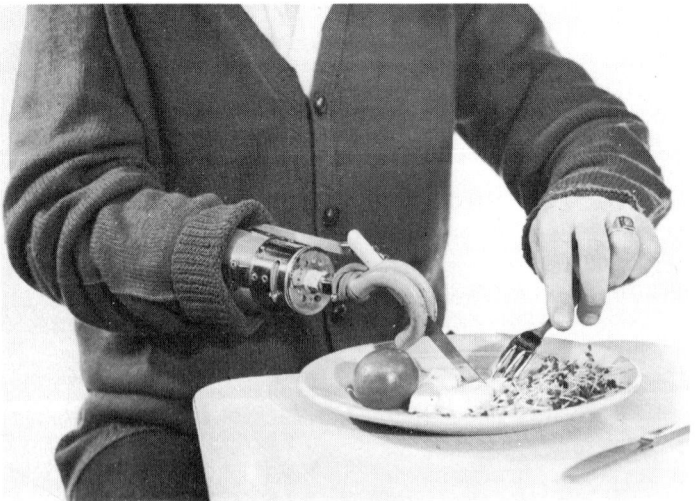

Fig. 160a. *Training the flail limb in bilateral activities.*

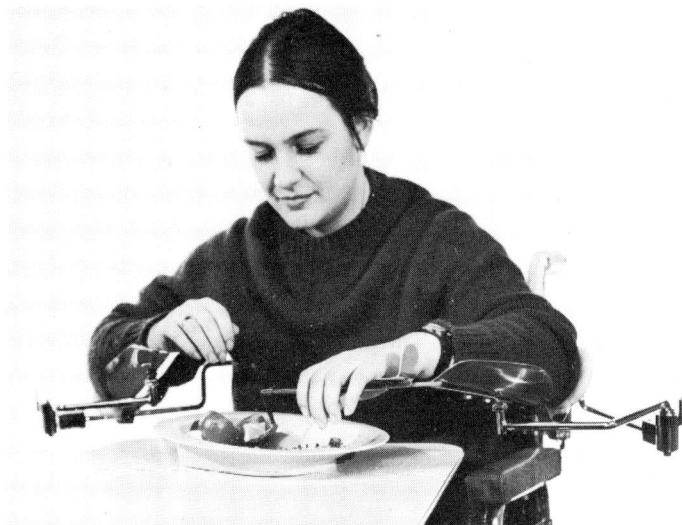

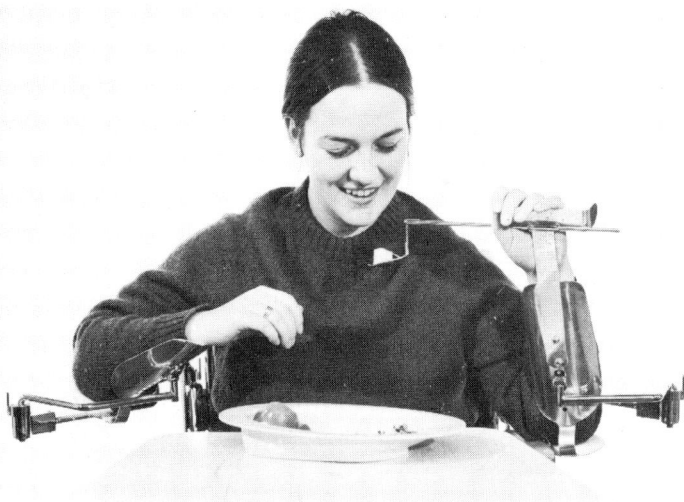

Fig. 160b. *Training the flail limb in bilateral activities using ball-bearing supports.*

ELECTRIC TREATMENT

Faradism and galvanism are seldom used.

OCCUPATIONAL THERAPY

The place of the occupational therapist in the rehabilitation of orthopaedic patients is often more difficult for the nurse to appreciate. The occupational therapist is more concerned with long-term care and the patient's ability to manage at home than with the acute care so dominant in a hospital ward. The occupational therapist nowadays is concerned with the functional day-to-day activities of patients. She is trained to assess their capabilities

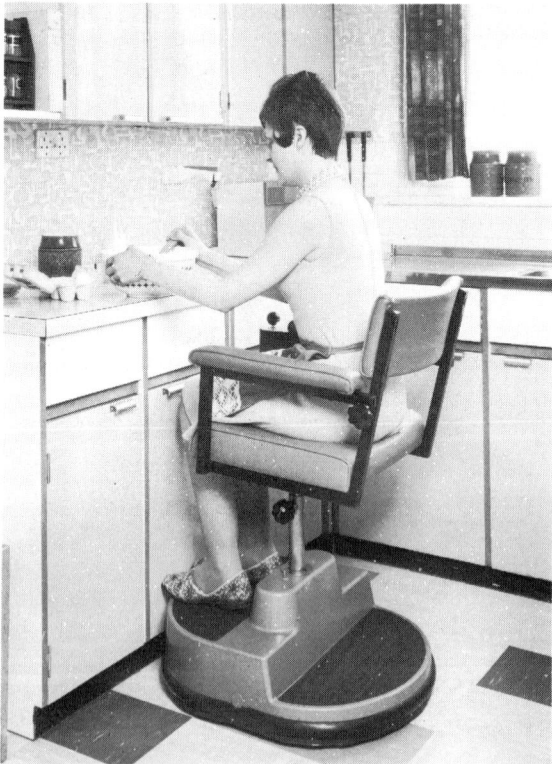

Fig. 161. *Assessment of a disabled in the working kitchen (by courtesy of Newton Aids Ltd).*

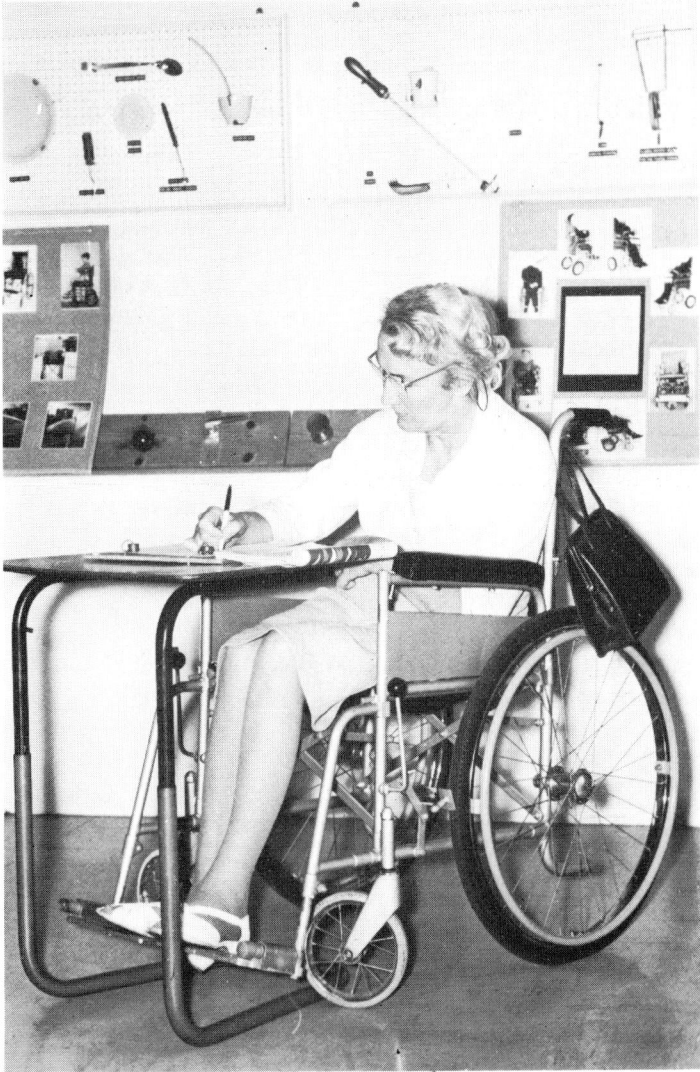

Fig. 162. *Assessment room in the disabled living research unit.*

in terms of activities of daily living (dressing, feeding, washing and toilet management). She is trained to teach patients to adapt to disabilities and to overcome them and she is trained to assess their capabilities in terms of return to work (pre-vocational assessment) and advise on retraining. As part of the assessment of functional capabilities she is concerned with the patient's home conditions and the need for altering the domestic arrangements or re-designing the home or work situation (Figs 161, 162). In the past, occupational therapists were more concerned with diversional activities, because there were many long-stay patients in hospital. Although such activity is still necessary for some patients the need is considerably less and in geriatric units and in the domiciliary sphere diversional activity is more directed toward productive and creative activities than the traditional craftwork.

It is much more important for a patient with a severe injury or illness to have a clear idea of his long-term rehabilitation programme, to understand what provisions, help and training are available and are planned, and to start to work towards such goals, than it is to provide him with the more traditional diversional activities. Diversional activities have their part to play, but long-term planning of resettlement in home and work are a far greater stimulant to active recovery. In this field the rehabilitation team has a large part to play in orthopaedics.

Medical Social Workers
With the complexity of legislation and the multiplicity of voluntary services available, the medical social worker's role becomes even more important. She will be concerned with social conditions, income, housing, transport, and retraining when necessary, all vital parts of rehabilitation.

If rehabilitation has been effective, the patient will be back with his family with his fullest physical, psychological and social potential. An inter-disciplinary approach is needed with all members of the team contributing their own special knowledge and skill in order to achieve the aim. The nurse has her place on the team in helping the patient to gain his maximum independence, his individuality, self respect, and dignity; bearing in mind that we are better at helping people than helping them to help themselves — 'Remembering that we should never push the disabled to the margins of our society but keep them as an integral part of the whole.'

Further Reading

Chapter 1

Le Vay, D. (1956) *Life of Hugh Owen Thomas*. Edinburgh: Churchill Livingstone.

Trueta, J. (1971) *Gathorne Robert Girdlestone*. Oxford: Oxford University Press.

Trueta, J. (1980) *Trueta: surgeon in war and peace*. London: Victor Gollancz.

Chapter 3

Kratz, C.R. (1979) *The nursing process*. London: Baillière Tindall.

Long, R. (1981) *Systematic nursing care*. London: Faber & Faber.

Nicoll, K.B. (1968) *Understanding traction*. A Nursing Times Publication.

Pembrey, S. (1980) *The ward sister — key to nursing*. London: RCN.

Rowe, J.W. & Dyer, L. (1977) *Care of the orthopaedic patient*. Oxford: Blackwell Scientific.

Royce, C.L. (1979) *Handbook of traction casting & splinting techniques*. Philadelphia, Pa: J.B. Lippincott.

Secretary of State for Social Services (1972) *Report of the committee on nursing. Chairman A. Briggs*. London: HMSO.

Stewart, J.D.M. (1975) *Traction in orthopaedic appliances*. Edinburgh: Churchill Livingstone.

Chapter 4

Fulford, G.E. & Hall, M.J. (1968) *Amputation & prosthesis.* Bristol: Wright.

Haward, J. (1979) Pain — psychological & social aspects. *Nursing, 1*: 1, 55.

Humm, W. & Rainey, A.E.S. (1977) *Rehabilitation of the lower limb amputee*, 3rd ed. London: Baillière Tindall.

Chapter 5

DHSS Training Council of Orthotists (1980) *Classification of orthosis.* London: HMSO.

Kennedy, J.M. (1979) *Orthopaedic splints and appliances.* London: Baillière Tindall.

Chapter 6

Farrell, J. (1982) *Illustrated guide to orthopaedic nursing*, 2nd ed. New York: Harper & Row.

Plaster of Paris techniques. Welwyn Garden City: Smith & Nephew.

Chapter 7

Adams, J. (1978) *Outline of fractures*, 7th ed. Edinburgh: Churchill Livingstone.

Bradley, D. (1980) *Accident and emergency nursing.* London: Baillière Tindall.

Wilson, J.N. (1982) *Watson Jones fractures and joint injuries.* Edinburgh: Churchill Livingstone.

Chapter 8

Bentley, G. & Duthie, R.B. (1975) Orthopaedic management of the haemophilias. In: *Recent advances in orthopaedics*, (Ed: B. McKibbin), Vol. 2. Edinburgh: Churchill Livingstone.

Duthie, R.B. & Bentley, G. (1983) *Mercer's orthopaedic surgery*, 8th ed. London: Edward Arnold.

Duthie, R.B., Mathews, J.M., Rizza, C.R. & Steel, W.M. (1972) *The management of musculo-skeletal problems in the haemophilias.* Oxford: Blackwell Scientific Publications.

Mowat, A.G. (1979) Physiotherapy. In: *Cash's textbook on medical conditions for physiotherapists*, (Ed. P.A. Downie), 6th ed. London: Faber & Faber.

Swinson, D.R. & Swinburn, W.R. (1980) *Rheumatology*. London: Hodder & Stoughton.

Chapter 9
Girdlestone, G.R. Somerville, E.W. & Wilkinson, M.C. (1965) *Tuberculosis of bone & joint*, 3rd ed. Oxford: Oxford University Press.

Chapter 10
Saunders, C.M. (1978) *The management of terminal disease*. London: Edward Arnold.

Chapter 11
Hollis, M. (1981) *Safer lifting for patient care*. Oxford: Blackwell Scientific Publications.

Chapter 12
Alderson, P. (1969) *What is a childrens ward?* National Association for the Welfare of Children in Hospital.
Allum, N. *The treatment and care of spina bifida children*. London: George Allen & Unwin Ltd.
Bates, S.M. (1979) *Practical paediatric nursing*, 2nd ed. Oxford: Blackwell Scientific Publications.
CIBA (1979) Clinical symposia. *Congenital dislocation of hip*. CIBA Laboratories, Horsham, Vol. 31, No. 1.
Duncombe, M. & Weller, B.F. (1979) *Paediatric nursing*, 5th ed. London: Baillière Tindall.
Hawthorn, P.J. (1974) *Nurse — I want my mummy*. London: RCN.
Keim, H.A. (1982) *The adolescent spine*, 2nd ed. Berlin:Springer-Verlag.
Menzies-Lyth, I. *The psychological welfare of young children making long stays in hospital*. Tavistock: The Tavistock Institute of Human Relations.
Ministry of Health, Central Health Services Council, Chairman Sir Harry Platt (1959). The welfare of children in hospital. London: HMSO.
Powell, M. (1982) *Orthopaedic nursing and rehabilitation*, 8th ed. Edinburgh: Churchill Livingstone.
Weller, B.F. (1980) *Helping sick children play*. London:Baillière Tindall.

Chapter 14

Goble, R.E.A. & Nichols, P.J.R. (1971) *Rehabilitation of the severely disabled.* London: Butterworth.

Johnstone, M. (1976) *The stroke patient, principles of rehabilitation.* Edinburgh: Churchill Livingstone.

Nichols, P.J.R. (1973) *Living with a handicap.* London: Priory Press.

Nichols, P.J.R. (1980) *Rehabilitation medicine*, 2nd ed.London: Butterworth.

Wilshire, E.R. (1978) *Equipment for the disabled: personal care*, 4th ed. Oxfordshire Area Health Authority.

Wilshire, E.R. (1980) Equipment for the disabled: disabled child, 4th ed. Oxfordshire Area Health Authority.

Woodhead–Faulkner (1975) *Handling the handicapped.*London: The Chartered Society of Physiotherapy.

Index

2/11/95

Dad :- Open excission
   of lateral clavical
   & decompression of (R) shoulder.

Osgood slatters syndrome - bones
in young boy grow quickly - football
injury?